Preterm Birth and Psychological Development

DEVELOPMENTAL PSYCHOLOGY SERIES

SERIES EDITOR
Harry Beilin

Developmental Psychology Program
City University of New York Graduate School
New York, New York

LYNN S. LIBEN. *Deaf Children: Developmental Perspectives*

JONAS LANGER. *The Origins of Logic: Six to Twelve Months*

GILBERTE PIERAUT-LE BONNIEC. *The Development of Modal Reasoning: Genesis of Necessity and Possibility Notions*

TIFFANY MARTINI FIELD, SUSAN GOLDBERG, DANIEL STERN, and ANITA MILLER SOSTEK. (Editors). *High-Risk Infants and Children: Adult and Peer Interactions*

BARRY GHOLSON. *The Cognitive-Developmental Basis of Human Learning: Studies in Hypothesis Testing*

ROBERT L. SELMAN. *The Growth of Interpersonal Understanding: Developmental and Clinical Analyses*

RAINER H. KLUWE and HANS SPADA. (Editors). *Developmental Models of Thinking*

HARBEN BOUTOURLINE YOUNG and LUCY RAU FERGUSON. *Puberty to Manhood in Italy and America*

SARAH L. FRIEDMAN and MARIAN SIGMAN. (Editors). *Preterm Birth and Psychological Development*

LYNN S. LIBEN, ARTHUR H. PATTERSON, and NORA NEWCOMBE. (Editors). *Spatial Representation and Behavior Across the Life Span: Theory and Application*

In Preparation

W. PATRICK DICKSON. (Editor). *Children's Oral Communication Skills*

EUGENE S. GOLLIN. (Editor). *Developmental Plasticity: Behavioral and Biological Aspects of Variations in Development*

Preterm Birth and Psychological Development

Edited by

SARAH L. FRIEDMAN

Laboratory of Developmental Psychology
National Institute of Mental Health
Bethesda, Maryland

MARIAN SIGMAN

Department of Psychiatry
School of Medicine
The Center for the Health Sciences
University of California, Los Angeles
Los Angeles, California

ACADEMIC PRESS **1981**

A Subsidiary of Harcourt Brace Jovanovich, Publishers

New York   London   Toronto   Sydney   San Francisco

ACADEMIC PRESS, INC.
111 Fifth Avenue, New York, New York 10003

United Kingdom Edition published by
ACADEMIC PRESS, INC. (LONDON) LTD.
24/28 Oval Road, London NW1 7DX

Library of Congress Cataloging in Publication Data
Main entry under title:

Preterm birth and psychological development.

(Developmental psychology series)
Includes bibliographies and index.
1. Infants (Premature)––Psychology. 2. Infants
(Premature)––Physiology. 3. Developmental psychology.
4. Infant psychology. I. Friedman, Sarah L.
II. Sigman, Marian. III. Series. [DNLM: 1. Infant,
Premature –Psychology. 2. Child development.
3. Growth. 4. Child behavior. WS 410 P942]
BF720.P7P73   155.4'5   80–980
ISBN 0–12–267880–X

PRINTED IN THE UNITED STATES OF AMERICA

81 82 83 84   9 8 7 6 5 4 3 2 1

Contents

I
Epidemiological and Medical Characteristics

1
Epidemiological Characteristics of Preterm Births
CARL A. KELLER

2
Medical Constraints to Optimal Psychological Development of the Preterm Infant
MILTON W. WERTHMANN, JR.

3
A Nonhuman Primate Model for Studying Causes and Effects of Poor Pregnancy Outcomes
GENE P. SACKETT

4

Perinatal Risks, Neonatal Deficits, and Developmental Crisis: A Review of Chapters 1-3

LEWIS P. LIPSITT

II

Neurophysiological Organization and Its Behavioral Implications

5

Animal Studies in Developmental Psychobiology: Commentary on Method, Theory, and Human Implications

GUENTER H. ROSE

6

Development of Vocal Communication in an Experimental Model

JENNIFER S. BUCHWALD

7

Auditory Function and Neurological Maturation in Preterm Infants

ARTHUR H. PARMELEE, JR.

8

Comparative Development of Feline and Human Cerebral Cortex: A Review of Chapters 5-7

DOMINICK P. PURPURA

III

Behavioral Patterns in the Neonatal Period

9

Sensory Processing in Pre- and Full-Term Infants in the Neonatal Period

SARAH L. FRIEDMAN, BLANCHE S. JACOBS, MILTON W. WERTHMANN, JR.

10

Mother-Infant Interactions in the Premature Nursery: A Sequential Analysis

PETER MARTON, KLAUS MINDE, JOHN OGILVIE

11

Sensory Responsiveness and Social Behavior in the Neonatal Period: A Review of Chapters 9 and 10

ANNELIESE F. KORNER

IV
Cognitive and Visual Development in the Early Months

16

Visual Development in Pre- and Full-Term Infants:
A Reveiw of Chapters 12-15

KEITH D. WHITE AND YVONNE BRACKBILL

V

Longitudinal Follow-up: Two Years and Above

17

Developmental Follow-up of Pre- and Postterm Infants

TIFFANY MARTINI FIELD, JEAN RYDBERG DEMPSEY, AND H. H. SHUMAN

18

The Relation of Early Infant Meausres to Later Development

MARIAN SIGMAN, SARALE E. COHEN, AND ALAN B. FORSYTHE

19

Predicting Intellectual Disorders in Childhood for Preterm Infants
with Birthweights below 1501 gm

JANE V. HUNT

20

Neonatal Compromise and Later Psychological Development:
A 10-Year Longitudinal Study

DANIEL V. CAPUTO, KENNETH M. GOLDSTEIN, AND HARVEY B. TAUB

List of Contributors

Numbers in parentheses indicate the pages on which authors' contributions begin.

YVONNE BRACKBILL (289), Department of Psychology, University of Florida, Gainesville, Florida 32611

JENNIFER S. BUCHWALD (107), Department of Physiology, Mental Retardation Research Center, BRI, School of Medicine, University of California, Los Angeles, Los Angeles, California 90024

DANIEL V. CAPUTO (353), St. Vincent's North Richmond Community Mental Health Center, and Queens College, City University of New York, Flushing, New York 11367

ALBERT J. CARON (219), National Institute of Mental Health, Mental Health Study Center, Adelphi, Maryland 20783

ROSE F. CARON (219), Department of Psychology, The George Washington University, Washington, D.C. 20052

LESLIE B. COHEN (241), Infant Research Laboratory, Institute for Child Behavior and Development, University of Illinois at Urbana, Champaign, Illinois 61820

SARALE E. COHEN (313), Division of Child Development, Department of Pediatrics, School of Medicine, University of California, Los Angeles, Los Angeles, California 90024

JEAN RYDBERG DEMPSEY (299), Neonatology Department, Baystate Medical Center, Springfield, Massachusetts 01107

JOSEPH F. FAGAN, III (417), Department of Psychology, Case Western Reserve University, Cleveland, Ohio 44106

TIFFANY MARTINI FIELD (299), Mailman Center for Child Development, University of Miami Medical School, Miami, Florida 33101

ALAN B. FORSYTHE (313), Department of Biomathematics, School of Medicine, University of California, Los Angeles, Los Angeles, California 90024

SARAH L. FRIEDMAN (159), National Institute of Mental Health, Laboratory of Developmental Psychology, Bethesda, Maryland 20205

KENNETH M. GOLDSTEIN (353), Staten Island Children's Community Mental Health Center, Staten Island, New York 10301

JANE V. HUNT (329), Institute of Human Development, University of California, Berkeley, Cardiovascular Research Institute, San Francisco, California 94720

ROSEMARY HUNTER (395), Department of Psychiatry and Pediatrics, School of Medicine, University of North Carolina, Chapel Hill, North Carolina 27514

BLANCHE S. JACOBS (159), National Institute of Mental Health, Laboratory of Developmental Psychology, Bethesda, Maryland 20205

CARL A. KELLER (3), National Institutes of Health, National Institute of Child Health and Human Development, Epidemiology and Biometry Research Program, Epidemiology Branch, Bethesda, Maryland, 20014

ANNELIESE F. KORNER (207), Department of Psychiatry and Behavioral Sciences, Stanford University School of Medicine, Stanford, California 94305

LEWIS P. LIPSITT (65), Department of Psychology and Child Study Center, Brown University, Providence, Rhode Island 02912

PETER MARTON (179), Department of Psychiatry, The Hospital for Sick Children, Toronto, Ontario M5G 1X8

KLAUS MINDE (179), Department of Psychiatry, The Hospital for Sick Children, Toronto, Ontario M5G 1X8

JOHN OGILVIE (179), Department of Psychology, University of Toronto, Toronto, Ontario M5G 1X8

ARTHUR H. PARMELEE, JR. (127), Division of Child Development, Department of Pediatrics, School of Medicine, The Center for the Health Sciences, University of California, Los Angeles, Los Angeles, California 90024

DOMINICK P. PURPURA (151), Department of Neuroscience, and Rose F. Kennedy Center for Research in Mental Retardation and Human Development, Albert Einstein College of Medicine, Bronx, New York 10461

CRAIG T. RAMEY (395), Frank Porter Graham Child Development Center, University of North Carolina, Chapel Hill, North Carolina 27514

GUENTER H. ROSE (73), Department of Psychology, Bowdoin College, Brunswick, Maine 04011

SUSAN A. ROSE (255), Department of Psychiatry, Albert Einstein College of Medicine, Bronx, New York 10461

GENE P. SACKETT (41), Regional Primate Research Center, University of Washington, Seattle, Washington 98105

ARNOLD J. SAMEROFF (387), Institute for the Study of Developmental Disabilities, University of Illinois at Chicago Circle, Chicago, Illinois 60680

H. H. SHUMAN (299), 689 Chestnut Street, Springfield, Massachusetts 01107

MARIAN SIGMAN (313), Department of Psychiatry, School of Medicine, Center for the Health Sciences, University of California, Los Angeles, Los Angeles, California 90024

LYNN TWAROG SINGER (417), Department of Psychology, Case Western Reserve University, Cleveland, Ohio 44106

EINAR R. SIQUELAND (271), Walter S. Hunter Laboratory of Psychology, Brown University, Providence, Rhode Island 02912

HARVEY B. TAUB (353), St. Vincent's North Richmond Community Mental Health Center, Staten Island, New York 10310, and Queens College, City University of New York, Flushing, New York 11367

MILTON W. WERTHMANN, JR. (17, 159), Perinatal / Neonatal Pediatrics, Washington Hospital Center, Washington, D.C. 20010

KEITH D. WHITE (289), Department of Psychology, University of Florida, Gainesville, Florida 32611

PHILIP SANFORD ZESKIND* (395), Frank Porter Graham Child Development Center, University of North Carolina, Chapel Hill, North Carolina 27514

* Present address: Mailman Center for Child Development, Departments of Psychology and Pediatrics, University of Miami, Miami Florida 33101

Preface

In the United States, about 10% of all infants are born before 37 weeks of pregnancy have been completed (see Chapter 2 by Werthmann and Chapter 9 by Friedman *et al.*). The immaturity of preterm infants at birth and in the weeks that follow may affect the rate and quality of their behavioral development. For example, it is possible that there are lower limits for critical periods in development such that a biological system may not be responsive to environmental stimulation before it reaches a minimum level of maturation. The poor health status of preterm infants in the neonatal period may also create developmental complications. The complications may be due to medical risk per se or to medical treatment that consists of irregular and noncontingent stimulation conditions.

Preterm birth is often a major crisis for the families of preterm neonates. The emotional, financial, and physical strains of dealing with such severe threats to life are enormous. For a time after birth, parents may not be allowed to interact with their infant. When this period of separation is over, their sense of confidence in handling even normal occurrences may be diminished. Once the medical situation has stabilized, the question of whether the early insult and complications have limited the infant's physical, neurological, and psychological development becomes critical.

Concern with psychological development stems, in part, from studies showing that children with cognitive and emotional problems are more likely to have been born preterm than are children without such problems. However, the basis for the high rates of handicapping conditions is unclear from these studies. Although it is often assumed that the medical and neurological complications associated with preterm birth damage the central nervous system, evidence is frequently lacking. Furthermore, many prospective studies of fullterm infants who suffer early medical and neurological complications do not identify future psychological limitations in their subjects. Since preterm birth is far more prevalent among poor families than in those who enjoy good medical care, nutrition, and social support systems, the effects of environmental factors cannot be overlooked.

The purpose of this volume is to review the psychological development of the preterm infant. The review is placed in a context suggesting the importance of epidemiological, medical, biological, and intervention issues.

The volume is divided into six parts. Part I (Epidemiological and Medical Characteristics) reviews the epidemiological factors (Chapter 1 by Keller) and medical complications (Chapter 2 by Werthmann). Chapter 3 (Sackett) presents an animal model for investigating genetic and environmental causes and effects of preterm birth. The fourth chapter (Lipsitt) is a review of the first three.

Chapters 5–8, by Rose, Buchwald, Parmelee, and Purpura, respectively, comprise Part II, Neurophysiological Organization and Its Behavioral Implications. These chapters suggest how animal models can be used to study the relationships between biological maturity, environmental stimulation, and behavioral development in preterm infants.

Part III, Behavioral Patterns in the Neonatal Period, is devoted to studies of preterm infants in the nursery and at expected date of birth. Chapter 9 (Friedman, Jacobs, and Werthmann) reviews the previous research on responses to sensory stimulation in preterm and full-term infants, and Marton, Minde, and Olgivie summarize prior research on the relation between parental factors, child abuse, and preterm birth in Chapter 10. Chapter 11 (Korner) reviews Chapters 9 and 10.

Although the early relationships of preterm infants and their caretakers have been investigated, most studies have focused on possible cognitive deficiencies reflected primarily in processing of visual information. Part IV, Cognitive and Visual Development in the Early Months, reviews the results of varying research strategies (Chapter 12 by Caron and Caron, Chapter 13 by Cohen, Chapter 14 by Rose, and Chapter 15 by Siqueland). Most of the investigations identify some differences between preterm and full-term infants, but the nature and extensiveness of these differences varies with the research method and sample characteristics. Brackbill and White (Chapter 16) discuss the findings presented in Part IV.

Longitudinal follow-up of preterm infants using standardized developmental measures and intelligence tests in infancy (Chapter 17 by Field, Dempsey, and Shuman, Chapter 18 by Sigman, Cohen, and Forsythe, Chapter 19 by Hunt) and the school years (Chapter 19 by Hunt, Chapter 20 by Caputo, Goldstein, and Taub) is the subject of Part V (Longitudinal Follow-Up: Two Years and Above). Most of these prospective studies find somewhat lower developmental scores for their preterm sample than for their full-term samples. However, as Sameroff points out in his review of these chapters, specific medical complications seem to have little direct effect on development, whereas environmental variables have a strong impact on outcome

(Chapter 21). Chapters 22 (Ramey, Zeskind, and Hunter) and 23 (Fagan and Singer), spell out implications for intervention from two different viewpoints.

A common feature of the studies surveyed in the present volume is the focus of the research methodology on processes of development. In the past, studies of the development of preterms have used measurements of school achievement, teachers' evaluations, and intelligence quotients. Current research both capitalizes and improves on knowledge gathered in the period between 1930 and 1960. Based on results indicating that preterm infants' performance on standardized measures is poorer than that of full-term individuals, researchers are now exploring the medical and social processes mediating this poor performance. At the same time, investigators are focusing on the sensory and cognitive processes that are likely to contribute to poor outcome. In attending to psychological processes, we have used research paradigms that are sensitive to age differences and to differences in central nervous system function. These research methodologies, together with relevant animal models, have the potential for specifying the nature of the differences between full- and preterm individuals. Only when we have identified the behavioral systems altered by preterm birth and the mechanisms that mediate or ameliorate the effects of preterm birth will we be ready to recommend effective psychological interventions for preterm infants.

Acknowledgments

The preparation of this volume was supported by The Center for Studies of Child and Family Mental Health and the Laboratory of Developmental Psychology, National Institute of Mental Health. We are particularly grateful to Joy Schulterbrandt and Marian Radke Yarrow, and to their respective staffs. We are also appreciative of the secretarial help and good humor of Luisa Castillo.

Finally, we would like to thank all the pre- and full-term infants and our children, Daphne, Hilary, and Daniel, who share their lives with us.

Sarah L. Friedman
Marian Sigman

Foreword

As the birthrate diminishes, each newborn acquires a greater value from the viewpoint of maintaining the qualitative and the quantitative stability of the population. Fortunately, even assuming no additional resources for the perinatal care of infants, society can assign a larger proportion of these resources to each pregnancy, birth, and infancy. In the recent past, substantial investments and advances have been made in the perinatal and postnatal survival of the newborn. Technological advances now enable industrial nations to assure the continuation of life for most preterm infants. These benefits have accrued not only to those who are born relatively well developed, but also have enabled newborns of smaller sizes to survive.

But maintenance of life is not enough. Each member of a birth cohort, including those born preterm, should also benefit through greater opportunities for a better quality of life. It is in this realm that physiological technology is essential but not sufficient. Quality of life depends not on mere survival and physical growth, but on adequate cognitive, emotional, social, and behavioral development as well. All these factors are highly interdependent and are constantly influenced by interactions between the infants and their environments, particularly those individuals who care for the highly dependent babies.

Preterm infants are at high risk for developmental deficits that may result from somatic, psychological, and social causes, or, as is usually the case, from a combination of them. Research and clinical practice have accomplished much in the areas of physiology and the maintenance of life, but we must advance our knowledge about all factors that influence development. Only in this fashion can we assure progress in the quality of life of these babies. It is in this context that I welcome this book and commend it highly to all those interested in the betterment of life for a particularly vulnerable group of infants.

George Tarjan, M.D.
Professor of Psychiatry
Director, Mental Retardation and Child Psychiatry Division
University of California, Los Angeles
Los Angeles, California

Preterm Birth and
Psychological Development

I

Epidemiological and Medical Characteristics

1

Epidemiological Characteristics of Preterm Births

CARL A. KELLER

The notion of a preterm birth implies that there exists some developmental stage of intrauterine fetal growth that could be considered an optimal time for birth of a healthy infant. A baby born before this stage has been reached can be considered a preterm birth and is generally assumed to be at elevated risk for present or future pathological sequelae. Unfortunately, it is often difficult to make a determination of maturity on clinical grounds either before or after birth, and such an assessment may be unreliable since it requires considerable subjective judgment. For epidemiologic and other research purposes, a more objective assessment based on available and reliable information must be selected to make a reasonable determination of what is to be considered a preterm birth.

The vast majority of human births in the United States occur at approximately 40 weeks after the beginning of the last menstrual period and weigh in the neighborhood of 3300 gm. In an evolutionary sense, this might be considered optimal, and the classification of preterm births on the basis of birthweight and/or gestational age has often been used. Although the word *term* seems to imply some function of the length of gestation, the concept of development might also be appropriately described as birthweight or as a function of both birthweight and gestational age.

If a single developmental pattern exists for all otherwise healthy human fetuses, then gestational age would be an accurate assessment of developmental maturity. On the other hand, if growth rates vary among individual fetuses, then birthweight may be a better measurement for classifying preterm babies. If both the developmental pattern and growth rates vary among individual fetuses, as is most likely the case, then neither measurement is suffi-

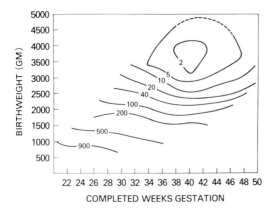

FIGURE 1.1. *Neonatal mortality rates per 1000 live births by gestational age and birthweight among total singleton births, California, 1966–1970. (Based on data from Cunningham et al., 1974.)*

cient for accurate classification. Perhaps the best measurement should be based on outcome in terms of health or disease.

One such outcome that has often been used as an indicator of health status for population groups is infant mortality. Utilizing over 1 million birth records from California for the years 1966–1970, the neonatal mortality rate by gestational age and birthweight has been computed by Cunningham, Williams, Hawes, Madore, Norris, and Phibbs (1974). Isopleths through points with similar neonatal mortality rates can be plotted as presented in Figure 1.1. These data indicate that the optimal survival in this population occurs among births of 3000–4250 gm at 37–42 weeks completed gestation. It should be noted that the isopleths tend to be strikingly more horizontal than vertical and indicate that birthweight is a better predictor of neonatal survival than gestational age, although the latter certainly has a significant effect. The isopleths begin a sharp rise below 2500 gm, the cutoff point generally used to designate the condition of low birthweight.

Fortunately, birthweight has most often been used as the criterion of prematurity in epidemiological studies (Berendes, 1963). An additional reason for this is that birthweight is more accurately reported than is gestational age. Apparently short gestational ages may be miscalculated following uterine bleeding during early pregnancy. Apparently long gestational ages can be the result of exceptionally long intervals between menstruation and subsequent ovulation (Boyce, Mayaux, & Schwartz, 1976).

The general magnitude of the proportion of preterm births is illustrated in Table 1.1, which gives the number and percentage of singleton births among white residents of Minnesota for the years 1967–1973. The births are divided into various birthweight and gestational age categories corresponding to most reported data. It is evident that 85% of these births occurred in the optimal birthweight and gestational age range, and this is generally true for white births in American and European populations.

Using linked birth and infant death records for all of the Minnesota births for the years 1967–1973, the infant mortality rates have been computed for

TABLE 1.1

Number and Percentage of White Singleton Births with Known Birthweight and Gestational Age.[a]

	< 37 weeks	37–43 weeks	44 + weeks
4501 + gm		7295	557
		(1.8)	(.1)
	16,405		
	(4.1)		
2501–4500 gm		342,304	14,320
		(85.2)	(3.6)
< 2500 gm	11,324	9187	350
	(2.8)	(2.3)	(.1)
401,742			
(100.0)			

[a] Minnesota, 1967–1973, residents of or born in Minnesota.

white singleton births among residents during that period. The availability of linked records makes it possible to calculate death rates in population groups defined by information included on the birth, but not on the death, certificate. Table 1.2 shows the numbers of deaths and rates per 1000 live births during the early neonatal period (less than 7 days) by gestation length and birthweight in the several groups defined in Table 1.1. The survival rate is optimal and the early neonatal mortality rate of the same order as that for California for a similar gestation length and birthweight group.

It should be noted that not only is the early neonatal mortality rate more than 100 times greater among the clearly premature (i.e., less than 37 weeks of gestation and under 2501 gm at birth) but over two-thirds of the deaths under 1 week occur in this group. These data are entirely consistent with what is generally known about the relationship between birthweight, gestation length, and neonatal mortality. Table 1.3 shows the numbers of deaths and rates dur-

TABLE 1.2

Number of Deaths and Rate per 1000 Live Births during Early Neonatal Period (Less than 1 Week)[a]

	< 37 weeks	37–43 weeks	44 + weeks
4501 + gm	223	20	5
	(13.6)	(2.7)	(9.0)
2501–4500 gm		690	69
		(2.0)	(4.8)
< 2500 gm	2733	319	22
	(241.3)	(34.7)	(62.9)
4081			
(10.2)			

[a] Minnesota, 1967–1973, white singleton residents of or born in Minnesota.

TABLE 1.3

Number of Deaths and Rate per 1000 Still Alive at End of First Week for Late Neonatal and Postneonatal Period (1 Week–1 Year) [a]

	< 37 weeks	37–43 weeks	44 + weeks
4501 + gm		21	2
		(2.9)	(3.6)
2501–4500 gm	119	1230	67
	(7.4)	(3.6)	(4.7)
$\leq$ 2500 gm	302	169	8
	(35.2)	(19.1)	(24.4)
1918			
(4.8)			

[a] Minnesota, 1967–1973, white singleton residents of or born in Minnesota.

ing the post-early neonatal period (1 week–1 year). Rates are per 1000 still alive at the end of the first week, and the total deaths from Tables 1.2 and 1.3 demonstrate that in this population, as in other recent United States populations, two-thirds of all infant deaths occur during the first week.

As can be seen in Table 1.3, the elevated risk among light and early babies, while substantial, is not nearly as dramatic as the risk during the early neonatal period. Unlike the first-week experience, the majority of post-early neonatal deaths occur in the optimal survival group defined by birthweight and gestation length; between 37–43 weeks and between 2501–4500 gm.

While birthweight and gestational age, the most practical methods for identifying prematurity, are excellent predictors of neonatal mortality, and therefore of total infant mortality, they are not nearly as useful in identifying the majority of potential deaths among older infants. This is particularly true of gestational age, and it may thus be fortuitous as well as more accurate that birthweight has most often been used as the measurement of prematurity for epidemiologic purposes. The remainder of this chapter will focus on the major risk factors associated with low birth weight (LBW).

Using published data from the National Center for Health Statistics (1973), Table 1.4 shows the amount of variation in the percentage of live births weighing less than 2501 gm (LBW) among different state populations in the United States. This variation indicates a near doubling of the proportion of LBW white babies in whole state populations—smaller areas would show an even greater variation. The three states with more than 8% white LBW are Colorado, New Mexico, and Wyoming; this probably reflects the effect of high altitude with reduced oxygen tension and slower growth (Abramowicz & Kass, 1966b).

Those states with low proportions of nonwhite LBW babies are either western states where the nonwhite populations are Asian or Native American, who tend to have larger babies, or states where the statistics are based on very small numbers of nonwhite births. Based on data from Placek (1977), Table

TABLE 1.4

Variation among the United States in Percentage of Low Birthweight, by Race (1973)[a,b]

Percentage LBW	Number of states	
	White	Nonwhite
< 5.0	1	1
5.0–5.9	12	1
6.0–6.9	31	2
7.0–7.9	4	4
8.0–8.9	3	3
9.0–9.9	—	4
10.0–10.9	—	6
11.0–11.9	—	5
12.0–12.9	—	13
13.0–13.9	—	10
14.0–14.9	—	1
15.0+	—	1
	51	51

[a] National Center for Health Statistics, 1977.
[b] Includes Washington, D.C.

1.5 shows that the South has the largest proportion of premature babies measured as birthweight less than 2501 gm or as gestation length less than 37 weeks. This is undoubtedly due to the much higher proportion of blacks, who have smaller babies. The proportion of black births weighing less than 2501 gm is about twice that found among white births in the United States. The discrepancy in actual prematurity may not be as great, since survival is better among black babies weighing less than 2501 gm than among whites in the same birthweight categories (Erhardt, Joshi, Nelson, Kroll, & Weiner, 1964).

While the variation in the percentage of babies born at 2500 gm or less in the United States is substantial considering the size and heterogeneity of state populations, much of this variation may be due to differences in the propor-

TABLE 1.5

Variation in Percentage of Low Birthweight and of Short Gestation by Region and Race from 1972 Natality Survey[a]

	Percentage LBW	Percentage less than 37 weeks
Northeast	6.3	9.3
North Central	6.4	9.3
South	8.4	10.9
West	6.2	8.4
U.S. White	6.2	9.0
U.S. Nonwhite	12.8	14.6

[a] Placek, 1977.

tion of high-risk groups in the different states. The more important individual risk factors that have been extensively investigated and that contribute to increases in the rate of low birthweight are mother's race, age, parity, previous pregnancy history, family income and education, cigarette smoking, weight gain during pregnancy, and prepregnancy weight (Abramowicz & Kass, 1966a, 1966b, 1966c, 1966d). Tables 1.6–1.12 present examples of the association between the percentage of babies weighing less than 2501 gm at birth and different levels of each of these factors. These data were derived from several studies in the United States, Canada, and Norway, and are referenced at the foot of each table.

Table 1.6 shows the effect of maternal age and birth order on the rate of low birthweight from two data sources. It is evident that the late twenties and the second birth are optimal for reduced risk of low birthweight in both races, as demonstrated in both data sets. The discrepancy in the 1972 Natality Survey may be due to the fact that it is based on a much smaller sample, and some selection may have occurred among those who answered a mailed questionnaire. The 1973 data are based on a 50% sample of all birth certificates in the United States and are consistent with previous years' data from the same source. Although the low-birthweight rate is less than 5% in the 25–29 year age group among the white population, the effect of increased rates among

TABLE 1.6
Low Birthweight by Maternal Age and Live Birth Order

Maternal age	Percentage LBW 1973 U.S. data[a]			1972 natality survey, all races[b]
	White	Black	Total	
< 15	11.6	17.3	15.1 ⎫	
15–17	8.2	14.4	10.3 ⎬	6.5
18–19	7.0	13.3	8.5	8.8
20–24	5.3	11.6	6.3	6.7
25–29	4.7	10.3	5.4	5.8
30–34	5.3	10.4	5.9	9.0
35–39	6.4	11.4	7.3 ⎫	
40–44	7.4	11.2	8.1 ⎬	7.7
45+	7.8	12.8	8.7 ⎭	
Birth order				
1	6.0	12.3	6.9	6.3
2	4.9	11.9	5.9	6.0
3	5.2	11.7	6.2	9.0
4	5.8	11.9	6.8	6.7
5+	6.6	11.7	7.8	10.5

[a] National Center for Health Statistics, 1977.
[b] Placek, 1977.

TABLE 1.7
Tendency to Repeat Low Birthweight

Previous LBW birth	Percentage LBW among second pregnancies	
	Norway [a]	Ontario [b]
Yes	15.2	13.5[c]
No	2.6	5.8

[a] Bakketeig, 1977.

[b] Meyer, Jonas, & Tonascia, 1976. Rates are adjusted for maternal smoking, hospital status, mother's birthplace, mother's height, prepregnant weight, sex of child, age, and parity.

[c] Previous pregnancy loss.

younger and older women is sufficient to raise the overall rate among whites to 6.2% for the same time period.

Table 1.7 shows a risk factor of considerable importance in some populations among multiparous women. In the Norwegian data, where subsequent births have been linked for the same mothers during the study period, the tendency to repeat low birthweight or preterm delivery, somewhat independently, accounted for 25% of low birthweight babies among second births in that population (Bakketeig, 1977). The relative importance of this factor is greater in populations with a lower rate of low-weight babies. In the Canadian data, a previous loss doubles the risk of having a low-birthweight baby.

Although the data are not presented here, it has often been noted that there is an association between prematurity and the timing of prenatal care. Among respondents to the 1972 Natality Survey (Placek, 1977), the rate of low birthweight among women who had received no prenatal care was nearly double that of other women, regardless of when care was started. Since this group may include a larger proportion of women whose first contact with the obstetrical service was at the time of a preterm delivery and who may have otherwise sought prenatal care later in their pregnancy, it is not a good measure of the effectiveness of prenatal care. On the other hand, the prematurity rate among women who seek prenatal care early during their pregnancy is often higher than among those first attending during the second and third trimesters. Since this group may include a significant proportion of women who are already having problems early in their pregnancy, it is likewise not a good measure of the ineffectiveness of early prenatal care. Thus, while prenatal care is universally considered to be good medical practice and public health programs aimed at reduction of perinatal mortality almost always encourage early utilization of antenatal care facilities, there is little epidemiological evidence to support the potential effectiveness of prenatal care in reducing prematurity.

TABLE 1.8
Low Birthweight by Socioeconomic Status

Family income (dollars)	Percentage LBW[a]	Per capita income (dollars)	Percentage LBW[b]
< 4000	10.9	600	7.0
4000–6999	7.6	1400	6.5
7000–9999	6.5	2200	6.0
10,000–14,999	6.0	3000	6.0
15000 +	6.5	3400 +	6.0

[a] Garn, Shaw, & McCabe, 1977.
[b] Placek, 1977.

Tables 1.8 and 1.9 show the relationship between income and education (as well as some data on cigarette smoking) to the risk for low birthweight. It is evident that both income and education are inversely associated with prematurity. Since these two variables are highly correlated with each other, the effects are probably not independent. However, the potential populations at elevated risk are large. Part of the data from a collaborative perinatal project containing information on smoking during pregnancy is included on the right-hand side of Table 1.9. The marked effect of mother's education among smoking women is consistent with other study results in which smoking is most strongly associated with low birthweight among women who are otherwise at increased risk.

It has been repeatedly demonstrated that cigarette smoking, particularly during the second half of pregnancy, is associated with a reduction in average birthweight of aproximately 200 gm at all gestational ages. The bottom line of Table 1.10 illustrates that, even when controlling for a number of other known risk factors, the effect of smoking one or more packs of cigarettes per day is to more than double the proportion of babies born under 2501 gm. It can be noted from the same table that the effect of decreased weight gain during pregnancy is at least as dramatic—and the risk factor has only recently been appreciated. That reduced weight gain may be partially responsible for the observed effects of cigarette smoking has been suggested by some investigators (Davies, Gray, & Ellwood, 1976; Rush, 1974). The importance of these two risk factors is made even more significant by the fact that both are at least potentially intervenable by health education efforts on an individual as well as community basis after pregnancy has been initiated.

Table 1.11 shows an association between prepregnancy weight and percentage low birthweight in both whites and blacks. These data show a significant gradient among substantial population groups from two perinatal studies.

Although a number of other factors have been associated with prematurity, they are either of lesser importance than those presented here or are outcomes of the pregnancy itself. Examples of the latter include breech delivery, bleeding during pregnancy, abruptio placenta, placenta praevia, incompetent

TABLE 1.9

Low Birthweight by Education of Parents

Years of education	Percentage LBW [a]
Mother	
≤ 8	9.7
9–11	7.2
12	6.6
13–15	6.5
16+	8.3
Father	
≤ 8	7.9
9–11	7.7
12	7.0
13–15	6.8
16+	6.4

	Percentage LBW [b]			
	White			
Years of education	All	Nonsmoker	Smoker	Black
Mother				
0–6	8.8	4.0	14.0	12.9
7–9	8.0	4.0	11.0	13.0
10–11	7.7	4.0	10.0	13.5
12–15	6.0	4.0	8.0	11.5
16+	4.0	3.0	6.0	10.5

[a] Placek, 1977.
[b] Garn, Shaw, McCabe, 1977.

TABLE 1.10

Low Birthweight by Maternal Weight Gain and Cigarette Smoking during Pregnancy [a]

	Percentage LBW (Ontario data) [b]		
Maternal weight gain (lb)	Nonsmoker	< 1 pack/day	> 1 pack/day
25+	2.2	3.3	5.9
10–24	5.4	9.3	13.8
< 10	13.8	21.2	33.7
Total	4.7	7.8	11.9

[a] Adjusted for prepregnancy weight, previous pregnancy history, hospital status, mother's birthplace, height, age, parity, and sex of child.
[b] Meyer, Jonas, & Tonascia, 1976.

11

TABLE 1.11
Low Birthweight by Prepregnancy Weight[a]

| | Percentage LBW | | | |
| Prepregnancy weight (lb.) | United States[b] | | Ontario[c], all races | Weight range |
	White	Black		
< 100	15	26 ⎫		
100–109	10	21 ⎬	8.5	< 120
110–119	9	17 ⎭		
120–139	6	13	5.8	120–139
140–159	5	10 ⎫		
160–179	4	9 ⎬	4.6	≥ 140
180–199	4	9 ⎪		
200 +	3	10 ⎭		

[a] Adjusted for maternal smoking, previous pregnancy history, hospital status, mother's birthplace, height, age, parity, and sex of child.
[b] Hardy & Mellits, 1977.
[c] Meyer, Jonas, & Tonascia, 1976.

cervix, premature rupture of the membranes, and toxemia and are best classified as obstetrical complications, which may in turn be the result of some of the risk factors presented here, as well as other and unknown factors.

While all of the factors included in this review show significant association with the risk of premature births measured as low birthweight, many of them are intercorrelated, and it is difficult to determine which are of more independent significance. In order to examine the contribution of many factors simultaneously while, in effect, adjusting for the others, a multiple regression analysis was applied to data from a collaborative perinatal project among multiparous women with births at 37 weeks or more (Weiss & Jackson, 1969). Table 1.12 shows the relative contribution of each of the variables included in this review as well as of a number of other factors. In addition to complications of pregnancy and labor and fetal conditions, it can be seen that weight gain during pregnancy, prepregnancy weight, last prior birthweight, previous pregnancy outcome, and smoking were the major independent contributors in this group. With the exception of having had a previous low-birthweight infant or a previous pregnancy loss, a similar result might be expected in an analysis of all births, since the results here are almost identical for both whites and blacks. However, it is somewhat surprising that mother's age, parity, and income do not independently contribute very much to the variation in birthweight among individuals, at least in multiparous women.

The extent to which all of the risk factors included in the present review explain interstate variation is unknown. An analysis of United States births during 1969–1971 indicates a standard deviation of .8% in low-birthweight rates among white state populations (Keller, 1977). Utilizing 22 physical, social,

TABLE 1.12

Percentage of Variance in Birthweight "Explained" by Various Factors among Multiparous Women [a]

Factors	Percentage of variance "explained"	
	White	Black
Weight gain	6.6	8.2
Prepregnancy weight	6.0	4.6
Last prior birthweight	6.0	4.6
Cigarettes/day	3.2	1.4
Previous pregnancy outcome	1.0	1.7
Parity	.3	.4
Age	0	0
Annual income	.1	.1
Height	0	0
Maternal diseases	.2	.4
Fetal attributes[b]	2.6	1.6
Complications of pregnancy and labor	7.3	6.5
Total "explained" variance (multiple R squared)	33.3	29.5

[a] Based on partial correlation and multiple correlation coefficients in a multiple linear regression analysis of 32 factors. (Weiss & Jackson, 1969).

[b] Includes sex, congenital malformations, and Coombs test.

and demographic characteristics based on information from the 1970 census as independent variables in a multiple linear regression model, two-thirds of this variation can be "explained" by a positive association with states average altitude above sea level and a negative association with the proportion of the foreign stock of Teutonic derivation. An additional 20% can be explained by statistically significant but minor contributions of several other characteristics, including positive associations with the proportion of first births and working mothers and negative associations with women's education, family income, urbanization, and the proportion of women in the labor force. Maternal age, industrialization, and several other social and demographic factors did not make a significant contribution in this simultaneous assessment of a number of variables. Unfortunately, appropriate data on prepregnancy weight, weight gains and cigarette smoking during pregnancy, and previous pregnancy outcome are not available for geographically definable populations on which this type of analysis is based. However, some of these variables, for example, prepregnancy weight and weight gain during pregnancy, may be related to ethnic or cultural identification, which appears to have a marked influence on birthweight.

In conclusion, while low birthweight is a measure of prematurity, which is also a good predictor of infant mortality, it is in itself the result of a number of other risk factors. A large number of potential risk factors have been evaluated; only a few of them appear to contribute independently and appreciably to the variation among individuals or groups. Although it has not been possible to assess the relative importance of all risk factors simultaneously, it is perhaps fortunate that two of the major contributors to low birthweight, cigarette smoking and weight gains, may be amenable to alteration via behavioral changes in pregnant women.

References

Abramowicz, M., & Kass, E. H. Pathogenesis and prognosis of prematurity. *New England Journal of Medicine,* 1966, *16,* 878-85. (a)

Abramowicz, M., & Kass, E. H. Pathogenesis and prognosis of prematurity. *New England Journal of Medicine,* 1966, *17,* 938-943. (b)

Abramowicz, M., & Kass, E. H. Pathogenesis and prognosis of prematurity. *New England Journal of Medicine,* 1966, *18,* 1001-1007. (c)

Abramowicz, M., & Kass, E. H. Pathogenesis and prognosis of prematurity. *New England Journal of Medicine,* 1966, *19,* 1053-1059. (d)

Bakketeig, L. S. The risk of repeated preterm or low birth weight delivery. In D. Reed & F. Stanley (Eds.), *The epidemiology of prematurity.* Baltimore: Urban and Schwarzenberg, 1977.

Berendes, H. Prematurity. *Transactions of the New England Obstetrical and Gynecological Society,* 1963, *7,* 205-206.

Boyce, A., Mayaux, M. J., & Schwartz, D. Classical and "true" gestational postmaturity. *American Journal of Obstetrics and Gynecology,* 1976, *125* (7), 911-914.

Cunningham, G., Williams, R., Hawes, W., Madore, C., Norris, F., & Phibbs, R. *Intrauterine growth and neonatal risk in California.* Unpublished manuscript, Community and Organizational Research Institute, University of California, Santa Barbara, and Infant Health Section, Maternal and Child Health, State of California Department of Health, Santa Barbara, Cal., 1974.

Davies, D. P., Gray, O. P., & Ellwood, P. C. Cigarette smoking in pregnancy: associations with maternal weight gain and fetal growth. *Lancet,* 1976, *1,* 385-387.

Erhardt, C. L., Joshi, G. B., Nelson, F. G., Kroll, B. H. & Weiner, E. E. Influence of weight and gestation on perinatal and neonatal mortality by ethnic group. *American Journal of Public Health,* 1964, *54,* 1841-1855.

Garn, S. M., Shaw, H. A., & McCabe, K. D. Effects of socioeconomic status and race on weight-defined and gestational prematurity in the United States. In D. Reed & F. Stanley (Eds.), *The epidemiology of prematurity.* Baltimore: Urban and Schwarzenberg, 1977.

Hardy, J. B., & Mellits, E. D. Relationships of low birth weight to maternal characteristics of age, parity, education, and body size. In D. Reed & F. Stanley (Eds.), *The epidemiology of prematurity.* Baltimore: Urban and Schwarzenberg, 1977.

Keller, C. A. Interstate variation in adverse pregnancy outcome. Paper presented at the 105th Annual Meeting of the American Public Health Association, Washington, D.C. 1977.

Meyer, M. B., Jonas, B. S., & Tonascia, J. A. Perinatal events associated with maternal smoking during pregnancy. *American Journal of Epidemiology,* 1976, *103,* 464-476.

U.S. Department of Health, Education and Welfare, Public Health Service, National Center for Health Statistics. *Vital statistics of the United States 1973, Vol. 1–Natality.* Washington, D.C.: U.S. Government Printing Office, 1977.

Placek, P. Maternal and infant health factors associated with low infant birth weight: Findings from the 1972 National Natality Survey. In D. Reed & F. Stanley (Eds.), *The epidemiology of prematurity*. Baltimore: Urban and Schwarzenberg, 1977.

Rush, D. Examination of the relationship between birthweight, cigarette smoking during pregnancy and maternal weight gain. *Journal of Obstetrics and Gynaecology of the British Commonwealth,* 1974, *81,* 746–752.

Weiss, W., & Jackson, E. C. Maternal factors affecting birth weight. In *Perinatal factors affecting human development*. Washington D.C.: Pan American Health Organization, 1969.

2

Medical Constraints to Optimal Psychological Development of the Preterm Infant

MILTON W. WERTHMANN, JR.

A normal, uneventful pregnancy and a healthy, robust, normal newborn are the desires of every expectant parent. Today's communications media and product advertisements reinforce this expectation with photographs of chubby, rosy-cheeked infants. Unfortunately, there are a significant number of newborn infants whose arrivals are ill timed, the result of maternal illness, placental malfunction, or problems in the infants themselves. These problems pose threats to the very survival of the newly born or to its subsequent normal growth and development. Until the last decade of the nineteenth century, survival of such tiny infants was rare. The well-known French obstetrician Pierre Budin and his student Martin Couney established and published guidelines for nursing care for such preterm infants (Budin, 1907). Somewhat later, Hess and Lundeen (1941) introduced concepts of isolation, specially trained nurses, and special equipment (incubators) and procedures that were effective in improving survival of these tiny infants. But it was not until the past 25 years that the attention of medical research has been so intensely focused on solving the problems of the fetus and newborn. The medical literature now abounds with etiologic mechanisms of newborn disorders, modalities of treatment, and devices to assist this tiny infant survive against what were once impossible odds.

Prematurity

Statistics traditionally have reported prematurity in terms of birthweight, with infants weighing less than 2500 gm being designated premature. While approximately accurate, this standard is misleading because it encompasses small-for-date term infants but not large-for-date infants who are, in fact, actually premature. Hence, comparison of survival data was difficult to interpret. Battaglia and Lubchenco (1967) defined the word *preterm* to distinguish any infant born before 37 completed gestational weeks dating from onset of last menses. Such infants, by weight, could therefore be small for gestation (below 10th percentile of the group), appropriate for gestation (between 10th and 90th percentile) or large for gestation (above 90th percentile). In 1977 in the United States, 3,167,788 births were recorded (U.S. Department of Health, Education, Welfare, Public Health Service, National Center for Health Statistics). Of these, 7.3% (231,248) weighed below 2500 gm (5 lb. 8 oz.) and 8.8% (278,765) were born before the completion of the thirty-seventh week of gestation.

The number of neonatal deaths occurring within 28 days of birth in the United States is between 34,000 and 40,000 per year (Behrman, 1977). There are approximately 250,000 preterm infants receiving care of various degrees in special-care nurseries across the country. As a result of the increased research and advances in this area since the mid-1960s, an endless array of neonatal devices have been developed to assist ventilation, monitor heart rate, treat jaundice, and control heat loss. Through utilization of the latest technology, risk of dying has been reduced in these preterm infants. However, medical problems still exist. There are some treatment-related iatrogenic problems as well. This chapter will relate factors of maternal, placental, and neonatal origin that may compromise normal development in the preterm infant.

Prenatal Factors

PREMATURE LABOR

Premature labor is the occurrence of frequent uterine contractions resulting in progressive cervical dilitation and/or effacement prior to completion of the thirty-seventh week of gestation. Premature labor occurs in approximately 10% of the pregnancies of white mothers and 20% of those of black mothers (Garn, Shaw, & McCabe, 1977). Breech presentation of the preterm fetus occurs in as many as 25% of births at or prior to 34 weeks gestation (Goldberg & Nelson, 1977). Although delivery of a breech at any gestation is accompanied by increased mortality and morbidity, the delivery of a preterm breech is accompanied by a much greater risk of asphyxia and low Apgar scores at birth because of the progressively larger body parts that must be delivered (Brenner, Bruce, & Hendricks, 1974). Vertex presentation is also accompanied by problems, since the small size of the fetal head allows for compound presentations or the umbilical cord to become trapped between the presenting fetal part and the bony pelvis of the mother. This condition results in fetal compromise and/or attempts to manipulate the fetus in the delivery process, during which the infant may be bruised or suffer fractured body parts. As a consequence of these potential problems, there is a definite trend toward a higher cesarean section rate for premature labor (Pritchard & MacDonald, 1976). The ever-increasing intact survival of smaller and smaller preterm infants poses another dilemma for the obstetrician. There are now widely divergent approaches to the basic problem of premature labor, which is, at what gestation should labor be halted or allowed to progress? Those favoring delivery without delay face the decision of cesarean versus vaginal delivery. If labor is desultory, oxytocin augmentation may increase the incidence of complicated deliveries and possible fetal trauma during a vaginal birth. Preterm infants delivered by cesarean section have a greater risk of pulmonary fluid retention and respiratory distress. Those favoring inhibition of labor face the increased risk of acute fetal distress if the cause of the labor was a problem in the fetal placental unit. They must also consider the possible untoward effect on the fetus of using many medical modalities, including analgesics, sedatives, tranquilizers, ethanol, beta-mimetic drugs, and xanthines, in an attempt to control premature labor (Dilts, 1970; Heymann, Rudolph, & Silverman, 1976; Mann, Bhakthavathsalan, Liu, & Makowski, 1975; Stander, Barden, Thompson, Pugh, & Werts, 1964; Wagner, Wagner, & Guerrero, 1970; Zuckerman, Reiss, & Rubenstein, 1974). Hepatic enzymes for drug detoxification in the fetus and preterm infant are functionally deficient, and drugs like sulfonamides, used in treating maternal urinary tract infection, are metabolized slowly, increasing the risk of neurotoxicity in some preterm infants born while the mother is on such treatment (Brown & Cevik, 1965).

PREMATURE RUPTURE OF MEMBRANES

Premature spontaneous rupture of membranes prior to the onset of labor occurs in 15-20% of preterm pregnancies compared to a rare instance in term pregnancies (Gunn, Mishell, & Morton, 1970; Russell & Cheung, 1974; Taylor, Morgan, Bruns, & Drose, 1961). Unfortunately, spontaneous labor within 24 hours of rupture of membranes occur in fewer than 50% of preterm pregnancies and only increases to 70% of preterm pregnancies within 72 hours post rupture of membranes (Gunn *et al.,* 1970). The risk of infection in preterm infants during such pregnancies is significantly increased with each day that delivery is delayed (Bada, Alojipan, & Andrews, 1977). As a result, maternal antibiotics are prescribed, usually including aminoglycosides, which have the potential for causing hearing loss or renal injury (McCracken & Nelson, 1977). Such infants also have complications, such as pneumonia and apnea, and often require respiratory support for the first few days of therapy.

TOXEMIA OF PREGNANCY

Toxemia (hypertensive disease of pregnancy) occurs in approximately 3-10% of pregnancies and poses risks of premature delivery, neonatal asphyxia (resulting from uterine hypoperfusion and / or antihypertensive drugs), drug depression (resulting from sedatives, tranquilizers), hypotonia and paralytic ileus (resulting from magnesium sulfate therapy), thrombocytopenia (resulting from thiazide diuretics), and intrauterine growth retardation (Babson, Benson, Pernoll, & Benda, 1975). In cases where maternal toxemia is present, preterm infants delivered in a tertiary perinatal center, who are promptly resuscitated, watched and treated for hypoglycemia, and managed for particular drug effects, do well in follow-up, although some limitation of physical growth may occur (Yogman, Speroff, Huttenlocher, & Kase, 1972).

ERYTHROBLASTOSIS FETALIS

Hepatosplenomegaly, edema, anemia, and heart failure as a result of relentless destruction of fetal cells coated with maternal antibody is known as hydrops fetalis—the stage prior to fetal death from erythroblastosis fetalis. Usually caused by Rh incompatibility but occasionally by other causes of hemolysis, this problem requires sequential assessment of maternal antibody titres and serial amniocenteses (Freda, 1965; Queenan & Goetschel, 1968) to assess the amount of bilirubin pigment accumulating in the amniotic fluid. Usually, significantly sensitized pregnancies require delivery of the infant prior to term to avoid fetal death *in utero*. Such infants may be or may become significantly anemic and/or jaundiced at birth, requiring treatment to avoid death or permanent brain damage (Queenan, 1967).

IATROGENIC FACTORS

Iatrogenic causes of premature births include the spontaneous onset of labor after amniocentesis (less than 1 in 1000 procedures) and after surgical procedures (Young, Matson, & Jones, 1976). Obstetric choice is the cause in Rh erythroblastosis with high amniotic fluid bilirubin or in maternal diabetes after 35 wks gestation. Error in correctly assessing length of gestation prior to elective repeat cesarean section without labor or induction of labor reportedly has been responsible for delivery of up to 10–15% of preterm infants (Behrman, 1977). Intrapartum management of preterm deliveries may be complicated by failure of the cervix to dilate and efface in a reasonable time after rupture of membranes. Pitocin used to stimulate labor and accomplish vaginal delivery in such cases may induce fetal head trauma with resultant bruising, fetal distress with passage of meconium and subsequent aspiration, fetal asphyxia, and intraventricular hemorrhage. Maternal hypotension resulting from epidural anesthesia adds yet another hypoxic insult to such a fetus.

Placental Factors

One of the placental factors leading to preterm delivery is retroplacental hemorrhage with partial or total abruption. In such cases, labor may commence spontaneously or delivery may be mandated by significant blood loss leading to maternal and/or fetal hypovolemia (Niswander, Friedman,

Hoover, Pietrowski, & Westphal, 1966). Frequently, such infants are also hypoxic at birth and may develop cerebral palsy subsequently (Schlesinger, Mazundar, & Logrillo, 1973). In view of current capabilities in neonatal intensive care, Goodlin (1979) recommends prompt delivery in such cases of placental hemorrhage to obtain the best baby physically and neurologically.

A placenta located in an area of poor uterine vascular supply, or with premature sinescence or significant infarction, may be unable to provide for adequate fetal nutrition, resulting in a small-for-date, low-birthweight, dysmature child. Often born prematurely, this child is at greater risk of developing hypoglycemia.

Neonatal Factors

Once past the hazards of the abnormal intrauterine milieu and the stresses of labor and delivery, the infant born preterm is cast forth into a hostile new environment for which it is incompletely prepared. The following are some of the postnatal challenges and problems with which the preterm infant must cope or be assisted by its caretakers if it is to survive. With expanding expertise to guide these caretakers, such infants are surviving with few handicaps at ever-smaller birth weights.

ASPHYXIA AND HYPOXIA

Neonatal asphyxia poses an immediate threat to survival. The incidence of asphyxia at birth increases from 5% of preterm infants near term to nearly 50% of tiny infants of less than 28 weeks gestation (O'Brien, Usher, & Maughan, 1966). Although it is generally accepted that newborn infants can utilize anaerobic metabolism and shift their circulation preferentially to critical areas (heart, brain) to extend their tolerance of asphyxia (Behrman, Lees, Peterson, DeLannoy, & Seeds, 1970), the infant depressed at birth may have already exceeded the tolerance level. One indicator of whether this point has been reached is the length of time it takes regular breathing to return during the resuscitation process. Since it takes approximately 2 min of resuscitative effort to reverse 1 min of asphyxia, lack of return of regular breathing after 16 min of resuscitative effort indicates asphyxia of at least 8 min duration (Adamsons, Behrman, Dawes, James, & Koford, 1964; James, 1964). In most cases, 8 min is the upper limit of anoxia tolerated by the preterm infant. Infants successfully resuscitated after longer asphyxia will show varying degrees of brain injury. In experimental animals, support of cardiac output and correction of acidosis during resuscitation has been shown to extend the time tolerated by the central nervous system prior to onset of permanent injury (Adamsons, Behrman, Dawes, Dawkins, James, & Ross, 1963; Dawes, Hibbard, & Windle, 1964). The acute obstruction of an endotracheal tube in a preterm infant on assisted ventilation also presents an asphyxial insult. However, such infants are usually attached to respiratory and heart-rate monitors and, in some centers, transcutaneous oxygen monitors. Such obstruction is rapidly detected, and the tube is removed and then replaced before the infant suffers anoxic insult.

Neonatal hypoxia is a partial deprivation of oxygen and poses a more subtle but equally dangerous threat to the central nervous system function. Well-oxygenated preterm infants with adequate circulating glucose have good cardiac glycogen stores and tolerate such procedures as change of endotracheal tube, weighing, and blood sampling without a decrease in heart rate. Conversely, gradual mucous accumulation causing narrowing of an endotracheal tube, too rapid weaning from oxygen, or too rapid reduction in respiratory support can result in an inadequate amount of oxygen reaching the tissues. In such cases, infants are depleted of cardiac glycogen and have minimal or no ability to sustain cardiac output during acute hypoxia (Dawes, Mott, & Shelley, 1959; Stafford & Weatherall, 1960). This fragility is evidenced by immediate bradycardia with even the slightest procedure (baby repositioning, endotracheal tube suctioning, etc.). Such infants gradually accumulate lactate as a result of incomplete metabolism, become acidotic as well as hypoxic, and begin gasping—a primitive response to oxygen deprivation. If hypoxic distress is not reversed, areas of microcirculation are irreversibly shut down with permanent loss of function of areas previously perfused (Ames, Wright, Kowada, Thurston, & Majno, 1968). The clinical picture of neonatal asphyxia–hypoxia compounded by episodes of recurrent hypoxia during the first few critical days results in a spectrum of effects ranging from severe (early seizures, hypotonia, or spasticity) to subtle ones not seen for several years (learning disabilities, behavior problems).

CIRCULATORY PROBLEMS

Intimately involved in the maintenance of all body organ functions is the cardiovascular system. Some problems that affect the preterm subsequent to birth include: (a) hypovolemia; (b) hypervolemia; (c) persistent fetal circulation; (d) patent ductus arteriosus; and (e) anemia.

Hypovolemia. Preterm infants are usually delivered in an environment anticipating neonatal problems. If the infant is in any way compromised, there is immediate cord clamping and delivery of the infant to the pediatric team for resuscitation. Cord clamping prior to the first breath deprives the preterm infant of the 25–50% increase in its circulating blood volume that would have been received in a cord clamping delayed 2–5 min (Saigal, O'Neill, Surainder, Chua, & Usher, 1972). Other causes of neonatal hypovolemia include umbilical cord tear, placental abruption, and fetal–maternal transfusion. Such infants are tachypneic, tachycardic, and pale with weak pulses. Restoration of circulatory volume and red cells relieves the symptoms and reduces the risk of organ injury. The combination of asphyxia and hypovolemia markedly decreases chances for intact neurologic survival. The clinical evolution of symptoms of hypoxic-ischemic encephalopathy together with neuropathologic correlates has been well reviewed by Volpe (1977).

Hypervolemia and polycythemia. Usher (1975) coined the term *symptomatic neonatal plethora* in the preterm infant to describe the acute clinical picture that results from delay in cord clamping 2–5 min postdelivery. This condition can also be caused iatrogenically by milking the cord toward the infant. Clinically, these infants are plethoric and tachypneic with shallow breathing and have pulmonary vascular congestion and edema on chest x-ray and expanded blood volumes in the range of 100–125 ml per kg. Because of volume overload, they have decreased cardiac output, metabolic acidosis, and hypotension (Moss & Monset-Couchard, 1976; Oh, Wallgren, Hannson, & Third, 1967). Phlebotomy results in rapid resolution of the symptoms.

Polycythemia (central hematocrit greater than 65%) can also result from delayed cord clamping, cord milking, or twin–twin transfusion (Rausen, Seki, & Strauss, 1965). The incidence has recently been determined to be 6% in preterm infants greater than 34 weeks gestation with weight approprate for gestational age (Wirth, Goldberg, & Lubchenco, 1979). Polycythemia due to placental transfusion is the principle cause of hyperviscosity (Bergqvist, 1974). Infants with hyperviscosity develop clinical cyanosis, hypoglycemia, hypocalcemia, hyperbilirubinemia, convulsions, and renal dysfunction (Aperia, Bergqvist, Broberger, Thodenius, & Vetterstrom, 1974; Stone, Thompson, & Schmidt-Nelson, 1968; Wood, 1959). Treatment for polycythemia–hyperviscosity is partial exchange transfusion with fresh frozen plasma. Currently, some preterm infants with central hematocrits of 62–65% are found to have hyperviscosity as well (Wirth *et al.*, 1979). Whether these borderline asymptomatic infants with hyperviscosity will have limitations in their future achievement potential is currently unknown.

Persistent fetal circulation. The fetus *in utero* tolerates its low-oxygen environment by preferentially shunting oxygenated blood to its brain and heart. Most oxygen-dependent fetal capabilities are not yet fully activated, and organ systems are in a standby status, allowing the placenta to perform the functions of liver, kidney, and lungs. Some preterm infants, postbirth and deprived of the placenta, fail to convert their circulation to obligate lung perfusion for oxygen uptake (Behrman, 1976; Gersony, Duc, & Sinclair, 1969). These preterm infants remain cyanotic and hypoxic, posing a true emergency state. Highly vasoactive drugs are then required to shift the circulation from fetal to adult configuration (Goetzman *et al.*, 1976). Occasionally, severe hypotension and shock, as a side effect of these drugs, further compromise the hypoxic cerebral perfusion. When successfully treated with appropriate improvement in systemic oxygenation, these infants seem to have no short-term evidence of central nervous system sequelae.

Patent ductus arteriosus. The ductus arteriosus (between the pulmonary artery and aorta) in preterm infants readily reopens when the preterm infant becomes hypoxic or acidotic (Danilowicz, Rudolph, & Hoffman, 1966; Siassi, Blanco, Cabal, & Coran, 1976). Persistent patency of the ductus arteriosus in preterm infants can lead to progressive left heart failure, pulmonary congestion, and pulmonary hypertension. Preterm infants with patent ductus arteriosus and respiratory distress syndrome are often unable to be weaned from the respirator. Medical treatment of such symptomatic patients may be successful in as many as 80% of cases (Friedman, Hirschklau, Printz, Pitlick, & Kirkpatrick, 1976; Heymann, Rudolph, & Silverman, 1976). When medical treatment is unsuccessful, surgical ligation of the patent ductus arteriosus will produce dramatic clinical improvement with low surgical mortality risk (Kitterman, Edmunds, Gregory, Heymann, Tooley, & Rudolph, 1972; Zackman, Steinmetz, Botham, Graven, & Ledbetter, 1974).

Anemia of prematurity. The preterm infant begins life with about the same amount of hemoglobin per kg as does the term infant (Burman & Morris, 1974). Before it leaves the nursery, however, the small preterm infant will have doubled or tripled its weight and its hemoglobin will have fallen to half or less than half of its birth value. The early anemia of prematurity has been associated with apnea, patent ductus arteriosus, and bronchopulmonary dysplasia (Usher, 1975). Yet in a recent review, Stockman (1977) shows very conclusively that even the apparently severe anemia of prematurity is indeed physiologic and iron deficiency plays no role in early anemia of prematurity. One is forced to conclude that early asymptomatic anemia of prematurity poses no threat to the asymptomatic preterm infant.

POOR THERMOREGULATION

The significance of heat control to the preterm infant, while recognized by Budin and Couney (1907), was lost to general medical awareness until the studies of Silverman, Fertig, and Berger (1958), Bruck (1961, 1968); and Scopes (1966). Since then, the physiology of thermal control, the effects of thermal stress, and the descriptions of various devices and procedures to maintain optimal environmental temperature have comprised ever larger chapters in textbooks on neonatology (Behrman, 1977; Klaus, Fanaroff, & Martin, 1979; Scopes, 1975).

The preterm infant magnifies the problem of maintaining thermal stability by its relatively high surface area to mass ratio, deficiency in subcutaneous insulating fat, and difficulty in consuming and assimilating sufficient calories to offset caloric expenditure. The iatrogenic quirks of medicine discussed in the following paragraphs add to these physical constraints. Hey (1971) described optimal thermal ranges for premature infants 1 kg or larger, nude or dressed, from birth to 30 days. The optimal thermal range (neutral thermal environment) is that set of thermal conditions at which heat production (measured as oxygen consumption) is minimal while maintaining a core temperature of 36.5–37.5°C (Oliver, 1977).

Hypothermia in the delivery room. Most delivery rooms are kept 20–25°C (67–76°F) for the comfort of adults (approximately the thermal neutral zone for typically dressed adults). The wet infant delivered into this environment has been estimated to lose 200 cal/kg/min (Oliver, 1977) unless provisions are taken to minimize this loss. When one considers 120 cal/kg/*day* as the goal of preterm nutrition, one can readily appreciate the magnitude of this stress. Oliver (1965) showed that the core temperature of any infant born under such thermal conditions falls by at least 2°C in the first 15 min after delivery and simultaneously oxygen consumption increases by 2.5 times. In an asphyxiated premature infant, this increased oxygen demand, combined with lack of adequate ventilation, rapidly removes essential available oxygen from the circulation.

Maternal anesthesia or drugs (e.g., diazepam) have been shown by Cree, Meyer, and Hailey (1973) to blunt the infant's thermogenic response. Hypothermia results in a severe metabolic acidosis, water loss, and hypoglycemia (Fisher, 1967; Gandy, Adamsons, & Cunningham, 1964; Kedes & Field, 1964). The failure to correct ongoing rapid heat loss leads to the syndrome of neonatal cold injury that affects preterm infants almost exclusively. It is characterized by a very slow metabolism with very cold skin, core temperature below 32°C (90°F), lethargy, central cyanosis or pallor, irregular slow respiration, bradycardia, and metabolic derangements including hyperkalemia.

Hypothermia in the nursery. Silverman *et al.*, (1958) showed the improvement in survival at all gestational ages achieved by maintaining environmental temperature in isolettes near 31.7°C (90°F). Mestyan, Jarai, & Bata (1964a, 1964b) showed an increase in metabolism and oxygen consumption when cool oxygen was blown over the trigeminal area of the face. Hence, oxygen hoods now have air deflectors. Scopes (1966) described the brown fat nonshivering thermogenesis mechanism by which newborn infants generate heat and showed how this thermogenesis was impaired by hypoxia. Plexiglas incubators were designed to maintain infant heat, but it was soon learned that placing incubators by a window or near an air conditioner or even in a cool room resulted in more radiant heat loss than the convected heat could replace (Hey & Mount, 1966). In spite of this, nursery temperature is still maintained for the comfort of the personnel. In addition, because the premature infant's breathing pattern needs to be observed, the infants are kept undressed in the incubator. Hey (1971) again showed that cot-nursed (dressed) premies had a lower ambient heat requirement and a wider range of tolerance than did naked premies. The evolution of apnea monitors and respiratory rate monitors has lessened (but not eliminated) the nurse's need to see the premie breathing.

Double-walled incubators and Plexiglas covers over the infant (Hey & Mount, 1966) have dramatically relieved this apparent stalemate. Erratic control of the on–off type heaters in incubators led Perlstein, Edwards, and Sutherland (1970) to demonstrate that this type of heater was a cause of apnea in premature infants. The servocontrol proportional heater, developed to solve this problem, introduced the next problem: elimination of skin temperature as a clinical determinant of body stress. With the skin temperature being held constant by a thermistor-controlled servomechanism, a baby who is becoming shocky or septic would receive an ever increasing ambient heat. Conversely, the febrile neonate would be subjected to an ever greater thermal stress as the servomechanism adjusts heat output lower and lower in response to the increased skin temperature. With this system, nurses must record incubator temperature to recognize these important changes. Dailey, Klaus, and Meyer (1969) showed that maintaining the ambient temperature at the low end of the thermoneutral zone significantly reduces the incidence of apnea attacks.

Such procedures as bathing, brain scans, x-ray studies, exchange transfusions, and surgery also cause significant thermal stress (Hey, Kohlinsky, & O'Connell, 1969). Transport of the preterm within a hospital or between hospitals requires significant attention to the thermal environment. Several devices utilizing heat-reflecting surfaces (Silver Swaddler) (Baum & Scopes, 1968) and air sacs trapped in laminated plastic (Besch, Perlstein, Edwards, Keenan, & Sutherland, 1971) have been utilized to reduce heat loss in transport.

RESPIRATORY PROBLEMS

The respiratory function of the preterm infant is a sensitive indicator of its well-being. Respiratory malfunction led to the development of most of the intensive care nursery monitoring and respiratory support equipment being used and increased numbers of personnel hours spent to preserve the infant intact. Immaturity of the lung poses anatomical and pathophysiologic problems (Stahlman, 1975) and functionally leads to a need for increased oxygen. This, in turn, requires either invasive (umbilical artery catheterization) (Baker, Berdon, & James, 1969; Larroche, 1970), radial (Adams & Rudolph, 1975) or temporal arterial punctures with determinations of values on blood-gas analyzers, or noninvasive transcutaneous oxygen monitoring (Huch, Huch, & Lubbers, 1973). These data must, in turn, result in oxygen administration controlled by oxygen-blending devices and oxygen monitors. All of these oxygen devices must be frequently evaluated for accuracy lest the child receive too much or too little oxygen. Beddis, Collins, Levy, Godfrey, and Silverman (1979) have recently introduced a method for servocontrolling blood-oxygen levels. Failure of the infant to breathe adequately may be due to central nervous system insensitivity resulting from immaturity (Rigatto & Brady, 1972a), birth anoxia (Rigatto & Brady, 1972b), hemorrhage, or drug-induced respiratory depression. Treatment may include oxygen or xanthines (caffeine or theophylline) to increase respiratory center activity (Lucey, 1975; Shannon, Gotay, Stein, Rogers, Todres, & Moylan, 1975). Too much oxygen results in retrolental fibroplasia (blindness) (James & Lanman, 1976) or pulmonary oxygen toxicity (Anderson & Stickland, 1971; Kapanci, Weibel, Kaplan, & Robinson, 1969; Kaplan, Robinson, Kapanci, & Weibel, 1969). Too little oxygen results in hypoxic encephalopathy (Volpe, 1975).

Monitoring oxygen, if done by transcutaneous electrode, causes usually insignificant areas of hyperemia under the electrode (Huch, Huch, & Albani, 1976) but requires site changes every 2–3 hours, which disturb the infant. If oxygen is monitored invasively, umbilical artery catheterization is usually performed. Difficulties in catheter insertion, circulatory compromise with blanching of the leg on the side of insertion (requiring repositioning or removal of the catheter), partial ischemia (Neal, Reynolds, Jarvia, & Williams, 1972) or embolism to organs perfused by blood vessels adjacent to the catheter, and infection (Krauss, Albert, & Kannan, 1970) are all occasional untoward occurrences that threaten intact survival of the infant.

Due to pulmonary surfactant deficiencies, atelectasis occurs (Avery & Mead, 1959). Because of a flexible chest wall, the premie cannot reexpand this lung well (or at all). The increased work involved in trying to breathe causes progressive acidosis. Finally, when arbitrary criteria are met, continuous positive airway pressure is initiated via nasal prongs (Kattwinkel, Fleming, Cha, Fanaroff, & Klaus, 1973), head hood, mask (Allen, Reynolds, Rivera, Le Souëf, & Wimberley, 1977), or endotracheal tube (Gregory, Kitterman, Phibbs, Tooley, & Hamilton, 1971). If ineffective, or if apnea occurs, mechanical ventilation is added to restore normal oxygenation and clearance of carbon dioxide. An infant who "fights" the ventilatory efforts of the respirator can develop a pneumothorax. Curare or pancuronium is used to paralyze the infant temporarily in such situations (Brady & Gregory, 1979).

With each successive step, control over its respiratory destiny is lost by the premature infant. Fortunately, the physiology of the respiratory mechanism and pathophysiology of respiratory malfunction have been very well elucidated and, when handled by competent caretakers, restoration of respiratory control to the infant's own feedback system results in no significant pulmonary morbidity (Lamarre, Linsao, Reilly, Swyer, & Levison, 1973). However, occasional complications do occur and include obstruction of the endotracheal tube, pulmonary interstitial emphysema, pneumothorax (Aranda, Stern, & Dunbar, 1972), bronchopulmonary dysplasia, pneumonia, sepsis, hypoventilation, hyperventilation, pneumomediastinum (Kuhns, Bednarek, Wyman, Roloff, & Borer, 1975), pulmonary hemorrhage, cerebral hemorrhage (Pope, Armstrong, & Fitzhardinge, 1976), hydrocephalus (Fitzhardinge et al., 1976), among others. Although some of these complications cause the death of the infant, most can be resolved with varying degrees of risk to the pulmonary or cerebral function of the premature thus affected (Johnson, Malackowski, Grobstein, Welsh, Dailey, & Sunshine, 1974; Outerbridge,

Ramsay, & Stern, 1974; Reynolds & Taghizadeh, 1974; Stahlman, Hedvall, Dolanski, Farelius, Burko, & Kirk, 1974).

FLUIDS AND NUTRITIONAL NEEDS

Because of their untimely birth, preterm infants have gastrointestinal and renal limitations that result in special nutritional and fluid needs and feeding procedures (Dweck, 1975). The previously described increase in heat loss compared to term babies necessitates larger expenditures of calories to maintain body temperature. There is also significant evaporative (4 ml/kg/hour) and insensible (15 ml/kg/24 hours) water loss (Babson et al., 1975). The stomach of the preterm infant is initially unable to accommodate either the volume of fluid or concentration of calories to accomplish a balanced caloric state (Fanaroff & Klaus, 1979). Attempts to utilize the gastrointestinal tract to its maximum potential are necessary but are accompanied by problems of residual formula (stomach has not emptied completely since last feeding), regurgitation or vomiting (attempt to introduce feedings in a volume greater than tolerable by the stomach), or pulmonary aspiration of gastric contents leading to acute respiratory distress, hypoxia, apnea, need for artificial ventilation, pneumonia, and other complications.

Attempts to accomplish adequate alimentary tract feedings include:

1. *Frequency of feedings.* Preterm infants are usually fed every 3 hours, but feedings every 2 hours or less are alternatives (Fanaroff & Klaus, 1979). Such feedings necessitate infant handling for the feeding period (10–30 min). It is not uncommon for infants after such feedings to have apneic episodes (Babson et al., 1975). This necessitates further handling. Thus, the less the stomach can tolerate, the less rest and sleep will be granted to such infants.

2. *Techniques of feedings.* Before 34 weeks gestation, the coordination of suck–swallow with esophageal peristalsis is poorly developed (Gryboski, 1973). Sucking and swallowing incoordination can easily lead to aspiration rather than ingestion of feeding. An orogastric or nasogastric feeding tube is utilized in such infants to avoid this hazard. The tube is either introduced and removed for each feeding or left in place. The feedings are either episodic or by continuous drip. In either case, periodic assessment of residual volume in the stomach is required to assess tolerance to the rate of feedings. Obviously, an excess feeding rate results in regurgitation and risk of aspiration. To avoid the latter problem, the technique of transpyloric (jejunal) feeding was developed (Cheek & Staub, 1973). In this procedure, the tube, by means of infant positional maneuvers, is induced to traverse the stomach and enter the upper part of the small intestine. Feedings can then be introduced with less concern for the potential of regurgitation. However, some formula will reflux into the stomach; hence, vomiting and regurgitation can still occur (Chen & Wong, 1974). Additionally, bypassing the stomach also bypasses its preparatory action on introduced feedings and the signals to the intestine to prepare for digestive processes. Such transpyloric feeding might be expected

to be in a form that would irritate or stress the intestine that received such feeding. This would impair assimilation of nutrients (Roy, Pollnitz, Hamilton, & Chance, 1976). Most predigested and regular infant formulas are hyperosmolar and can cause abdominal distention (Rhea, Ahman, & Mange, 1975). This in turn leads to regurgitation and vomiting, diarrhea, or distention injury–paralysis of the intestine. The latter is often followed by ischemia, infection of the intestinal wall, and necrosis—an entity known as necrotizing enterocolitis (NEC) (Heird, 1974). NEC often leads to gangrene and/or perforation with need for surgical intervention. If the infant survives, there is an extended period of time when no feedings can be given. Such infants require parenteral nutrition.

3. *Type of feedings.* Currently, because of limited volumes tolerable by the infant, premature infant formulas have been evolved to provide the infant with carbohydrate, fat, protein, and minerals in proportions more appropriate to the preterm and in formulations designed to accomplish better absorption. Breast milk adds the additional dimension of antibacterial action via its secretory immunoglobulin (Pittard, Polmar, Fanger, & Fanaroff, 1976) and macrophage content (Pitt, Barlow, & Heird, 1977). Breast milk feeding alone in the tiny preterm infant has also been shown to cause defective skeletal mineralization (Shaw, 1976). Therefore, based on the work of Ziegler (1976), some neonatal services now add glucose, medium chain triglycerides, and/or calcium to augment breast milk value to the preterm infant. But breast milk is not always available, and the risk of transmission of cytomegalovirus by breast milk to susceptible premies cannot be ignored. Furthermore, breast milk is not a standardized product. High salt content in breast milk has also been reported (Connor, 1979; Sevy, 1972).

The amount of fluid required by the preterm infant must be reviewed frequently. Since the preterm kidney is functional but less efficient and effective than that of the term infant or child, its limited ability to excrete water load can lead to edema if administered fluids exceed this excretory capacity (Leake, 1977). The increased salt excretion of the preterm kidney can easily result in hyponatremia and convulsions if sodium is not carefully monitored and replaced (Roy, Chance, Radde, Hill, Willis, & Sheepers, 1976). Consequently, the small preterm infant is usually found with intravenous infusion and limb constraints for several days postbirth.

INFECTION

The preterm infant has an incidence of neonatal sepsis four to five times that of the term infant (McCracken & Shinefield, 1966). The passage through the birth canal and residence in the intensive care nursery provide the bacterial contamination. At the time of birth, the preterm infant receives less transplacental antibodies than its term peer to protect it or limit bacterial invasion (Rothberg, 1969). Its leukocytes are less responsive to bacterial stimuli, do not ingest bacteria well, and are deficient in killing those bacteria ingested

(Coen, Grush, & Kander, 1969; Miller, 1971; Miller & Stiehm, 1973). Thus, generalized rather than localized infection is to be expected. This decreased resistence to infection is further characterized by a 30% incidence of meningitis in infants with septicemia (Speck, Fanaroff, & Klaus, 1979). Once symptoms are well established, a high mortality rate is the rule.

Initial symptoms may be as subtle as a nurse's perception that the infant is acting a "bit different." Gottoff and Behrman (1970) have published a table of symptoms by systems (central nervous, respiratory, gastrointestinal, circulatory, hemopoietic, and epidermal) that demonstrates the multiple manifestations and presenting symptoms. Sepsis is not an easy diagnosis to make early, since these symptoms are also found in several other diagnoses affecting the neonate. Over the past 20 years, changing nursery procedures, treatment, and antibiotic availability have changed the organism most likely to cause illnesses. The current organism threatening the neonate is Group B streptococcus (Aber, Allen, Howell, Wilkenson, & Facklam, 1976; Baker & Barrett, 1973). A high index of suspicion and early initiation of treatment while awaiting confirmatory studies is the hallmark of successful treatment. Once seriously symptomatic, such complications as pneumonia, disseminated intravascular coagulopathy, meningitis, shock, apnea, and convulsions, together with potential drug treatment side effects, result in significant incidence of long-term neurologic sequelae (Baker, 1977).

HYPERBILIRUBINEMIA

One of the most common and potentially dangerous problems that confront the preterm infant is neonatal jaundice (hyperbilirubinemia). This results from the catabolism of hemoglobin to bilirubin, which must then be metabolized by the liver and excreted via the bile. Approximately 50% of all preterm infants will experience neonatal jaundice (Maisels, 1975). These infants will require sequential bilirubin determinations and/or treatment. The preterm infant produces about 2.5 times the amount of bilirubin an adult does, probably in part because of its decreased red blood cell life span (Maisels, Pathak, Nelson, Nathan, & Smith, 1971). Other causes of increased bilirubin in the preterm infant include decreased transport Y-protein in the hepatocyte (Levi, Gatmaitan, & Arias, 1970), shunting of blood past the liver via the ductus venosus (Ogawa, 1965), and the presence of a significant amount of beta glucuronidase in the stool (Poland & Odell, 1971). Perinatal problems that result in decreased gastric motility and failure to pass meconium within 12 hours of birth also cause significant increase in bilirubin (Seligman, 1977). Recent reports from British literature have related oxytocin used to induce labor with significant increase in neonatal jaundice (Beazley & Alderman, 1975). Since premature rupture of membranes leading to prolonged rupture without labor is a common problem of the preterm pregnancy, oxytoxic agents are frequently employed to induce labor and effect delivery of the preterm infant before ascending infection jeopardizes the life of the infant and mother.

Concern about levels of bilirubin began first with the association of kernicterus with bilirubin levels in 1952 (Hsia, Allen, Gellis, & Diamond, 1952). The typical picture of progressive kernicterus occurs on the third or fourth day of life and includes lethargy, hypotonia, poor feeding, vomiting, increased irritability, high-pitched cry, fisting, oculogyric crises, opisthotonus, convulsions, hemorrhage, and often death (Maisels, 1975; Poland & Ostrea, 1979). The gross pathologic findings of yellow staining of basal ganglia and hippocampus by unbound bilirubin, which are typical findings in kernicterus, are also found in some preterm infants who have shown few or none of these symptoms antemortum (Claireaux, Cole, & Lathe, 1953; Diamond, 1969). The term infant usually is not at risk until the bilirubin level exceeds 20 mg%. Preterm infants have been reported to develop kernicterus at less than one-half that value (Stern & Denton, 1965). Factors that increase the risk of kernicterus at lower levels in preterm infants include decreased bilirubin binding by albumin (Kapitulnik, Valaes, Kaufmann, & Blondheim, 1974), acidosis (Nelson, Jacobsen, & Wennberg, 1973), increased hematin from hemolysis (Bratlid, 1972), anoxia (Lucey, Hibbard, Behrman, Esquivel, & Windle, 1964), and inadequate nutrition with elevated plasma-free fatty acids (Lee & Gartner, 1978). Unbound (free) bilirubin, in addition to being neurotoxic as described, is also nephrotoxic (Odell, Natzschka, & Storey, 1967) and affects platelet function (Maurer & Caul, 1972) and white blood cell function (Rola-Pleszczynski, Heusen, Vincent, & Bellanti, 1975). Preterm infants with symptomatic hyperbilirubinemia have sequelae that include various degrees of spasticity, chorioathetosis, visual difficulties, deafness, and mental retardation. Some preterm infants with apparently asymptomatic courses and mild jaundice, followed 8 months to 5 years, still develop characteristics of minimal brain dysfunction (short memory and attention span, learning and reading disabilities, etc.) (Boggs, Hardy, & Frazier, 1967; Odell, Storey, & Rosenberg, 1979).

Since neurotoxicity is nonreversible (Poland & Ostrea, 1979), it is necessary to anticipate its appearance and minimize its elevation to these dangerous levels.

One form of treatment is phototherapy (Cremer, Perryman, & Richards, 1958)—use of light in the blue-light range of 420–460 nm (Mims, Estrada, Gooden, Caldwell, & Kotas, 1973). The toxic form of bilirubin is photodegraded to nontoxic isomers and rapidly eliminated from the body (Ostrow, 1972). Increased insensible fluid loss, one side effect of phototherapy, can be significant, requiring substantial increase in fluids that must be ingested or administered (Oh & Karecki, 1972). Diarrhea, another side effect of phototherapy (Rubaltelli & Largajolli, 1973), causes loss of additional water and electrolytes from the body. Phototherapy on infants with hyperbilirubinemia has been shown to decrease intestinal lactase activity (Bakkan, 1976). The hyperbilirubinemic infants fed formula or breast milk containing lactose while receiving phototherapy are subject to lactose intolerance and increase in diarrhea. The possibility of retinal toxicity necessitates use of eye patches for the duration of the treatment (Seligman, 1977).

Exchange transfusion, a second form of treatment for hyperbilirubinemia of the preterm infant, is a rapidly effective modality of treatment in which the baby's bilirubin-laden blood is "exchanged" in small aliquots for donor blood free of bilirubin. This procedure removes about 87% of fetal cells, replacing them with longer lived adult cells (Valaes, 1963). It also reduces serum bilirubin acutely to about one-half of its previous value, allowing the donor albumin to pull bilirubin out of tissue back into the bloodstream for processing by the liver. Some reported complications (infrequent) that can occur with exchange transfusions are dislodging of emboli during insertion of the umbilical vein catheter (through which the exchange will be done), infection, necrotizing enterocolitis, graft-versus-host reaction, electrolyte imbalance, thrombocytopenia, and hypoglycemia (Hardy, Savage, & Shirodaria, 1972; Odell, Bryan, & Richmond, 1962; Parkman, Mosier, Umanski, Cochran, Carpenter, & Rosen, 1974; Poland & Ostrea, 1979).

Summary

The premature infant enters this world ill prepared for its challenges. The great medical advances of the past decade have made it possible for the frontier of viability to be pushed back to 24–26 weeks gestation. Neonatology is in a period of rapid growth. Special care and intensive care nurseries are being established and placed into operation in almost every hospital with a significant obstetric population. Adequate in-depth knowledge and training for physicians and nurses who are responsible for provision of care to premature infants in these settings is an obvious necessity but difficult to achieve. The few (by no means all-inclusive) examples of complex interrelated and often simultaneous medical problems that have been presented serve to illustrate the precarious balance between intact survival and survival with handicaps. In this medical milieu, the nurses, doctors, parents, and infants attempt to interrelate. This is often done under emotional strain and with time constraints induced by episodically short nurse–doctor–patient staffing ratios. Only in the past few years has the field of neonatology begun to concentrate on evolving a technique to evaluate the effect of these medical constraints on optimum psychological development in the preterm·infant. These investigations will, no doubt, result in modification of many current nursery practices to minimize the negative aspects of care and identify those infants destined to need early psychophysiologic intervention.

References

Aber, R., Allen, N., Howell, J., Wilkenson, H. W., Facklam, R. R. Nosocomial transmission of group B streptococci. *Pediatrics,* 1976, *58,* 346.

Adams, J., & Rudolph, A. The use of indwelling radial artery catheters in neonates. *Pediatrics,* 1975, *55,* 261.

Adamsons, K., Jr., Behrman, R., Dawes, G., Dawkins, M., James, L., & Ross, B. The treatment of acidosis with alkali and glucose during asphyxia in foetal rhesus monkeys. *Journal of Physiology,* 1963, *169,* 679.

Adamsons, K., Behrman, R., Dawes, G. S., James, L. S., & Koford, C. Resuscitation by positive pressure ventilation and tris-hydroxmethylaminomethane of rhesus monkeys asphyxiated at birth. *Journal of Pediatrics,* 1964, *65,* 807.

Allen, L., Reynolds, E., Rivers, R., LeSouëf, P., & Wimberley, P. Controlled trial of continuous positive airway pressure given by face mask for hyaline membrane disease. *Archives of Disease of Children,* 1977, *52,* 373.

Ames, A., Wright, L., Kowada, M., Thurston, J., & Majno, G. Cerebral ischemia. The no-flow phenomenon. *American Journal of Pathology,* 1968, *52,* 437.

Anderson, W. R., & Strickland, M. B. Pulmonary complications of oxygen therapy in the neonate. *Archives of Pathology,* 1971, *91,* 506.

Aperia, A., Bergqvist, G., Broberger, O., Thodenius, K., & Vetterstrom, R. Renal function in newborn infants with high hematocrit valves before and after isovolemic haemodilution. *Acta Paediatrica Scandinavica,* 1974, *63,* 878.

Aranda, J. V., Stern, L., & Drenbar, J. D. Pneumothorax with pneumoperitoneum in a newborn infant. *American Journal of Diseases of Children,* 1972, *123,* 163.

Avery, M. E., & Mead, J. Surface properties in relation to atelectasis in hyaline membrane disease. *American Journal of Diseases of Children,* 1959, *97,* 517.

Babson, S. G., Benson, R. C., Pernoll, M. L., & Benda, G. I. *Management of high-risk pregnancy and intensive care of the neonate.* St. Louis: Mosby, 1975.

Bada, H. S., Alojipan, L. C., & Andrews, B. F. Premature rupture of membranes and its effect on the newborn. *Pediatric Clinics of North America,* 1977, *24,* 492.

Baker, C. Summary of the workshop on perinatal infections due to Group B streptococcus. *Journal of Infectious Diseases,* 1977, *136,* 137.

Baker, C., & Barrett, F. Transmission of Group B streptococci among parturient women and their neonates. *Journal of Pediatrics,* 1973, *83,* 919.

Baker, D., Berdon, W., & James, L. Proper localization of umbilical arterial and venous catheters by lateral roentgenograms. *Pediatrics,* 1969, *43,* 34.

Bakkan, A. F. Intestinal lactase deficiency as a factor in the diarrhea of light-treated jaundiced infants. *New England Journal of Medicine,* 1976, *294,* 615. (Letter to editor)

Battaglia, F. C., & Lubchenco, L. O. A practical classification of newborn infants by weight and gestational age. *Journal of Pediatrics,* 1967, *51,* 159.

Baum, D. S., & Scopes, J. W. The Silver Swaddler. *The Lancet,* 1968, *1,* 672.

Beazley, J. M., & Alderman, B. Neonatal hyperbilirubinemia following the use of oxytocin in labour. *British Journal of Obstetrics and Gynecology,* 1975, *82,* 265.

Beddis, I. R., Collins, P., Levy, N. M., Godfrey, S., & Silverman, M. A new technique for servo control of arterial orxygen tension in preterm infants. *Archives of Disease in Childhood,* 1979, *54,* 278.

Behrman, R. Persistence of fetal circulation. *Journal of Pediatrics,* 1976, *89,* 636–637.

Behrman, R. E. *Neonatal-perinatal medicine* (2nd ed.). St. Louis: Mosby, 1977.

Behrman, R., Lees, M., Peterson, E., DeLannoy, C., & Seeds, A. Distribution of the circulation in the normal and asphyxiated fetal primate. *American Journal of Obstetrics and Gynecology,* 1970, *108,* 956.

Bergqvist, G. Viscosity of the blood in the newborn infant. *Acta Paediatrica Scandivica,* 1974, *63,* 858.

Besch, N. J., Perlstein, P. H., Edwards, N. K., Keenan, W. J., & Sutherland, J. M. The transport baby bag. *New England Journal of Medicine,* 1971, *284,* 121.

Boggs, T. R., Jr., Hardy, J. B., & Frazier, T. M. Correlation of neonatal serum total bilirubin concentrations and developmental status at age eight months. *Journal of Pediatrics,* 1967, *71,* 553.

Brady, J. P., & Gregory, G. A. Assisted ventilation. In M. H. Klaus & A. A. Fanaroff (Eds.), *Care of the high-risk neonate.* Philadelphia: Saunders, 1979.

Bratlid, D. The effect of free fatty acids, bile acids and hematin on bilirubin binding by human erythrocytes. *Scandinavian Journal of Clinical and Laboratory Investigation,* 1972, *30,* 107.

Brenner, W. E., Bruce, R. D., & Hendricks, C. H. The characteristics and perils of breech presentation. *American Journal of Obstetrics and Gynecology,* 1974, *118,* 700.

Brown, A. K., & Cevik, N. Hemolysis and jaundice in the newborn following maternal treatment with sulfamethoxypyridazine. *Pediatrics,* 1965, *36,* 742.

Bruck, K. Temperature regulation in the newborn infant. *Biology of the Neonate,* 1961, *3,* 65.

Bruck, K. Which environmental temperature does the premature infant prefer? *Pediatrics,* 1968, *41,* 1027.

Budin, P. [The nursling: The feeding and hygiene of premature and full term infants] (W. J. Maloney, Trans.). London: Caxton, 1907.

Burman, D., & Morris, A. F. Cord hemoglobin in low birth weight infants. *Archives of Disease in Childhood,* 1974, *49,* 382.

Cheek, J. A., & Staub, G. F. Nasojejunal alimentation for premature and full-term newborn infants. *Journal of Pediatrics,* 1973, *82,* 955.

Chen, J., & Wong, P. Intestinal complication of nasojejunal feeding in low-birth-weight infants. *Journal of Pediatrics,* 1974, *85,* 109.

Claireaux, A. E., Cole, P. G., & Lathe, G. H. Icterus of the brain in the newborn. *The Lancet,* 1953, *2,* 1226.

Coen, R., Grush, O., & Kander, E. Studies of the bacterial activity and metabolism of the leucocyte in full term neonates. *Journal of Pediatrics,* 1969, *75,* 400.

Conner, A. E. Elevated levels of sodium and chloride in milk from mastitic breast. *Pediatrics,* 1979, *63,* 910.

Cree, J. E., Meyer, J., & Hailey, D. M. Diazepam in labour, its metabolism and effect on the clinical condition and thermogenesis of the newborn. *British Medical Journal,* 1973, *4,* 251.

Cremer, R., Perryman, P., & Richards, D. Influence of light on the hyperbilirubinemia of infants. *Lancet,* 1958, *1,* 1094.

Dailey, W., Klaus, M., & Meyer, H. Apnea in premature infants: Monitoring incidence, heart rate changes, and effect of environmental temperature. *Pediatrics,* 1969, *43,* 510.

Danilowicz, D., Rudolph, A., & Hoffman, J. Delayed closure of the ductus arteriosus in premature infants. *Pediatrics,* 1966, *37,* 74.

Dawes, G., Hibbard, E., & Windle, W. The effect of alkali and glucose infusion on permanent brain damage in rhesus monkeys asphyxiated at birth. *Journal of Pediatrics,* 1964, *65,* 801.

Dawes, G. S., Mott, J. C., & Shelley, H. J. The importance of cardiac glycogen for the maintenance of life in foetal lambs and newborn animals during anoxia. *Journal of Physiology,* 1959, *146,* 516.

Diamond, I. Bilirubin binding and kernicterus. In I. Shulman (Ed.), *Advances in Pediatrics.* Chicago: Yearbook Publishers, 1969.

Dilts, P. V. Effect of ethanol on uterine and umbilical hemodynamics and oxygen transfer. *American Journal of Obstetrics and Gynecology,* 1970, *108,* 221.

Dweck, H. S. Feeding the prematurely born infant. *Clinics in Perinatology,* 1975, *2,* 183-202.

Fanaroff, A., & Klaus, M. Resuscitation of the newborn infant. In M. H. Klaus & A. A. Fanaroff (Eds.), Care of the high-risk neonate. Philadelphia: Saunders, 1979.

Fisher, D. M. Cold diuresis of the newborn. *Pediatrics,* 1967, *40,* 636.

Fitzhardinge, P. M., Pope, K., Arstikaitis, M., Boyle, M., Ashby, M., Rowley, A., Netley, C., & Swyer, P. R. Mechanical ventilation of infants of less than 1501 gms. Birth weight; health, growth, and neurologic sequelae. *Journal of Pediatrics,* 1976, *88,* 531.

Freda, V. J. The Rh problem in obstetrics and a new concept of its movement using amniocentesis and spectrophotometric scanning of amniotic fluid. *American Journal of Obstetrics and Gynecology,* 1965, *92,* 341.

Friedman, W., Hirschklau, M., Printz, M., Pitlick, P., & Kirkpatrick, S. Pharmacologic closure of patent ductus arteriosus in the premature infant. *New England Journal of Medicine,* 1976, *295,* 526.

Gandy, G., Adamsons, K., Jr., & Cunningham, N. Thermal environmental and acid-base homeostasis in human infants during the first few hours of life. *Journal of Clinical Investigation,* 1964, *43,* 751.

Garn, S. M., Shaw, H. A., & McCabe, K. D. Effects of social-economic status and race on weight defined and gestational prematurity in the U. S. A. In E. M. Reed & S. J. Stanley (Eds.), *Epidemiology of prematurity.* Baltimore: Urban and Schwarzenberg, 1977.

Gersony, W., Duc, G., & Sinclair, J. "PFC" syndrome (persistence of fetal circulation). *Circulation,* 1969, *39,* 111.

Goetzman, B., Sunshine, P., Johnson, J., Wennberg, R., Hackel, A., Merten, D., Bartoletti, A., & Silverman, N. Neonatal hypoxia and pulmonary vasospasm: Responses to tolazoline. *Journal of Pediatrics,* 1976, *89,* 617.

Goldenberg, R. L., & Nelson, K. G. The premature breech. *American Journal of Obstetrics and Gynecology,* 1977, *127,* 240.

Goodlin, R. C. *Care of the fetus.* New York: Masson, 1979.

Gotoff, S., & Behrman, R. Neonatal septicemia. *Journal of Pediatrics,* 1970, *76,* 142.

Gregory, G., Kitterman, J., Phibbs, R., Tooley, W., & Hamilton, W. Treatment of the idiopathic respiratory-distress syndrome with continuous positive airway pressure. *New England Journal of Medicine,* 1971, *284,* 1333.

Gryboski, J. Suck and swallow in the premature infant. *Pediatrics,* 1969, *43,* 96.

Gunn, G. C., Mishell, D. R., & Morton, D. C. Premature rupture of the fetal membranes. *American Journal of Obstetrics and Gynecology,* 1970, *106,* 469.

Hardy, J. D., Savage, T. R., & Shirodaria, C. Intestinal perforation following exchange transfusion. *American Journal of Diseases of Children,* 1972, *124,* 136.

Heird, W. C. Nasojejunal feeding: A commentary. *Journal of Pediatrics,* 1974, *85,* 111.

Hess, J. H., & Lundeen, E. C. *The premature infant: Its medical and nursing care.* Philadelphia: Lippincott, 1941.

Hey, E. The care of babies in incubators. In D. Hull & D. Gairdner (Eds.), *Recent advances in pediatrics.* Edinburg: Livingstone, 1971.

Hey, E. N., Kohlinsky, S., & O'Connell, B. Heat losses from babies during exchange transfusion. *Lancet,* 1969, *1,* 335.

Hey, E. N., & Mount, L. Temperature control in incubators, preliminary communications. *The Lancet,* 1966, *2,* **202.**

Heymann, M. A., Rudolph, A. M., & Silverman, N. H. Closure of the ductus arteriosus in premature infants by inhibition of prostaglandin synthesis. *New England Journal of Medicine,* 1976, *295,* 530.

Hsia, D. Y-Y, Allen, F. H., Gellis, S. S., & Diamond, L. K. Erythroblastosis fetalis studies on serum bilirubin in relation to kernicterus. *New England Journal of Medicine,* 1952, *247,* 668.

Huch, R., Huch, A., & Albani, M. Transcutaneous PO_2 monitoring in routine management of infants and children with cardiorespiratory problems. *Pediatrics,* 1976, *57,* 681.

Huch, R., Huch, A., & Lubbers, D. W. Transcutaneous measurements of blood PO_2 (T_c PO_2): Method and applications in perinatal medicine. *Journal of Perinatal Medicine,* 1973, *1,* 183.

James L. Onset of breathing and resuscitation. *Journal of Pediatrics,* 1964, *65,* 807.

James, L., & Lanman, J. (Eds.). History of oxygen therapy and retrolental fibroplasia. *Pediatrics,* 1976, *57* (suppl.), 591.

Johnson, J. D., Malackowski, N. C., Grobstein, R., Welsh, D., Daily, W. J. R., & Sunshine, P. Prognosis of children surviving with the aid of mechanical ventilation in the newborn period. *Journal of Pediatrics,* 1974, *84,* 272.

Kapanci, Y., Weibel, E., Kaplan, H., & Robinson, F. Pathogenesis and reversability of the pulmonary lesions of oxygen toxicity in monkeys. II. Ultrastructural and morphometric studies. *Laboratory Investigation,* 1969, *20,* 101.

Kapitulnik, J., Valaes, T., Kaufmann, N. A., & Blondheim, S. H. Clinical evaluation of sephadex gel filtration in estimation of bilirubin binding in serum in neonatal jaundice. *Archives of Disease in Childhood,* 1974, *49,* 886.

Kaplan, H., Robinson, F., Kapanci, Y., & Weibel, E. Pathogenesis and reversability of the pulmonary lesions of oxygen toxicity in monkeys. I. Clinical and light microscopic studies. *Laboratory Investigation,* 1969, *20,* 94.

Kattwinkel, J., Fleming, D., Cha, C., Fanaroff, A., & Klaus, M. A device for administration of continuous positive airway pressure by the nasal route. *Pediatrics,* 1973, *52,* 131.

Kedes, L. H., & Field, J. B. Hypothermia; a clue to hypoglycemia. *New England Journal of Medicine,* 1964, *271,* 785.

Kitterman, J. A., Edmunds, L. H., Jr., Gregory, G. A., Heymann, M., Tooley, W., & Rudolph, A. Patent ductus arteriosus in premature infants. Incidence, relation to pulmonary disease, and management. *New England Journal of Medicine,* 1972, *287,* 473.

Klaus, M., Fanaroff, A., & Martin, R. The physical environment. In M. H. Klaus & A. A. Fanaroff (Eds.), *Care of the high-risk neonate.* Philadelphia: Saunders, 1969.

Krauss, A. N., Albert, R. F., & Kannan, M. M. Contamination of umbilical catheters in the newborn infant. *Journal of Pediatrics,* 1970, *77,* 963.

Kuhns, L., Bednarek, F., Wyman, M., Roloff, D., & Borer, R. Diagnosis of pneumothorax or pneumomediastinum in the neonate by transillumination. *Pediatrics,* 1975, *56,* 355.

Lamarre, A., Linsao, L., Reilly, B. J., Swyer, P. R., & Levison, H. Residual pulmonary abnormalities in survivors of idiopathic respiratory distress syndrome. *American Review of Respiratory Disease,* 1973, *108,* 56.

Larroche, J. Umbilical catheterization: Its complications. *Biology of the Neonate,* 1970, *16,* 101.

Leake, R. D. Perinatal nephrobiology: A developmental perspective. *Clinical Perinatology,* 1977, *4,* 323.

Lee, K., & Gartner, L. M. Transport of bilirubin in plasma by free fatty acids. *Pediatric Research,* 1978, *7,* 338. (Abstract)

Levi, A. J., Gatmaitan, Z., & Arias, I. M. Deficiency of hepatic organic anion-binding protein, impaired organic anion uptake by liver and "physiologic" jaundice in newborn monkeys. *New England Journal of Medicine,* 1970, *283,* 1136.

Lucey, J. F. The xanthine treatment of apnea of prematurity. *Pediatrics,* 1975, *55,* 584.

Maisels, M. J. Neonatal jaundice. In G. B. Avery (Ed.), *Neonatology: Pathophysiology and management of the newborn.* Philadelphia: Lippincott, 1975.

Maisels, M. J., Pathak, A., Nelson, N., Nathan, D., & Smith, C. Endogenous production of carbon monoxide in normal and erythroblastotic newborn infants. *Journal of Clinical Investigation,* 1971, *50,* 1.

Mann, L. I., Bhakthavathsalan, A., Liu, M., & Makowski, P. Placental transport of alcohol and its effect on maternal and fetal acid-base balance. *American Journal of Obstetrics and Gynecology,* 1975, *122,* 837.

Maurer, H., & Caul, J. Influence of bilirubin on human platelets. *Pediatric Research,* 1972, *6,* 136.

McCracken, G. H., & Nelson, J. D. *Antimicrobial therapy for newborns.* New York: Grune & Stratton, 1977.

McCracken, G. & Shinefeld, H. Changes in the pattern of neonatal septicemia and meningitis. *American Journal of Diseases of Children, 1966, 112,* 33.

Mestyan, J., Jarai, I. B., & Bata, G. The significance of facial skin temperature in the chemical heat regulation of premature infants. *Biology of the Neonate,* 1964, *7,* 243. (a)

Mestyan, J., Jarai, I. B., & Bata, G. Surface temperature versus deep body temperature and the metabolic response to cold of hypothermic premature infants. *Biology of the Neonate,* 1964, *7,* 230. (b)

Miller, E. Chemotactic function in the human neonate: Humoral and cellular aspects. *Pediatric Research,* 1971, *5,* 487.

Miller, E., & Stiehm, E. Phagocytic opsonic and immunoglobulin in newborns. *California Medicine,* 1973, *119,* 43.

Mims, L. C., Estrada, M., Gooden, D. S., Caldwell, R. S., & Kotas, R. U. Phototherapy for neonatal hyperbilirubinemia—a dose: Response relationship. *Journal of Pediatrics,* 1973, *83,* 658.

Moss, A. J., & Monset-Couchard, M. Placental transfusion: Early versus late clamping of the umbilical cord. *Pediatrics,* 1967, *40,* 109.

Neal, W. A., Reynolds, S. W., Jarvis, C. W., & Williams, H. J. Umbilical artery catheterization: Demonstration of arterial thrombosis by aortography. *Pediatrics,* 1972, *50,* 6.

Nelson, T., Jacobsen, J. B., & Wennberg, R. P. pH and bilirubin toxicity. *Pediatric Research,* 1973, 7, 334. (Abstract)

Niswander, K. R., Friedman, E. A., Hoover, D. B., Pietrowski, H., & Westphal, M. C. Fetal morbidity following potentially anoxigenic obstetric conditions. I. Abruptio placentae. *American Journal of Obstetrics and Gynecology,* 1966, *95,* 838.

O'Brien, J. R., Usher, R. H., & Maughan, G. B. Causes of birth asphyxia and trauma. *Canadian Medical Association Journal,* 1966, *94,* 1077.

Odell, G. B., Bryan, W. B., & Richmond, M. D. Exchange transfusion. *Pediatric Clinics of North America,* 1962, *9,* 605.

Odell, G., Natzschka, J., & Storey, G. Bilirubin nephropathy in the Gunn strain of rat. *American Journal of Physiology,* 1967, *212,* 931.

Odell, G. B., Storey, G. N. B., & Rosenberg, L. A. Studies in kernicterus III. The saturation of serum proteins with bilirubin during neonatal life and its relationship to brain damage at five years. *Journal of Pediatrics,* 1970, *76,* 12.

Ogawa, J. Post-natal circulatory observations of liver and intestine in newborn infants. In *Proceedings of the XI International Congress of Pediatrics,* 1965.

Oh, W., & Karechi, H. Phototherapy and insensible water loss in the newborn infant. *American Journal of Diseases of Children,* 1972, *124,* 230.

Oh, W., Wallgren, G., Hannson, J. S., & Third, J. The effects of placental transfusion on respiratory mechanics of normal term newborn infants. *Pediatrics,* 1967, *40,* 6.

Oliver, T. K., Jr. Temperature regulation and heat production in the newborn. Pediatric Clinics of North America, 1965, *12,* 765.

Oliver, T. K. Thermal regulation. In R. Behrman (Ed.), *Neonatal-perinatal medicine.* St. Louis: Mosby, 1977.

Ostrow, J. O. Mechanisms of bilirubin photodegradation. *Seminars in Hematology,* 1972, *9,* 113.

Outerbridge, E. W., Ramsay, M., & Stern, L. Developmental follow-up of survivors of neonatal respiratory failure. *Critical Care Medicine,* 1974, *2,* 23.

Parkman, R., Mosieg D., Umanski, Cochran, W., Carpenter, C., & Rosen, F. S. Graft-versus-host disease after intrauterine and exchange transfusions for hemolytic disease of the newborn. *New England Journal of Medicine,* 1974, *290,* 359.

Perlstein, P. H., Edwards, N. K., & Sutherland, J. M. Apnea in premature infants and incubator–air-temperature changes. *New England Journal of Medicine,* 1970, *282,* 461.

Pitt, J., Barlow, B., & Heird, W. Protection against experimental necrotizing enterocolitis by maternal milk. I. Role of milk leukocytes. *Pediatric Research,* 1977, *11,* 906.

Pittard, W., Polmar, S., Fanger, M., & Fanaroff, A. Identification of immunoglobulin bearing lymphocytes in fresh human breast milk. *Pediatric Research,* 1976, *10,* 359.

Poland, R. L., & Odell, G. B. Physiologic jaundice: The enterohepatic circulation of bilirubin. *New England Journal of Medicine,* 1971, *284,* 1.

Poland, R. L., & Ostrea, E. M. Neonatal hyperbilirubinemia. In M. Klaus & A. Fanaroff (Eds.), *Care of the high-risk neonate.* Philadelphia: Saunders, 1979.

Pope, K., Armstrong, D., & Fitzhardinge, P. Central nervous system pathology associated with mask ventilation in the very low birth weight infant: A new etiology for intracerebellar hemorrhages. *Pediatrics,* 1976, *58,* 473.

Pritchard, J. A., & MacDonald, P. C. (Eds.). *Williams Obstetrics* (15th ed.). New York: Appleton-Century-Crofts, 1976.

Queenan, J. T. *Modern management of the Rh problem.* New York: Hoeber, 1967.

Queenan, J. T., & Goetschel, E. Amniotic fluid analysis for erythroblastosis fetalis. *Obstetrics and Gynecology,* 1968, *32,* 120.

Rausen, A. R., Seki, M., & Strauss, L. Twin transfusion syndrome. *Journal of Pediatrics,* 1965, *66,* 613.

Reynolds, E. O. R., & Taghizadeh, A. Improved prognosis for infants mechanically ventilated for hyaline membrane disease. *Archives of Disease in Childhood,* 1974, *49,* 505.

Rhea, J. W., Ahman, M. S., & Mange, M. S. Nasojejunal (transpyloric) feeding: A commentary. *Journal of Pediatrics,* 1975, *86,* 451.

Rigatto, H., & Brady, J. P. Periodic breathing and apnea in preterm infants. I. Evidence for hypoventilation possibly due to central respiratory depression. *Pediatrics,* 1972, *50,* 202. (a)

Rigatto, H., & Brady, J. P. Periodic breathing and apnea in preterm infants. II. Hypoxia as a primary event. *Pediatrics,* 1972, *50,* 219. (b)

Rola-Pleszczynski, M., Heusen, S., Vincent, M., & Bellanti, J. A. Inhibitory effects of bilirubin on cellular immune response in man. *Journal of Pediatrics,* 1975, *86,* 690.

Rothberg, R. Immunoglobulin and specific antibody synthesis during the first weeks of life of premature infants. *Journal of Pediatrics,* 1969, *75,* 391.

Roy, N., Pollnitz, R., Hamilton, R., & Chance, G. Impaired assimilation of nasojejunal feeds in very low-birth-weight infants. *Pediatric Research,* 1976, *10,* 359.

Roy, R. N., Chance, G. W., Radde, I. C., Hill, D., Willis, D., & Sheepers, J. Late hyponatremia in very low birth weight infants (< 1.3 kilograms). *Pediatric Research,* 1976, *10,* 526.

Rubaltelli, F. F., & Largajolli, G. Effect of light exposure on gut transit time in jaundiced newborns. *Acta Paediatrica Scandivica,* 1973, *62,* 146.

Russell, K. P., & Cheung, J. Treatment of patients with premature rupture of the fetal membranes: (a) Prior to 32 weeks: (b) After 32 weeks. The management of premature rupture of fetal membranes—a continuing controversy. In D. E. Reid & C. D. Christian (Eds.), *Controversy in obstetrics and gynecology* (Vol. 2). Philadelphia: Saunders, 1974.

Saigal, S., O'Neill, A., Surainder, Y., Chua, L., & Usher, R. Placental transfusion and hyperbilirubinemia in the premature. *Pediatrics,* 1972, *49,* 406.

Schlesinger, E. R., Mazundar, S. M., & Logrillo, V. M. The impact of placenta previa on survivorship of offspring to four years of age. *American Journal of Obstetrics and Gynecology,* 1973, *116,* 657.

Scopes, J. W. Metabolic rate and temperature control in the human body. *British Medical Bulletin,* 1966, *22,* 88.

Scopes, J. W. Thermoregulation in the newborn. In G. B. Avery (Ed.), *Neonatology, pathophysiology and management of the newborn.* Philadelphia: Lippincott, 1975.

Seligman, J. W. Recent and changing concepts of hyperbilirubinemia and its management in the newborn. *Pediatric Clinics of North America,* 1977, *24,* 509–527.

Sevy, S. Acute emotional stress and sodium in the breast milk. *American Journal of Diseases of Children,* 1972, *122,* 459.

Shannon, D., Gotay, F., Stein, I., Rogers, M., Todres, I., & Moylan, F. Prevention of apnea and bradycardia in low birthweight infants. *Pediatrics,* 1975, *55,* 589.

Shaw, J. Evidence for defective skeletal mineralization in low birth weight infants: The absorption of calcium and fat. *Pediatrics,* 1976, *57,* 16.

Siassi, B., Blanco, C., Cabal, L., & Coran, A. Incidence and clinical features of patent ductus arteriosus in low birth weight infants: A prospective analysis of 150 consecutively born infants. *Pediatrics,* 1976, *57,* 347.

Silverman, W. A., Fertig, J. W., & Berger, A. P. The influence of the thermal environment upon the survival of newly born premature infants. *Pediatrics,* 1958, *22,* 876.

Speck, W. T., Fanaroff, A. A., & Klaus, M. Neonatal infections. In M. Klaus & A. Fanaroff (Eds.), *Care of the high-risk neonate.* Philadelphia: Saunders, 1979.

Stafford, A., & Weatherall, J. A. C. The survival of young rats in nitrogen. *Journal of Physiology,* 1960, *153,* 457.

Stahlman, M. T. Acute respiratory disorders in the newborn. In G. B. Avery (Ed.), *Neonatology, pathophysiology and management of the newborn.* Philadelphia: Lippincott, 1975.

Stahlman, M., Hedvall, G., Dolanski, E., Farelius, G., Burko, H., & Kirk, V. A six-year follow-up of clinical hyaline membrane disease. *Pediatric Clinics of North America,* 1973, *20,* 433.

Stander, R. W., Barden, T. P., Thompson, J. F., Pugh, W. R. & Werts, C. E. Fetal cardiac effects of maternal isoxuprine infusion. *American Journal of Obstetrics and Gynecology,* 1964, *89,* 792.

Stern, L., & Denton, R. L. Kernicterus in small premature infants. *Pediatrics,* 1965, *35,* 483.

Stockman, J. A., III. Anemia of prematurity. *Clinics in Perinatology,* 1977, *4,* 239.

Stone, H. O., Thompson, H. K., Jr., & Schmidth-Nelson, K. Influence of erythrocytes on blood viscosity. *American Journal of Physiology,* 1968, *214,* 913.

Taylor, E. D., Morgan, R. L., Bruns, P. D., & Drose, V. Spontaneous premature rupture of the fetal membranes. *American Journal of Obstetrics and Gynecology,* 1961, *82,* 1341.

U.S. Department Health, Education and Welfare, Public Health Service, National Center for Health Statistics. Personal communication, 1979.

Usher, R. H. The special problems of the premature infant. In G. B. Avery (Ed), *Neonatology, pathophysiology and management of the newborn.* Philadelphia: Lippincott, 1975.

Valaes, T. Bilirubin distribution and dynamics of bilirubin removal by exchange transfusion. *Acta Paediatrica Scandivica,* 1963, *52* (Suppl.) 149 .

Wirth, F. H., Goldberg, K. E., & Lubchenco, L. O. Neonatal hyperviscosity: I. Incidence. *Pediatrics,* 1979, *63,* 833.

Wood, J. L. Plethora in the newborn infant associated with cyanosis and convulsions. *Journal of Pediatrics,* 1959, *54,* 143.

Yogman, M. W., Speroff, L., Huttenlocher, P. R., & Kase, N. G. Child development after pregnancies complicated by low urinary estriol excretion and preeclampsia. *American Journal of Obstetrics and Gynecology,* 1972, *114,* 1069.

Young, P. E., Matson, M. R., & Jones, O. W. Amniocentesis for antenatal diagnosis. *American Journal of Obstetrics and Gynecology,* 1976, *125,* 495.

Zackman, R., Steinmetz, G., Botham, R., Graven, S., & Ledbetter, M. Incidence and treatment of the patent ductus arteriosus in the ill premature neonate. *American Heart Journal,* 1974, *87,* 697.

Ziegler, E., O'Donnell, A., Nelson, S., & Fomon, S. Body composition of the reference fetus. *Growth,* 1976, *40,* 329.

Zuckerman, H., Reiss, U., & Rubinstein, I. Inhibition of human premature labor by indomethacin. *Obstetrics and Gynecology,* 1974, *44,* 787.

developed a complete repertoire of species-normal behaviors, including copulation, without any special therapy other than contact with socially reared peers. For rhesus macaques, however, similar overall levels of recovery have been found only for animals that receive special therapy with much younger infants immediately after termination of isolation rearing (Novak, 1979; Suomi & Harlow, 1972). To add to this apparent lack of generality in isolation effects between these two macaque species, no gender differences were found for pigtail isolates on any postrearing measure.

These gender and species differences in response to presumably catastrophic events in infancy point to the conclusion that important nonenvironmental factors play a role in determining risk for developing abnormal behavior. Such factors may involve differential maturation rates, with important systems maturing prenatally for some individuals or species, thereby making these systems relatively immune to later environmental influences. Genetic differences in reactivity, emotionality, tolerance for ambiguity or change, or ability to inhibit maladaptive or inappropriate responses could also result in differential vulnerability. In order to attack the problem of differential vulnerability for abnormal development following inadequate rearing experiences, it seems essential to devise methods to study the actual interaction of genetic and prenatal factors with postnatal environmental variables. The remainder of this chapter describes an approach to research on these interactions in a nonhuman primate species. The purpose of this research model is to identify the correlates and actual mechanisms underlying both deviant and species-typical primate development.

The Primate Resource

Our subjects are pigtail macaques (*Macaca nemestrina*) living among the 1100 animals in the Regional Primate Research Center at the University of Washington, Seattle, Washington. There are about 650 breeding females, producing 250–300 conceptions each year. Of these conceptions, 15–20% result in fetal and perinatal loss, 5–10% in neonatal death, and 5% in maternal rejection or abuse. The liveborns include about 5% infants that are premature or small for date. Monkeys are considered to be premature if their gestational age at birth is under 150 days, which is more than 2.5 standard deviations from the mean gestational age of 170 days. Studies of respiratory system development also show that lung anatomy and biochemistry are relatively normal after 150 days of gestation, with increasing probability for respiratory distress at earlier gestational ages (Woodrum, Guthrie, & Hodson, 1978). Infants are considered small for date if they achieve a birthweight at or below the 10th percentile for their gestational age or have much less developed bone ossification centers than would be expected from gestation-specific norms (Newell-Morris, 1977). These neonates almost all die if left with their mothers, whereas 80–85% survive when hand raised by humans in a high-risk monkey infant nursery (Ruppenthal & Reese, 1979). In the nursery, at-risk monkey newborns receive almost identical care to that of at-risk human babies. This includes isolette housing, respiratory assistance, and tube feeding when necessary, and round-the-clock surveillance by veterinary personnel.

A major resource of our primate center consists of computerized colony records containing 16 years of information on breeding and pregnancy outcome, growth, clinical treatments, and causes of death. These records were used to generate birthweight and growth norms for colony-born pigtail macaques (Sackett, Holm, Davis & Fahrenbruch, 1975). The liveborn birthweight distributions for 950 males and 865 females are shown in Figure 3.1. Males average 50 gm heavier at birth than females, yet the heaviest individuals are females and the lightest are males. The colony records show gestation is typically 170 days, with a standard deviation of 6 days. Although this estimate is probably adequate for overall norms, most pregnancies are detected by manual palpation and can be off by as much as 30 days unless the palpation is done in the first month. Therefore, the records are generally not adequate to obtain accurate gestational ages at birth for most newborns, with the exception of about 5% that were produced by timed matings.

The cumulative birthweight distributions were used to define low birthweight for each sex, with the criterion set at or below the 10th percentile. Figure 3.2 shows 4½-year growth curves as a function of birth percentile ranges for males and females. Males and females that weigh less than normal

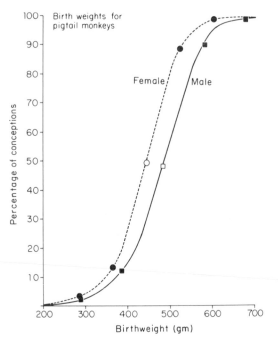

FIGURE 3.1. *Cumulative probability distributions for birthweights of liveborn male and female pigtail macaques. Broken line shows female; solid line shows male; open symbols show mean; closed symbols show ± 1 and 2 S.D.*

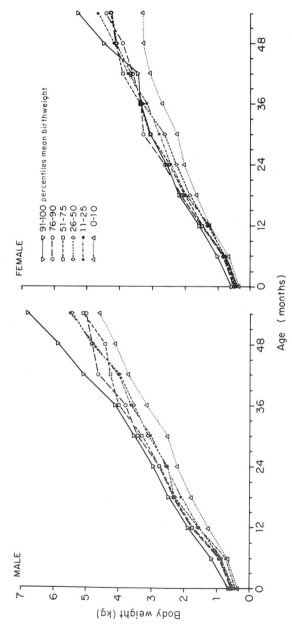

FIGURE 3.2. *Average body weight for male and female pigtail macaques grouped according to their birthweight percentile scores, mixed cross-sectional longitudinal data.*

at birth (low birthweight) remain the lightest animals up to 4½ years of age, the time of reproductive maturity. Males that weigh more than normal at birth (high birthweight) remain heaviest and show an adolescent growth spurt sooner than low-birthweight animals. High-birthweight females lose their weight advantage after the first postnatal year, although they may again become heaviest after reproductive maturity. Unfortunately, the female sample size for these latter ages is still small ($N = 23$ for the high-birthweight females at 48 months of age), so this effect is tentative.

Development of Nursery-Raised Low-Birthweight Infants

Over 80 sick, maternally rejected or abused, premature, and very small infants have been hand reared in the Infant Primate Laboratory at the University of Washington. About half of these newborns were at or below the 10th percentile low-birthweight criterion, and some of these were premature, based on timed gestational age estimates or radiograph norms on development of bone ossification centers (Newell-Morris & Tarrant, 1978). Among a large battery of measures taken on these newborns were (a) daily bodyweight and formula intake; (b) rating of sleep–wakefulness state once every 30 min, 24 hours per day; and (c) pulse and respiration rate and rectal temperature taken every 4 hours, 24 hours per day. These infants and physically normal controls live in an environment-controlled isolette for the first 10–14 days. They are held up to a nipple attached to a feeding box until they are able to feed without assistance. They continue to live in the nursery in individual wire cages until they are 28–30 days old. In addition to 80 normal controls, we have also studied 26 newborns delivered by cesarean section at or close to full term. This group represents a control for possible trauma induced by the birth process.

Figure 3.3 presents age at attaining self-feeding ability for our four neonate groups. Although normal, cesarean section, and maternally rejected infants did not differ in this developmental milestone, low-birthweight animals took over twice as long to achieve self-feeding compared with the overall mean of the other groups ($t(76) = 10.05$, $p < .001$). Figure 3.4A shows weight gain for normal and low-birthweight infants over the first 16 weeks of postnatal age. Low-birthweight animals remained lighter during this period, and males showed no trend toward catching up with the normals. Differences in intake (Figure 3.4B) were much smaller proportionately than in weight, suggesting that caloric differences do not account for the failure of low-birthweight monkeys to reach normal weight ranges (Sackett, Holm, & Fahrenbruch, 1979).

While in the nursery, our subjects were observed once every 30 min around the clock. The observer recorded whether the animal was behaviorally asleep, awake but inactive, or awake and active. The data were summarized for each

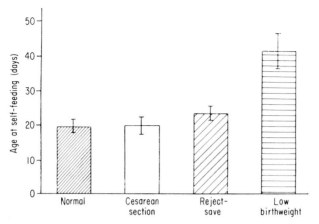

FIGURE 3.3. *Average day of age on which infants required no further assistance in feeding from a formula bottle attached to their living cage. Bars give standard error of mean.*

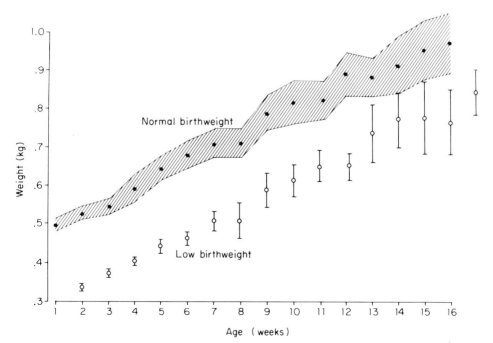

FIGURE 3.4A. *Weight gain for low-birthweight males (upper graph) and females compared with physically normal infants. Shaded area shows mean ± S.E.M. for normal infants; bars show S.E.M about the mean for low-birthweight infants.*

47

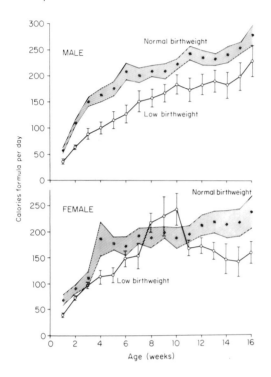

FIGURE 3.4B. *Caloric intake for the animals whose weight gains were plotted in Figure 3.4A. Shaded area shows mean ± S.E.M. for normal infants; bars give standard error of mean about the mean for low-birthweight infants.*

animal on a weekly basis in six 4-hour time blocks beginning with the observation after midnight. With 8 observations per day per time block, a total of 56 observations per week constituted a complete data set for each animal during any given 4-hour time period. The percentage of these 56 observations spent in each of the three sleep–wakefulness states is plotted in Figure 3.5 for normal, cesarean section, and low-birthweight neonates.

Regression analyses involving the six time-of-day blocks (T) and T^2, T^3, and T^4 (quadratic, cubic, and quartic trend components) were used to assess development of cyclicity for each behavior state percentage measure. Birth group and week of age were dummy coded in these analyses, and terms were also included for all interactions among birth group, age, and time-of-day components (Cohen & Cohen, 1975). Statistical significance employed alpha at or beyond the .01 level. The normal group differed from the other two groups in at least one nonlinear trend component of time of day on each of the 4 weeks for both the sleep and active states. Sleep cyclicity was more pronounced in the normal group than in the other two groups on all 4 weeks, with both cesarean section and low-birthweight neonates exhibiting a significantly higher overall percentage of sleep on all weeks. The normal animals had more pronounced cyclicity of the active state from week 2 on and had a higher overall percentage of observations spent in the active state. Trend components for the awake-but-inactive state did not differ reliably between groups,

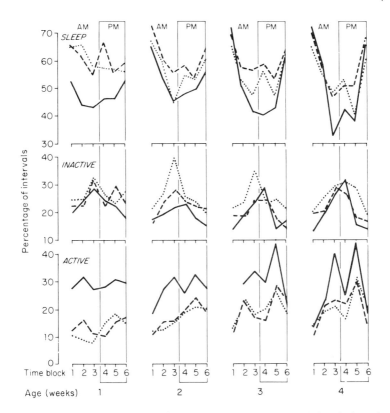

FIGURE 3.5. *Development of sleep–wakefulness state cyclicity in normal, low-birthweight, and nearly term cesarean section infants. Animals were observed once each 30 min around the clock, yielding 56 samples for each of the 4-hour time blocks plotted in each weekly curve. Upper graph shows sleep; middle graph shows awake but inactive; lower graph shows awake and active. Solid line shows normal, broken line shows low-birthweight, and dotted line shows cesarean section infants.*

although cesarean section and low-birthweight animals were observed in the inactive state more than normals.

Every 4 hours, we measured respiration rate (by counting chest wall movements), heart rate (by stethoscope), and rectal temperature (by electronic thermometer). Each of these measures, averaged for each 4-hour time block per week, served as a dependent variable for a regression analysis. Independent variables were the time-of-day, age, and birth group comparisons described above for behavioral state cyclicity. Diurnal cycle curves for each group on each week are shown in Figure 3.6. The temperature cyclicity of the low-birthweight group was similar to that of the other two groups, but the average daily values for each week were lower. Diurnal cyclicity of respiration differed between all groups after week 1, with low-birthweight animals initially lower in average daily respiration rate but achieving markedly higher

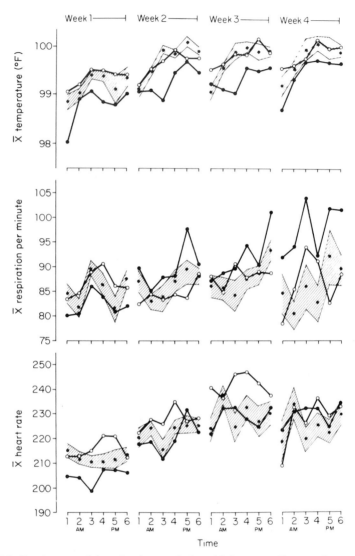

FIGURE 3.6. *Development of diurnal cyclicity in the basic life functions of heart and respiration rate and rectal temperature for normal, low-birthweight, and cesarean section infants. Means for each 4-hour time block are based on longitudinal data with seven points per week for each infant. Shaded area shows normal (mean ± S.E.); closed circles show low birthweight; and open circles show cesarean section.*

respiration rates on week 4. Heart rate cyclicity differed reliably between all groups on weeks 3 and 4, with low-birthweight animals having lower average daily heart rates on weeks 1–3 and cesarean section neonates having reliably higher heart rates on these weeks. (Sackett, Fahrenbruch, & Ruppenthal, 1979, present a detailed discussion of test methods and results used in these studies of diurnal cycle maturation.)

These data concern growth, basic adaptive abilities, and ability to regulate basic life functions. The results suggest that low-birthweight infants are markedly deviant from normal monkey newborns in ways remarkably similar to those in which human low-birthweight newborns are deviant from normal human newborns (e.g., Stern, Parmelee, & Harris, 1973). Unfortunately, only a few of the low-birthweight monkey infants were produced by timed matings, so their exact gestational ages were generally unknown. For those of known gestational ages, developmental lags in self-feeding and physiological cyclicity were greater than their degree of prematurity, indicating that these functions were actually retarded in maturation rate. Eleven low-birthweight subjects had an average known gestational age at birth of 21.7 weeks, compared with the normal value of 24.3 weeks. They achieved self-feeding at 31.4 weeks on the average, compared with 27.1 weeks for normal infants. This yields a developmental lag of 1.6 weeks (self-feeding at 4.3 postnatal weeks minus 2.7 weeks preterm gestation). These premature infants did not achieve the normal week 4 values in trend components across the six 4-hour time-of-day blocks for sleep and active states until week 7. The developmental lag for sleep–wakefulness cyclicity was thus 1 week greater than the degree of prematurity.

Various behaviors of nursery infants in isolettes and individual cages were recorded daily, using a digital data acquisition system yielding measures of response frequency, duration, and sequences (Sackett, Stephenson, & Ruppenthal, 1973). Figure 3.7 presents observational data for normal and low birthweight newborns in isolettes during the first week after birth. Low-

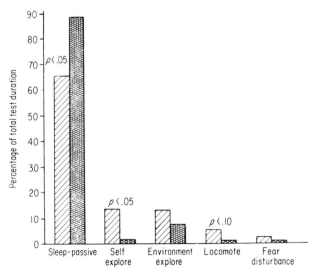

FIGURE 3.7. *Behavior of normal and low-birthweight newborns during week 1 after birth. All animals lived in isolettes controlled for temperature, oxygen, and humidity. Lined bars show normal-birthweight newborns, shaded bars show low-birthweight newborns.*

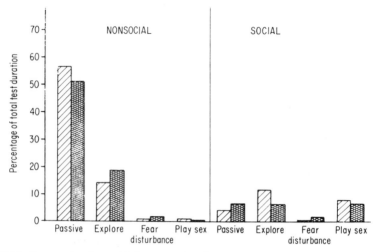

FIGURE 3.8. *Nonsocial and social behavior profiles for normal and low-birthweight infants during their first month of social experience in a playroom with four to six other animals of the same age. Lined bars show normal, shaded bars show low-birthweight newborns.*

birthweight monkeys slept more and spent less time in self-exploration and self-manipulation.

Upon leaving the nursery at 28–30 days of age, infants live in individual cages in a large rearing room. For 30 min, 5–6 days each week, animals are socialized in groups of four to six in a playroom. Figure 3.8 shows behavior profiles for low-birthweight and normal infants during their first month in the playroom (31–60 days of age). Nonsocial behaviors did not differ reliably between groups. However, normal animals did show more exploration of and physical contact with other monkeys and less socially elicited fear behavior. These data suggest that low-birthweight infants may be somewhat retarded in their social development. Ongoing work will determine whether these differences can be replicated and whether they persist into later life.

In sum, for pigtail infants low birthweight is related to a syndrome of deviant behavioral, physiological, and physical development. Such infants seem to be at high risk for developmental retardation and therefore should be an excellent comparison group in which to study the interaction of high and low risk for poor development with rearing under deprived versus enriched conditions.

Breeders at High and Low Risk for Poor Pregnancy Outcome

Our problem, at this point, concerns how to produce low-birthweight and/or premature infants that would be good models for human conditions. Although such animals could be delivered prematurely by cesarean section, our interest is in producing spontaneously delivered high-risk offspring. To solve this problem, we used the computerized colony records to predict which female and male breeders were most likely to produce poor pregnancy outcomes.

Poor pregnancy outcomes were defined as abortions, stillbirths, neonatal deaths, and low-birthweight offspring. A regression analysis was performed on over 3200 conceptions. The dependent variable was coded "1" if pregnancy outcome was in any of the categories described above and "0" for offspring not of low birthweight surviving the neonatal period (days 0–30). Independent variables included (*a*) age for colony-born breeders; (*b*) age estimates and time in colony for wild-born breeders; (*c*) colony parity; (*d*) various blood and other biochemistry values contained in the records; (*e*) prior history of poor pregnancy outcomes; (*f*) social stress prior to conception, measured by the number of treatments for bite wounds while living in the standard harem breeding group; and (*g*) change in body weight in the 6 months before conception (Sackett *et al.,* 1975). The results yielded a probability from 0 (low) to 1.00 (high) of risk for having a poor pregnancy outcome on the next conception. The equation was tested on 100 consecutive births and was found to predict with better than 90% accuracy for probabilities between .01–.20 (low risk) and .80–.99 (high risk). The most important predictor was prior history of poor pregnancy outcomes, with maternal age and parity next in importance. Interestingly, males contributed independently of females to the prediction, based on their prior history of poor pregnancy outcomes. Two of the 60 breeding males had over 65% poor outcomes, compared with overall norms of 30%.

In 1974 we applied this equation to the records of all current breeding females with a minimum of three prior conceptions and males with a minimum of 20 prior inseminations. Our goal was to identify, for selective breeding, those animals at highest and lowest risk for poor pregnancy outcomes. Table 3.1 shows the characteristics of this initial set of high- and low-risk female breeders, compared with data on the remaining 110 females of parity 3 or more actively breeding in the colony at that time. Low-risk females had over 90% viable offspring that survived the neonatal period and produced only 3.9% low-birthweight (10th percentile) offspring among their term infants. Average breeders had 66% surviving offspring and of course a 10% low-birthweight rate. The high-risk females had only 35.7% surviving offspring with 46.3% of term infants at low birthweight.

High-risk females formed four subgroups according to type of poor pregnancy outcome (Table 3.2). One group specialized in abortions, with their rate of 63.6% well above the 15.1% value for average breeders. A second group had 38.1% stillbirths and 47.9% neonatal deaths, compared with 9.5% for these outcomes by average breeders. A third group had a mixture of each poor outcome in their breeding history, being well above average in fetal, perinatal, and neonatal losses as well as in low-birthweight offspring. The

TABLE 3.1

Pregnancy Outcomes for 29 Low-Risk, 37 High-Risk, and 110 Average Breeding Females,
Identified from Colony Records among Females Having Three or More Prior Conceptions

	Pregnancy outcome					
Risk group	Viable	Aborted	Stillborn	Neonatal death	Total N^a	Low-birth-weight term infants
Low						
N^a	150	6	1	4	161	6
Percentage of total	93.2	3.7	.6	2.5	—	3.9
Mean/female	5.2	.2	0	.1	5.6	.2
High						
N^a	66	51	38	30	185	62
Percentage of total	35.7	27.6	20.5	16.2	—	46.3
Mean/female	1.8	1.4	1.0	.8	5.0	1.7
Average						
N^a	376	86	54	54	570	49
Percentage of total	66.0	15.1	9.5	9.5	—	10.1
Mean/female	3.4	.8	.5	.5	5.2	.4

$^a N$ = number of conceptions.

fourth group did not differ from average in mortality but had a 55.9% rate of low-birthweight offspring, although only one of these seven breeding females was herself small in stature and low in weight.

Table 3.3 presents pregnancy outcome data for the three high- and low-risk males in our initial breeding population. High-risk males exceeded low-risk males in each category except "viable," yet both groups were mated to a random assortment of females whose overall pregnancy outcomes did not differ from those of average breeders. This, like our regression analysis results, suggests that pigtail males make a contribution to poor pregnancy outcomes that is independent of female factors. Males are almost never considered as a source of poor pregnancy outcomes in human studies, so we cannot compare our monkey data with those for humans.

We began selectively breeding these monkeys in 1974. Animals of like risk were time mated for 1–2 days at the female's expected date of ovulation. Subjects were housed in individual cages before and during pregnancy, with hormone and other biochemical measures taken at periodic intervals during this time. Positive pregnancy was determined by palpation and hormone measurement 30 days after mating. Unfortunately, this procedure does not discriminate between early abortion and failure to conceive, so our abortion estimates presented in the following discussion may be conservative.

Each female was scheduled to have two pregnancies, one under minimal stress and the other under high stress, with order counterbalanced within each

TABLE 3.2

Types of Poor Pregnancy Outcomes among the 37 High-Risk Female Breeders

Poor outcome group	Pregnancy outcome					Low-birth-weight term infants
	Viable	Aborted	Stillborn	Neonatal death	Total N^a	
Aborted ($n = 10^b$)						
N^a	6	28	6	4	44	6
Percentage of total	13.6	63.6	13.6	9.1	—	33.5
Mean/female	.6	2.8	.6	.4	4.4	.6
Perinatal–neonatal death ($n = 6)^b$						
N^a	4	0	8	9	21	12
Percentage of total	19.0	0	38.1	42.9	—	57.1
Mean/female	.7	0	1.3	1.5	3.5	—
Mixed ($n = 14)^b$						
N^a	27	20	19	17	83	25
Percentage of total	32.5	24.1	22.9	20.5	—	39.7
Mean/female	1.9	1.4	1.4	1.2	5.9	1.8
Low birthweight ($n = 7)^b$						
N^a	29	3	5	0	37	19
Percentage of total	78.4	8.1	13.5	0	—	55.9
Mean/female	4.1	.4	.7	0	5.3	2.7

^{a} N = number of conceptions.

^{b} n = number of females.

risk condition. Stress was produced by hand capturing the female and confining her in a small cage for 5 min. This method was chosen because pigtail macaques exhibit clear signs of distress and disturbance when undergoing hand capture and do not habituate over repeated captures except for animals reared by humans in a nursery.

This procedure was followed for 26 of the 39 females contributing offspring to the study, with almost half of the first pregnancies for these 26 animals under the high-stress condition. Unfortunately, some females failed to conceive a second time, and several in each risk group became ill or died before achieving a second pregnancy. Therefore, 13 females produced only one pregnancy, with 7 under low-stress and 6 under high-stress conditions.

Pregnancy outcome results for these 66 conceptions are shown in Table 3.4, which gives the total number of pregnancies and the percentage of abortions in each risk–stress group. High-risk females had 55% abortions, a significant increase over their prior rate of 35.7%. Stress had no differential effect on the abortion rate of high-risk females. Low-risk females had an overall abortion

TABLE 3.3

Pregnancy Outcome Data for Three High- and Three Low-Risk Males Inducing 10 or More Prior Conceptions

Risk group	Subject	Pregnancy outcome				Total N^a	Low-birth-weight term infants
		Viable	Aborted	Stillborn	Neonatal death		
High							
	1	14	4	5	20	43	12
	2	4	10	7	1	22	5
	3	10	14	4	4	32	8
N^a		28	28	16	25	97	25
Percentage of total		28.9	28.9	16.5	25.8	—	36.2
Low							
	1	20	5	1	2	28	1
	2	29	5	2	4	40	2
	3	24	2	2	2	30	2
N^a		73	12	5	8	98	5
Percentage of total		74.5	12.2	5.1	8.2	—	5.8

$^a N$ = number of known conceptions.

rate of 15%, a highly reliable difference from the high-risk rate ($\chi^2 = 11.28$, $df = 1$, $p < .001$). Among nonstressed low-risk females, there was 1 abortion, a result consistent with our expectation of 1 in about 26 conceptions. Among stressed low-risk females there were 4 abortions, a significant deviation from an expected 3.7% rate when tested against the poisson distribution

TABLE 3.4

Percentage of Abortions for within-Risk-Group Matings of High- and Low-Risk Females Subjected to Minimal and High Stress during Pregnancy

Risk	Stress				Overall Percentage abortion
	High		Minimal		
	N^a	Percentage abortion	N^a	Percentage abortion	
High	15	53	18	56	55
Low	18	22	15	7	15
Overall	—	36	—	33	—

$^a N$ = total number of conceptions.

($p = .02$). These results suggest that stress during pregnancy may affect only low-risk females, an outcome currently under study in 12 additional low-risk–high-stress subjects.

These results validated the predicted risk characteristics of our high- and low-risk population, even in animals living in single cages under systematic experimental procedures rather than in social groups of 8–12 monkeys. Unfortunately, even under almost constant observations, aborted fetuses were not recovered from our monkeys. Therefore, the remainder of this study concerned characteristics of live- and stillborn offspring and development of surviving infants. Because of the excessive abortion rate in high-risk breeders, only 15 surviving infants could be studied from this group, compared with 28 from low-risk breeders. On the other hand, it seems reasonable to assume that these high-risk survivors are the most biologically fit offspring from the high-risk population, so differences between them and low-risk offspring probably underestimate their true potential for abnormal development.

Development of Offspring Differing in Parental Risk and Prenatal Stress

A number of developmental measures were taken on our offspring, including (*a*) birthweight, ponderal growth, and neurological and behavioral reflexes; (*b*) hormone and nutritional assays; and (*c*) physiological, social and exploratory behavior, and learning parameters. Only a few of these measures will be reported here; a more detailed account of growth, neonatal, and physiological results can be found in Ruppenthal and Reese (1979).

Physical Maturity

Radiographs of bone ossification centers were taken periodically from birth through month 6, when full ossification occurs (Fahrenbruch, Burbacher, & Sackett, 1979). Using a regression analysis to control for sex and gestational age differences, we found that low-risk offspring had significantly more mature skeletal systems at birth and developed postnatally at a faster rate than did high-risk offspring. The slowest rate of bone maturity was found for offspring of high-risk females that were stressed during pregnancy (risk-times-stress interaction significant below .025 level). Birthweight percentiles for the four groups are presented in Table 3.5. These were generated by converting each birthweight to its corresponding cumulative proportion in the sex-specific norms for all colony liveborn infants. This procedure eliminates the real sex difference of 50 gm between males and females from these comparisons. Low-risk offspring had reliably higher birthweight percentiles than those from the high-risk group ($p < .025$). A significant risk-times-stress interaction ($p < .04$) revealed that high-risk offspring from prenatally stressed

TABLE 3.5

Average Birthweight Percentiles for Surviving Offspring of High- and Low-Risk Females Subjected to Minimal and High Stress during Pregnancy

		Stress			
		High		Low	
Risk	N^a	Birthweight percentile	N^a	Birthweight percentile	Overall birthweight percentile
High	6	41	9	60	51
Low	11	75	17	80	78
Overall	—	58	—	70	—

$^a N$ = total number of conceptions.

mothers were lowest in birthweight percentiles among the four groups. These data indicate that high-risk breeders produce generally less mature offspring for a given gestational age and that these offspring mature skeletally at a slower rate than those produced by low-risk breeders. Further, the addition of stress during pregnancy retards high-risk offspring even more, although stress does not apparently affect low-risk offspring on these measures.

Learning and Performance

A number of learning and performance measures were taken on these infants between the third and seventh postnatal months, including adaptation to a Wisconsin General Test Apparatus (WGTA) (Harlow, 1959), black-and-white discrimination learning and reversal, set breaking, and object quality discrimination learning.

WGTA adaptation consisted of a series of steps in which the subject (a) took a food reward off a wooden tray; (b) removed the food reward from a depression (food well) in the tray after watching the food being placed in the well; (c) displaced a wooden object covering the food well after watching the food being put in the well and the well being covered with the object; and (d) displaced the object to obtain the food after an opaque screen was raised that had blocked the monkey's view of the tester and baiting of the food well. Subjects were given 25 trials per day at each step until they took the food on 23 of the 25 trials. Response latencies (time to obtain the food after food baiting or raising of the screen) did not differ between risk or prenatal stress conditions on trials when food was actually taken. However, number of trials per test day on which no effort was made to get the food (balks) did show effects in steps *b–d*. Analysis of variance revealed a reliable interaction between risk and stress ($p < .01$) that resulted from high-risk stress offspring averaging 7.8,

6.2, and 6.5 balks per day during steps *b, c,* and *d* of the procedure. The other three risk–stress conditions did not differ from each other at any step, with the overall averages for these groups being 2.2, 2.4, and 2.6 balks per day at each of these three adaptation phases. This suggests that offspring of high-risk females that were stressed during pregnancy are either less motivated to obtain food rewards and/or are more distracted or frustrated by changes in test procedures.

Black-and-white discrimination was studied by presenting the subject with two wooden objects, one black and one white. One object, randomly determined for each subject, covered a food reward, while the other covered an empty food well. The side on which each object was presented was randomly determined on each of the 25 daily trials. The learning criterion was 22 correct (food-rewarded) responses in 25 daily trials. The day after the monkey achieved criterion, reversal trials were begun, with the previously incorrect object now covering the food. Again, criterion was 22 correct choices in 25 trials.

Days to reach criterion did not differ between any of the four risk–prenatal stress conditions in either original acquisition or reversal phases. However, stressed animals as a group had twice the balk rate of nonstressed offspring during original learning (mean = 6.2 trials per day in which no response was made toward the objects within a 3-min period after the opaque screen was raised). This difference was reliable by ANOVA at the .01 level. Risk yielded no significant effects on original learning balks. Days to criterion on the reversal phase also yielded no differences between the four groups. However, stressed offspring had 2.4 times more balks (mean = 7.5 per day) than nonstressed offspring ($p < .01$). A reliable risk-times-stress interaction ($p < .01$) was produced because offspring of high-risk females that were stressed during pregnancy had a reliably higher balk rate (mean = 9.2 per day) than any of the other three risk–stress groups. These results again suggest that motivation to perform on these simple discrimination tasks is affected by stress to the mother during pregnancy, with especially strong effects resulting from stress to high-risk females.

Two-choice learning set problems, with six trials per problem, were presented at a rate of five problems per day. Each problem differed by presenting a totally new pair of "junk" three-dimensional objects, with one randomly designated as correct. The objects covered food wells in a movable tray. The incorrect object covered an empty well, while the correct object covered a raisin or grape. A total of 240 problems were given, requiring 48 test days. Objects were randomly placed on the left or right on each trial. A learning set is said to occur when the subject can use the information from the first trial, when objects are correct on a random basis, to perform at successfully higher correct probabilities on trial 2 of each six-trial problem. An optimal strategy is a win–stay, lose–shift approach, which can lead to 100% correct responses on trial 2 if the subject continues to choose the correct object or

TABLE 3.6

Percentage Correct Responses on Trials 2–6 during the Last Block of 30 Learning Set Problems for Offspring of High- and Low-Risk Breeders

Risk group	N^a	Trial				
		2	3	4	5	6
High	13	59.7	68.4	74.2	77.5	79.9
Low	25	69.1	73.4	77.8	81.0	85.7

^{a} N = total number of conceptions.

switches away from an incorrect object chosen on trial 1. Monkeys and young children find this task quite difficult, and rhesus macaques do not approach even 90% correct trial 2 performance until they reach 3–4 years of age.

Table 3.6 presents results for the final block of 30 problems, comparing high- with low-risk offspring (risk-time-trial interaction significant below the .025 level). Low-risk infants had almost 10% higher probability of correct responses on trial 2 than did high-risk infants. Even on the final trial, the low-risk exceeded the high-risk monkeys ($p < .05$). These data provide some preliminary evidence that parental risk factor may affect the intellectual development of monkey offspring. With animals studied to date, prenatal stress has failed to affect learning set performance.

However, evidence from a set breaking *einstellung*-type test has supported the hypothesis that prenatal stress can affect adaptive behavior. In this test series, subjects were given a number of trials using the Hamilton search procedure (Harlow, 1959). Four identical boxes with hinged lids were presented to the subject. On each trial, one of the boxes was randomly baited with a food reward, so the subject had no clue as to which box contained the reward. The subject could lift the box lids repeatedly until it found the food morsel. Over trials, monkeys developed a systematic search pattern resulting in a strong trend toward opening each box only once per trial. We presented 25 trials on each test day. When the subject stabilized in mean number of lid openings to reward, we stopped this set forming procedure and went on to the main set breaking test. In set breaking, the box that was least preferred as a first choice during the set forming trials was always baited, so that the infant had to stop responding with its previous pattern and could gain the reward by simply lifting the same box lid on each trial.

The number of trials to reach a criterion of 18/20 correct responses (reward box opened first) for offspring of minimally stressed females was 22.5. These infants thus broke set on the first day of 25 test trials. Offspring of high-stressed females averaged 73.4 trials to this same criterion, and 6 of 15 subjects failed to reach criterion by the end of their fifth test day. Thus, stress during pregnancy appears to affect the offspring's willingness or ability to alter learned behavior that is no longer appropriate for situational contingencies. Parental risk, however, did not reliably affect performance on this task.

This suggests that the performance dimensions affected by the risk variable (e.g., learning set concept formation) are different from those affected by prenatal stress (e.g., inhibition of inappropriate behavior).

Current Research Using this Nonhuman Primate Model

In addition to replication studies of our original findings, we are currently working on four major problems using high- and low-risk breeders. In one study, females are mated with males from the opposite risk condition to estimate the contribution of the male to poor pregnancy outcomes and to deviant offspring development. In a second study, fetuses are delivered by cesarean section at the end of the first trimester of pregnancy in an effort to determine the role of fetal and placental factors in causing abortions in the high-risk group. The goal of this work is to prevent abortions and thereby obtain a greater number of full-term high-risk offspring for postnatal developmental studies. In a third experiment, infants are delivered by cesarean section both prematurely and close to term. These offspring are to be reared in socially enriched versus isolated conditions to study the interactive effects of parental risk and birth condition with quality of rearing experiences.

In a fourth endeavor, we will more directly investigate the genetic versus prenatal causes of poor pregnancy outcomes. We are developing procedures for performing embryo transfers in our breeding female population. Embryo transfer has been highly successful in rodents, cattle, sheep, and goats. Fertilized preimplantation blastocysts are recovered from a donor female and transferred into recipient females that are hormonally synchronized with the donors. Using another procedure, we will recover unfertilized ova from the donor, fertilize the egg *in vitro,* and transfer it to appropriate recipients after 4–5 days of *in vitro* development. *In vitro* fertilization has been successful in humans (Steptoe & Edwards, 1978), while a healthy baboon has been produced using the fertilized blastocyst technique (Kraemer, Moore, & Kramen, 1976). Our aim is to separate genetic from prenatal factors by prenatal cross-fostering. Transfers will be made between females of high and of low risk for poor pregnancy outcomes. As in postnatal cross-fostering, we can then determine whether pregnancy outcomes and offspring development follow the course expected for the biological mother or for the pregnant host female.

In summary, we believe that our high- and low-risk breeding population harbors sufficient similarities with high- and low-risk humans to provide a reasonably valid model for studying genetic, physiological, biochemical, and anatomical factors related to poor pregnancy outcomes in both monkeys and humans. Our results on growth and development of low-birthweight monkeys are similar to reports concerning human infants. Thus, this aspect of the research model seems appropriate for studying a number of significant human development problems with monkey subjects. Finally, the addition of the embryo transfer technique to research on nonhuman primates should aid in clarifying old controversies concerning nature versus nurture and may lead to the discovery of fundamental mechanisms underlying both normal and abnormal pregnancy and offspring development.

References

Clark, D. L. *Immediate and delayed effects of early, intermediate, and late social isolation in the rhesus monkey.* Unpublished doctoral dissertation, University of Wisconsin, 1968.

Clarke, A. M., & Clarke, A. D. *Early experience: Myth and evidence.* New York: Free Press, 1977.

Cohen, J., & Cohen, P. *Applied multiple regression/correlation anaylsis for the behavioral sciences.* Hillsdale, N.J.: Erlbaum, 1975.

Farenbruch, C. E., Burbacher, T. M., & Sackett, G. P. Assessment of skeletal growth and maturation of premature and term *Macaca nemestrina*. In G. C. Ruppenthal & D. A. Reese, (Eds.), *Nursery care of nonhuman primates.* New York: Plenum, 1979.

Harlow, H. F. The nature of love. *American Psychologist* 1958, *13,* 673–685.

Harlow, H. F. The development of learning in the rhesus monkey. *American Scientist,* 1959, *47,* 485–479.

Harlow, H. F. Sexual behavior in the rhesus monkey. In F. A. Beach (Ed.), *Sex and behavior.* New York: Academic Press, 1965.

Harlow, H. F., & Harlow, M. K. The affectional systems. In A. M. Schrier, H. F. Harlow, & F. Stollnitz (Eds.). *Behavior of nonhuman primates* (Vol. 2). New York: Academic Press, 1965.

Harlow, H. F., & Suomi, S. J. Nature of love—simplified. *American Psychologist,* 1970, *25,* 161–168.

Hinde, R. A., & Spencer-Booth, Y. Effects of brief separation from mothers on rhesus monkeys. *Science,* 1971, *173,* 111–118.

Kraemer, D. C., Moore, G. T., & Kramen, M. A. Baboon infant produced by embryo transfer. *Science,* 1976, *192,* 1246–1247.

Mineka, S., & Suomi, S. J. Social separation in monkeys. *Psychological Bulletin,* 1978, *85,* 1376–1400.

Newell-Morris, L. Growth and development parameters associated with gestational age in *Macaca nemestrina* fetus. *American Journal of Physical Anthropology,* 1977, *47,* 152.

Newell-Morris, L. N., & Tarrant, L. H. Ossification in the hand and foot of the macaque *(M. nemestrina).* I. General features. *American Journal of Physical Anthropology,* 1978, *48,* 441–453.

Novak, M. A. Social recovery of monkeys isolated for the first year of life. II. Long-term assessment. *Developmental Psychology,* 1979, *15,* 50–61.

Rosenblum, L. A., & Kaufman, I. C. Variations in infant development and response to maternal loss in monkeys. *American Journal of Orthopsychiatry,* 1968, *38,* 418–426.

Ruppenthal, G. C., & Reese, D. A. (Eds.). *Nursery care of nonhuman primates.* New York: Plenum, 1979.

Sackett, G. P. Isolation rearing in monkeys: Diffuse and specific effects on later behavior. In R. Chauvin, (Ed.), *Animal models of human behavior.* Paris: Colleques Internationaux du C.N.R.S., 1972.

Sackett, G. P. Sex differences in rhesus monkeys following varied rearing experiences. In R. C. Friedman, R. M. Richart, & R. L. Vende Wiele (Eds.), *Sex differences in behavior.* New York: Wiley, 1974.

Sackett, G. P., Fahrenbruch, C. E., & Ruppenthal, G. C. Development of basic physiological parameters and sleep-wakefulness patterns in normal and at-risk neonatal pigtail macaques. In G. C. Ruppenthal & D. A. Reese (Eds.), *Nursery care of nonhuman primates*. New York: Plenum, 1979.

Sackett, G. P., Holm, R. A., Davis, A. E., & Fahrenbruch, C. E. Prematurity and low birth weight in pigtail macaques: Incidence, prediction, and effects on infant development. In S. Kondo, M. Kawai, A. Ehara, & S. Kawamura (Eds.), *Symposia of the Fifth Congress of the International Primatological Society*. Tokyo: Japan Science Press, 1975.

Sackett, G. P., Holm, R. A., & Fahrenbruch, C. D. Ponderal growth in colony- and nursery-reared pigtail macaques. In G. C. Ruppenthal & D. A. Reese (Eds.), *Nursery care of nonhuman primates*. New York: Plenum, 1979.

Sackett, G. P., Holm, R. A., Ruppenthal, G. C., & Fahrenbruch, C. E. The effects of total social isolation rearing on behavior of rhesus and pigtail macaques. In R. N. Walsh & W. T. Greenough (Eds.), *Advances in behavioral biology* (Vol. 17) *Environments as therapy for brain dysfunction*. New York: Plenum, 1976.

Sackett, G. P., Stephenson, E., & Ruppenthal, G. C. Digital data acquisition systems for observing behavior in laboratory and field settings. *Behavior Research Methods and Instrumentation*, 1973, *5*, 344–348.

Sameroff, A. J. Early influences on development: Fact or fancy? *Merrill–Palmer Quarterly*, 1975, *21*, 267–294.

Steptoe, P. C., & Edwards, R. G. Birth after the reimplantation of a human embryo. *Lancet*, 1978, *2*, 366.

Stern, E., Parmelee, A. H., & Harris, M. A. Sleep state periodicity in prematures and young infants. *Developmental Psychobiology*, 1973, *6*, 357–365.

Suomi, S. J., & Harlow, H. F. Social rehabilitation of isolate-reared monkeys. *Developmental Psychology*, 1979, *6*, 487–496.

Woodrum, D. E., Guthrie, R. D., & Hodson, W. A. Development of respiratory control mechanisms in the fetus and newborn. In W. A. Hodson (Ed.), *The development of the lung*. New York: Marcel Dekker, 1978.

Perinatal Risks, Neonatal Deficits, and Developmental Crises: A Review of Chapters 1-3

LEWIS P. LIPSITT

Perinatal risks produce neonatal deficits that result in developmental crises. If this statement sounds like hyperbole, let it be understood that we are truly living in an age of superlatives. Never has so much attention been paid to the phenomena of pregnancy wastage and human developmental insufficiencies. If an obstetrician or pediatrician who retired 20 years ago (and that is a very short period of time in the history of humanity!) were to return to his local lying-in hospital today, he would be astounded at the change of conditions and attitudes: mothers not having to use the stirrups during delivery; fathers routinely in the delivery room—taking pictures, snipping the umbilicus; mothers sitting up holding their babies to their bare bosoms minutes after delivery.

If 20 years seems like a short time in which to get over the tetanizing effect that institutionalized childbirth had come to have, consider that it was less than 100 years ago when anesthetized deliveries were introduced (Wertz & Wertz, 1979). And that, too, is a short period in the history of mankind.

We have come a long way, along several routes and not without travel tensions all around. While the care of the normal newborn is now quite routine and even relaxed, the scientific and medical technologies of the century have all converged upon the neonatal intensive care unit and upon the baby at risk. Never have people, including people in the maternal and child care health professions, been so engrossed with the survival of the baby, with the study of perinatal factors that influence birth outcome, with the role of genetics and of early experiences in determining the developmental growth and learning achievements of the youngster, or with the plasticity of the birthing milieu, and even of the special-care nursery.

PRETERM BIRTH AND
PSYCHOLOGICAL DEVELOPMENT

Most people today, at least those with a high school education or more, are aware that heredity is a factor in certain types of infantile blood diseases; that congenital aberrations are involved in Down's syndrome; that excessive alcohol consumption or smoking can be hazardous to the welfare of the fetus; that amniocentesis can determine before birth whether a baby will be in poor condition from a genetic defect; that humans have options with regard to the utilization of reasonably safe abortion procedures if the fetus is found defective or if the parents consider their own lives to be jeopardized by the birth; and that the birth of a risky infant need not be the end of the world, especially for parents who are intent on optimizing the child's development by offering exceptional environmental opportunities.

All the new concern for the delivery of viable and wanted infants and for the optimization of the quality of life for children and parents alike, along with the proliferation in recent years of personnel in the field of neonatology, has placed a great empirical burden upon the medical sciences associated with birth and development. Obstetricians, neonatologists, developmental psychologists, and parents all want to know more about the relationships between perinatal risk events and neonatal outcomes. Similarly, we are woefully lacking in important information concerning the newborn's condition and the implications of this for later development. If maternal alcoholism produces a jittery and cantankerous baby, must this mean that the child of the alcoholic mother will inevitability be retarded, mean, or alcoholic himself? If birth asphyxia and eventual resuscitation through modern methods yield a bluish baby with lethargic responses to respiratory threats, does this mean his or her risk of dying of crib death (sudden infant death syndrome) some 2–4 months hence is greater than that of the child born uneventfully? Were infants the focus of insurance consumer attentions, these are questions that responsible insurance companies would want to have answered and on which they would probably be avidly collecting data, just as they collect data for adults on the medical–environmental conditions that correlate with longevity and viability. Indeed, insurance companies would surely have been more significantly involved by now in the sponsorship of pregnancy-outcome and neonatal research than they are. The task has fallen instead to the health care and allied research disciplines to rally and often to pursue this information under conditions of inadequate financial support, poor staffing, and less than well-standardized conditions.

Contributors to the task of better understanding the conditions of fetal, neonatal, and childhood stresses that take their toll on optimal development are Werthmann, Keller, and Sackett (see Chapters 1, 2, and 3, this volume). Each has come up with a different kind of work, a different research design, to illuminate the descriptive verities that are the first step toward a deeper understanding of the processes and mechanisms whereby one developmental condition or event produces another. The ultimate study of antecedent–consequent relations in this area of developmental jeopardy is of paramount importance. The study of causation should be the objective of descriptive or epidemiological or actuarial studies, which should be regarded as only the first step toward the documentation of causes.

Keller's meticulous chapter on epidemiological characteristics (Chapter 1, this volume) has a number of important messages for us. We find that there is a close relationship among birthweight, gestation length, and neonatal mortality. The major and best-documented consequent of very low birthweight or profound prematurity is death in the first week of life. But very interestingly and importantly, among babies who survive the first week of life, the majority of subsequent deaths "occur in the optimal survival group defined by birthweight and gestation length: between 37 and 43 weeks and between 2501 and 4500 gm [p. 4]." This finding has vast implications, not the least of which is that our attentions as researchers and clinicians must be turned toward the apparently normal offspring whom we have tended to assume are "safe" and therefore not needy of extensive developmental monitoring. In fact, the histories of infants succumbing to crib death suggest, on close examination, that these infants, while ostensibly normal, had in their backgrounds a number of soft signs. Certain perinatal events and conditions each taken by itself may be no cause for alarm at the time the infant is discharged from the hospital, but the sum of them, taken as a constellation of risk factors, might dispose the child to developmental jeopardy (Lipsitt, 1979; Protestos, Carpenter, McWeeny, & Emery, 1973; Swift & Emery, 1973). As clinical resources and research attentions in the field of neonatology are intensified for the care of the clearly high-risk infant, it will become increasingly important to keep in close touch with the data on developmental outcomes of essentially normal infants.

In many studies, and those discussed by Keller are no exception, race and socioeconomic level show up as significant variables in relation to prematurity and low birthweight and thus to developmental deficits of many kinds (Niswander & Gordon, 1972). While it is scientifically inelegant to think of correlations in terms of cause–effect relations, it is high time that we did appreciate and acknowledge that race and socioeconomic level are themselves highly intercorrelated with such birth risk factors as mother's age, previous pregnancy history, and other variables that do have known causative mechanisms underlying hazardous birth and development. Lack of prenatal care, and all the neglect of one's physical and mental well-being that this implies, is in turn highly related to these variables, and it is perhaps in that area that we need to look for "hidden causes." This is a plea, as will be realized, for greater attention on the part of perinatal risk researchers to the psychological, the behavioral aspects of pregnancy, birthing, and the mother–infant cohabitation. Keller has properly called our attention to the fact that two of the major contributors to the infant's low birthweight, cigarette smoking and weight gain of the mother, are conditions that are subject to behavioral manipulation.

The title of Werthmann's chapter (Chapter 2, this volume), calls our attention to *medical* constraints on the *psychological* development of the preterm child. Especially when one gets into the substance of his chapter, it becomes apparent that this is a litany of conditions that seems to travel a one-way street. The presentation is all about frank physiological conditions of the pregnancy and birthing process that could result in problems (mostly unspecified) later. The fact is that the chapter could equally well have been titled, with a slight bit of expansion, "Psychological constraints to optimal fetal development," for many of the risk conditions cited have behavioral roots. This is not to deny their physical reality but only to point out that how one chooses to, or must, live during pregnancy, how culture dictates the conditions of birth, and what kinds of prophylactic, resuscitative, and other remedial techniques are available to the birthing mother are largely under environmental control and behavioral instigation. How much she eats during pregnancy, whether she uses drugs or smokes or drinks excessively, whether she has been vaccinated against rubella, whether her diabetes is adequately controlled during pregnancy, and whether vulnerable parents have Tay-Sachs screening or amniocentesis for the detection (and possible abortion) of an affected fetus—these are all environmentally manipulable matters. They are, in short, of a psychological nature. Not so surprisingly, many of these facets of pregnancy and childbirth have a great deal to do with one's socioeconomic level, education, and personal information about and attitudes toward pregnancy and children. One would think that our society—and other societies as well—would be concentrating on psychological aspects of birthing and early child development that are in principle remediable. It will not be easy, of course, but it has been neither easy nor inexpensive to come to this point in the history of medicine and child development where the physical constraints on optimal fetal and neonatal outcome are known (Stratton, 1977). It is only 100 years since 20% of the patients in a major American lying-in hospital died of puerperal fever (a higher rate than occurred, incidentally, among births outside the hospital). As it turned out, it was largely a matter of education and change of behavior, principally of the attending physicians, that brought the mortality rate down to today's low level (Wertz & Wertz, 1979).

Additional behavioral aspects of pregnancy and childbirth are underscored by Sackett (Chapter 3, this volume). Drawing upon the classic studies of the Harlow and the Hinde laboratories, he shows that social and maternal isolation of the infant female monkey results in the development of an aberrant adolescent and a young adult that has difficulty conceiving. When she does conceive and bears an infant herself, she is, to put it truthfully, a lousy mother. Moreover, studies of Harlow and of Sackett have shown that males are even more vulnerable than females when raised under conditions of isolation or by surrogates; whereas about half of females so reared do go on to procreate and become at least some kind of mothering individual, males seem almost uniformly affected, showing anomalous sexual behavior for protracted periods of time into adolescence and adulthood even under ordinarily ideal conditions of mating. Sex differences. coupled with species differences well documented by Sackett, are suggested by him to reveal the importance of "nonenvironmental factors . . . in determining risk for developing abnormal behavior [p. 43]. At the same time, he points out that any paradigm designed to reveal the causes of abnormal behavior in development must deal with the inevitable interactions between genetic or constitutional variables, on the one hand, and environmental factors, on the other.

When we look at the particulars of the Sackett study, which serves as an excellent animal model for the exploration of conditions presumed in humans to be of great consequence in pregnancy outcome, it becomes obvious that had an interaction paradigm not been used, some very important data would have been lost. The animal model has the advantage, of course, that the mothers and the pregnancies can be subjected to a range of risk manipulations to determine differential outcomes under varying degrees of fetal stress. In an ambitious study design, Sackett scheduled each female to undergo two pregnancies, one under an environmental–psychological stress condition and the other under essentially normal conditions. Although high-risk females produced many more abortions (55 %) than the low-risk females (15%), just as one could easily expect from human data, it was the interaction between risk and stress that proved so illuminating. Whereas stress did not affect the rate of abortion in the high-risk group, perhaps because this population was already in such jeopardy for fetal demise, it increased the rate of abortion fourfold in the low-risk group.

A look at the surviving infants in the Sackett study, of which there were a greater number in the low-risk than in the high-risk group, also produced some edifying results, particularly about the continuing impact of hazardous pregnancies. The design enabled comparisons between level of risk, level of stress, and the interaction between them. High risk and stress acting together yielded the slowest growing group of offspring; the double insult of a high-risk history plus a stressful event during pregnancy produces the greatest apparent damage. Further to the point about the importance of the interaction design, some learning tasks showed effects of prenatal risk, some the effects of pregnancy stress, some the effects of neither, and some the effects of both. The study of pregnancy outcome under different historical conditions will undoubtedly turn out to be even more complex and subtle than is immediately implied by these data. This is all the more reason for an aggressive research approach to these difficult empirical issues that are of such great social importance.

References

Lipsitt, L. P. Critical conditions in infancy: A psychological perspective. *American Psychologist,* 1979, *34,* 973–980.

Niswander, K. R., & Gordon, M. *The women and their pregnancies: The collaborative perinatal study of the National Institute of Neurological Diseases and Stroke.* Philadelphia: Saunders, 1972.

Protestos, C., Carpenter, R. McWeeny, P., & Emery, J. Obstetric and perinatal histories of children who died unexpectedly (cot death). *Archives of Disease in Childhood,* 1973, *48,* 835–841.

Stratton, P. M. Criteria for assessing the influence of obstetric circumstances on later development. In T. Chard & M. Richards (Eds.), *Benefits and hazards of the new obstetrics.* London: Spastics International Medical Publications, 1977.

Swift, P. G. F., & Emery, J. L. Clinical observations on response to nasal occlusion in infancy. *Archives of Disease in Childhood,* 1973, *48,* 947–951.

Wertz, R. W., & Wertz, D. C. *Lying-in: A history of childbirth in America.* New York: Schocken, 1979.

II

Neurophysiological Organization and Its Behavioral Implications

5

Animal Studies in Developmental Psychobiology: Commentary on Method, Theory, and Human Implications

GUENTER H. ROSE

Developmental psychobiology, although a relatively new field, has shown a phenomenal growth rate in recent years; over 400 animal studies have been published since the mid-1970s alone. Their theoretical and research concerns are focused on the biological basis of behavioral development, both learned and unlearned, that emerge during pre- and postnatal maturation. The studies range from neurochemical, physiological, and anatomical investigations that briefly mention behavioral implications, to those emphasizing behavioral analyses while suggesting neural–hormonal correlates. The vast majority, however, are truly interdisciplinary, with both behavioral and biological factors as independent or dependent variables or measures.

It is not my intention to review this vast literature. The reader will find several recent publications that accomplish this task, especially those by Ellis (1975), Gottlieb (1973, 1974, 1976, 1978), Himwich (1970), Jacobsen (1978), Riesen (1975), and Sterman, McGinty, and Adinolfi (1971), to mention a few. Instead, using a limited sample of visual evoked potential and neurobehavioral studies in neonatal animals, I wish to illustrate, as well as critique, the general nature of developmental (sensory) studies, especially as they may contribute to the understanding of normal and aberrant processes in early human infancy. Therefore, a brief section will also be devoted to the current status of evoked potential recording in adult and infant humans. It is important that those working primarily with human infants appreciate the complex issues surrounding the nature, usefulness, as well as the limitations, of animal models beyond the obvious factors involved in cross-species comparisons.

A major point of concern, one that will be stressed repeatedly, regards the

PRETERM BIRTH AND
PSYCHOLOGICAL DEVELOPMENT

paucity of normative or baseline[1] neurophysiological and especially behavioral data in young animals necessary for the appropriate interpretation of so-called early-experience studies that overwhelmingly dominate the field. A secondary concern is that more emphasis be placed on the role of the entire central nervous system when discussing the development of sensory–perceptual capabilities instead of the current practice of focusing almost exclusively on the classical sensory pathways.

Historical Background

The issues outlined in the preceding paragraphs may best be placed in some perspective by a brief historical synopsis of developmental psychobiology (including behavioral embryology), which most would agree began with the studies of William Preyer (1841–1897). The relevance of Preyer to these issues as well as to this volume is that not only did he publish the first modern comprehensive text on the psychobiology of prenatal development, *Specielle Physiologie des Embryo* (Preyer, 1885), but 3 years earlier he wrote *Die Seele des Kindes (The Mind of the Child,* Preyer, 1882), a volume with considerable influence in stimulating the field of developmental psychology (see Gottlieb's 1973 essay on Preyer).

Beginning with Preyer and until the late 1940s, one finds the majority of studies concentrating on the delineation of normative–baseline data in young pre and postnatal animals and children (see, for example, Carmichael, 1946). Most of the theoretical–conceptual battles of that era dealt with the question of whether eventual complex behaviors began as total patterns of activity followed by subsequent differentiation (e.g., Coghill, 1929; Hooker, 1952; Humphrey, 1969) or as isolated reflexes that eventually integrated into complex patterns (e.g, Windle, 1944.) Another major early conceptualization of the maturation process was Anokhin's (1964) theory of systematogenesis (first introduced in 1948), which emphasized heterochronic maturation. This concept focused attention on the role of the differential development of neural subsystems at particular ages, as the basis of behavioral repertoires emerging during a particular stage of development. It was basically a predeterministic viewpoint, however, as was that of many of the behavioral biologists, in that it stressed preprogrammed (genetic) systems, deemphasizing environmental influences.

Then in 1949 Donald Hebb published *The Organization of Behavior,* a most significant reevaluation of the role of early influences particularly with regard to perceptual development. It precipitated a head-on rush by most

---

[1] I suggest we use the term *normative development* to refer to species-typical behavior, whether in the field or laboratory (e.g., imprinting), and use *baseline development* to refer to behaviors primarily elicited by the laboratory, experimental situation, or apparatus (e.g., bar pressing).

psychologists into studies in support of the external environmental influences. It likewise added renewed fuel to the persistent nature–nurture controversy.

What, then, is the current emphasis in animal developmental psychobiology studies? In the field of visual perception, for example, one finds that (*a*) an overwhelming emphasis is placed on the effects of early experience, including manipulations of the internal milieu (lesions, hormones, etc.) or of the external milieu (sensory deprivation, selective stimulation, etc.), on later behavioral and/or biological processes; (*b*) most assessments are undertaken later in maturation or adulthood, often without adequate experimental design (e.g., Solomon & Lessac, 1968); (*c*) the effects of the interaction between internal and external milieu manipulations have not been extensively studied (e.g., the effects of the external environment on lesion recovery); (*d*) there is a relative decrease in normative–baseline studies, especially in the early neonatal period, with the accompanying result that few studies examine the effect of experimental manipulations on the maturational process itself; (*e*) most neurophysiological studies place a large emphasis on single-unit recordings of the "primary" cortical regions as the predominate electrophysiological measure; and finally (*f*) the theoretical battles concerning nature–nurture continue unabated around such specific issues as whether the effects of visual deprivation on later neurobehavioral functions are due to inappropriate stimulation of genetically determined neural patterns fixed at birth (functional validation hypothesis) or whether the effects are due to lack of appropriate stimulation of neurons only loosely genetically specified at birth and hence malleable by external stimulation (functional specification hypothesis). For a modern synopsis of these controversies and attempts at their resolution, the reader is referred to the recent series by Gottlieb (1973, 1974, 1976, 1978) and the publication by McCleary (1970).

Given that this is the *zietgeist* in animal psychobiological studies, what is the current emphasis in human infant studies for which the animal studies are to serve as models? Here we find (*a*) a heavy emphasis on the analysis of normative processes (habituation, discrimination, etc.) studied both cross-sectionally and longitudinally; (*b*) the utilization, in the neonatal period, of a complex and sophisticated battery of observational–experimental assessment techniques; and (*c*) the use of the evoked potential and EEG as the primary electrophysiological measures.

Thus, studies on the development of normative or baseline behaviors, although common to ethologists, behavioral biologists, child psychologists, and pediatricians, are studied to a far lesser degree by animal developmental psychobiologists. It is obvious that to a large extent the differences in technique are due to ethical, scientific, and practical considerations. These, however, can be independent of the question of research emphasis or zeitgeist, especially with regard to such issues as biological constraints, to be discussed later.

Methodological Considerations

There is no question of the great value of much of the early-experience infant animal research; I have also undertaken such studies (Rose & Gruenau, 1973). My primary suggestion with regard to our topic is that we reexamine some of our assumptions and priorities, particularly in the light of recent advances in the study of human adult and infant neurophysiological events as well as the increasing sophistication of current human infant behavioral studies. I am devoting considerable emphasis to methodological considerations because there is a danger (usually unspoken) when one is unfamiliar with infant animal psychobiological studies to assume or propose relevance uncritically to the human infant when either extreme caution is necessary or a different question, species, or design would have been more appropriate.

Such publications as those by Gottlieb (1976, 1978), Seligman and Hager (1972), and Rose (1971, 1975) attempt to establish a more complete conceptualization of the interaction of biological and environmental influences in animals, on the one hand, and the role of normative or baseline developmental data in interpretation of the manipulations or early experience, on the other. A number of significant questions emerge, which the reader should consider in examining such studies for possible human infant relevancy. For example, what are the limits in the interpretation of early-experience studies that are ignorant of normative developmental sequences and different maturation rates within and between biological systems and within and between species; that ignore biological constraints; that use developmentally inappropriate measures; etc.? We know that there are transient events unique to particular stages of development (e.g., protospines on cell bodies of neurons, age-related activity peaks); how much do they contribute to the manifestations of our early interventions? Since neural regions as well as functional systems mature at different rates, to what extent can we apply adult neurological models of behavior, based on established connections, to the emerging processes when considering developmental neurobiological interventions? Under the term *early experience,* why not include normal developmental strategies (e.g., light avoidance) that vary with age between and even within species, with possible later consequences during behavioral assessment (Rose & Collins, 1975b)? To paraphrase Gottlieb (1976), do our experimental manipulations maintain, facilitate, or induce various processes and are our experiments designed to reflect these options? What other systems (e.g., endocrine) influenced by the early experience (e.g., light) may influence the neural mechanisms of concern (e.g., visual)? Some of these issues will be referred to again in subsequent sections.

In the remainder of this chapter, I will (*a*) briefly review some of our early evoked potential studies on kittens; (*b*) discuss newer combined behavioral-physiological studies on neonatal animals that emphasize early baseline data; and (*c*) suggest possible implications of such animal studies for human infant research, especially with regard to recent advances in human evoked potential recording and analysis.

Animal Neurophysiological Studies

An evoked potential (EP) represents the synchronous electrical activity of many neurons in response to an intended or known input; in the following studies, this consists of an electrocortical potential to a brief focused light flash.

Figure 5.1 illustrates the developmental sequence of visually evoked potentials recorded with implanted electrodes from the striate cortex of unanesthetized, awake kittens. The earliest response, obtained at approximately 4 days of age, consists of a long latency negative wave (N_2) recorded over a wide cortical region, as well as from the primary visual cortex. By age 5 days, a shorter latency negative wave (N_1) appears resulting in a N_1N_2 configuration (not shown in Figure 5.1). Subsequently, a yet shorter latency positive component (P_1) emerges. Both latter components (N_1P_1) are obtained only from the primary visual cortex. By 2 weeks, an obvious $P_1N_1N_2$ pattern is evident. Subsequently, whereas in anesthetized kittens the N_2 component disappears resulting in a simple adultlike P_1N_1 waveform at 4 weeks, the progressive sequence in the unanesthetized kitten cumulates in a complex w-shaped adultlike wave in the same time period (weeks 2-4). In addition to the more

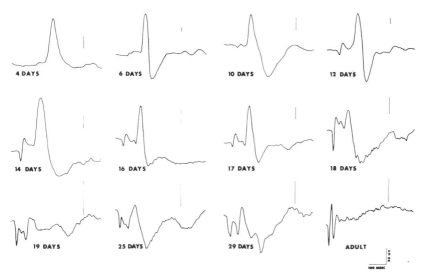

FIGURE 5.1. *Computer-summated evoked potentials from contralateral visual cortex of unanesthetized kittens at age 4-29 days and of one adult. Focused monocular stimulation occurred at onset of trace. Monopolar recordings; neck reference. Traces are summations of 25 responses. (From Rose, Gruenau, & Spencer, 1972.)*

complex waveform changes, a transitory wave (*NA*) of unknown origin appears at approximately 2 weeks, to disappear by 4 weeks.

Outside of the primary visual cortex, the long latency negative wave (N_2) gradually takes on the characteristics (longer latency, longer duration) of visual association responses (Rose, Gruenau, & Spencer, 1972), as also suggested by Marty (1962). Whether alternatively, they are the precursors of polysensory region responses (Thompson, Johnson, & Hoopes, 1963) is in need of further investigation. For example, Mayers, Robertson, Rubel, and Thompson (1971) recorded visual unit responses in association response area PMSA (posterior middle suprasylvian area) at 8 days (kitten). Thereafter, there was a substantial decrease in the unimodel responses (visual), with a subsequent increase in multimodel responses (visual, auditory, somesthetic) until approximately 3 weeks, followed by a more gradual increase in the latter until 50 days.

The developmental sequence of the kittens' visual evoked potential (VER) has also been obtained in the rat (Rose, 1968) and dog (Fox, 1968), as well as in the premature human infant (Ellingson, 1967; Umezaki & Morrell, 1970; Watanabe, Iwase & Hara, 1973), shown as Figure 5.2. As in all species, the earliest response of premature human infants, obtainable at approximately 25 weeks gestational age, is always a single negative wave, followed by a sequence of waveform changes that eventually achieve adultlike characteristics, usually a w-shaped wave, as seen at 39 days (approximately 1 month in kittens).

The above finding, that the premature human infant's VEP developmental

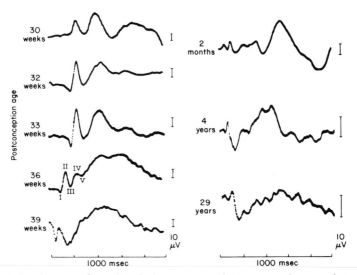

FIGURE 5.2. *Development of visual evoked responses in the premature human infant at various post-conception ages. (From Umezaki & Morrell, 1970.)*

sequence is very similar to that of other species, especially the kitten, has important implications. Most human infant evoked potential studies to date concentrate on latency, and to a lesser degree amplitude, especially as related to behavioral variables, while merely mentioning waveform alterations. This is because (*a*) the waveform may be quite variable due to various factors (behavioral state, light intensity, etc.), which adds to problems of interpretation; (*b*) until recently the types of analyses to separate out these factors have not been available (this will be discussed in the section on human neurophysiological studies later in this chapter); and (*c*) we are only beginning to obtain the necessary information from animal research (especially on kittens) as to what the various components recorded from the premature as well as the normal postnatal infant signify.

Upon obtaining the normative kitten EP data, the assumption was made that the various components that emerged probably reflect the corresponding development of increasingly complex underlying neural mechanisms. Indeed, further VEP differentiation on the basis of recording topography, manipulation of stimulus parameters, subcortical lesions, and responsiveness to anesthetics and biochemical agents (Anohkin, 1964; Rose, 1971) suggests the contribution of several neural mechanisms and/or regions in the development of visual processes.

First, as previously mentioned, the early-appearing long latency negative wave is recordable over a wide cortical area including the occipital region in kittens as well as human infants. Second, in kittens this component is selectively affected by manipulations such as light adaptation, as well as by subcortical lesions, all suggesting involvement of indirect and/or nonspecific pathways (Rose *et al.,* 1972). Third, early unilateral pretectal collicular lesions in kittens result in permanent visual field defects (Atwell & Lindsley, 1975).

In contrast, the later-appearing shorter latency complex, which is limited to the striate visual cortex, is relatively unaffected by dark adaptation but is reduced by lesions of the lateral geniculate, suggesting the involvement of the direct geniculostriate system. Visual field defects seen in kittens as a result of early unilateral lateral geniculate lesions recovered by 3 months of age. Atwell and Lindsley (1975) suggest that the behavioral recovery differences seen after the two types of lesions reflects the earlier functional status or more fixed "degree of commitment" of the superior colliculus at the ablation age.

A differential pathway system is also supported by comparing evoked potential development in unanesthetized versus anesthetized kittens (Rose *et al.,* 1972). Barbituate anesthesia selectively eliminates those later components in the primary visual cortex felt to be mediated or influenced by the nonspecific system.

At this writing, the exact genesis of the N_2 wave is still uncertain. Suggestions include activity (*a*) in an extraprimary pathway involving reticular formation and/or nonspecific thalamus (Anokhin, 1964: Rose & Lindsley, 1965, 1968); (*b*) via a more direct route, involving the pretectum, the posterolateral nucleus, and possibly also the superior colliculus (Rose, 1971; Rose *et al.*, 1972); or (*c*) involving only the lateral geniculate and optic radiations (Myslivecek, 1970). The fact that barbituate anesthesia does not alter EP waveform in the first 2 weeks and such subsequent alterations first occur at the time of initial EEG arousal to light (Marley & Key, 1963; Rose *et al.*, 1972) poses a problem for the first suggestion unless one assumes that barbituate anesthesia has an age-unique effect on other regions in early maturation.

If we consider only the cerebral cortical response to light in the adult animal, we can cite evidence of the involvement of the specific geniculostriate system, the nonspecific reticular mechanisms, the lateroposteriorpulvinar complex, the association cortex, the polysensory regions, the inferotemporal cortex, and the motor cortex, as well as other regions to a lesser degree (see Figure 5.3 and reviews by Graybiel, 1974, and Jones, 1974). Perhaps, as Jones (1974) suggests, the various areas are so intimately connected that it is difficult to conceive of separate alternate pathways that do not involve some degree of interaction. Furthermore, the degree and complexity of the interaction is probably unique at various stages of development, initially constantly changing.

Thus, the original flash evoked potential studies, as well as more recent investigations utilizing a variety of complex stimuli, with the addition of intra- and extracellular recordings, have all supported the viewpoint that the visual system, and its behavioral manifestations, is a complex interaction of many neural regions. Yet, there is a tremendous paucity of normative–baseline developmental information regarding these cortical systems, other than the striate cortex, with far less known of subcortical mechanisms, in spite of am-

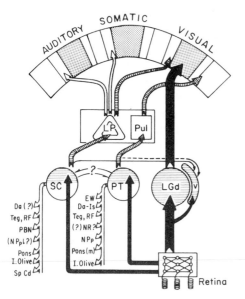

FIGURE 5.3. *Highly schematic diagram summarizing vision-related pathways discussed in the text.* Right: *classic retinogeniculostriate pathway.* Left: *tectal and pretectal channels. SC = superior colliculus; PT = pretectal region; LGd, v = dorsal and ventral nuclei of lateral geniculate body; LP = nucleus lateralis posterior; Pul = pulvinar; EW = nucleus of Edinger-Westphal; Da = nucleus of Darkschewitsch; Is = nucleus interstitialis of Cajal; Teg, RF = tegmentum, reticular formation, NR = nucleus ruber, perirubral fields; NP_p = nucleus papilioformis; Sp Cd = spinal cord; I. Olive = inferior olive. (From Graybiel, 1974.)*

ple evidence of their involvement in adult visual functions and their use in models of human infant perception (as seen in Figure 5.4 from Bronson, 1974).

However, as previously mentioned, we cannot assume that this kind of model, excellent but derived primarily from adult animal studies, can be easily applied to developing behaviors. To cite one reason, the various implicated subcortical structures in kittens develop at different rates, which would suggest differential functional capability of these structures at various ages as well (Rose & Goodfellow, 1973).

Thus, there is an obvious need for a more complete analysis of the physiological and biochemical basis of visual activity in developing cortical and subcortical regions other than the primary sensory regions studied to date as well as for a more complete analysis of the immature cortical evoked potential per se. Again, in both cases, the kitten is especially useful because of its availability and possible relevance to the human premature infant. However,

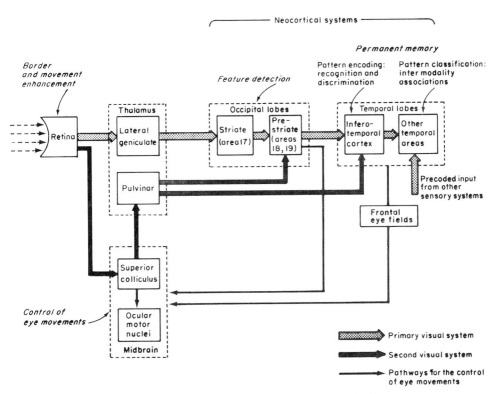

FIGURE 5.4. *A simplified representation of information processing in the human visual system. (From G. W. Bronson, The postnatal growth of visual capacity,* Child Development, *1974, 45, 873-890.)*

analysis of other species, such as ferrets who are born in yet a more immature state, may prove to be useful (Rose, in press).

The first suggestion with regard to subcortical mechanisms should be obvious. The usefulness of further analysis of visual responses in various cortical regions is illustrated by Glass's study (1973) in which he attempted to resolve some of the discrepancy between behavioral recovery to monocular deprivation, on the one hand, and the lack thereof in striate neurons, on the other, by looking outside of the primary visual cortex. He found that although VEPs recorded from the primary visual, association, and motor regions of the cortex were all initially affected by the deprivation, deficits persisted after behavioral recovery only in the marginal gyrus, suggesting involvement of the other regions in the recovery process.

Why, however, do I suggest additional evoked potential analysis instead of an increased concentration on unit studies as the current zeitgeist, as well as problems in the interpretation of the evoked potential (Schlag, 1973), suggests? The reason is primarily that a growing amount of increasingly sophisticated human evoked potential analyses are beginning to be applied to infants, and single-unit recording is obviously impossible in the average human infant at this time.

Later in this chapter, I will provide some illustrations of current human evoked potential data for which the kinds of animal studies described above may provide information regarding underlying neural mechanisms. First, however, I wish to give examples of infant animal studies regarding neurobehavioral analysis that also provide animal models of human infant phenomena.

Animal Neurobehavioral Studies

Recently, we initiated a program to obtain behavioral data on early neonatal kittens, both to correlate with neurophysiological maturation and to provide baseline data necessary for adequate evaluation of early experience effects on these physiological and behavioral processes during maturation.

Figure 5.5 illustrates the kind of visual behavioral information available for the kitten. The VEP data shown in the top portion of the figure is used only as a developmental index, with no assumption of cortical involvement in the functions below, many of which are probably mediated by subcortical structures. These studies suggest that in the very young kitten, with cloudy ocular media and an immature visual system, visual input serves to arouse and alert the kitten rather than convey specific visual information. Later when the media clears and the system matures, the animal is better able to respond to specific features of the visual environment. This conclusion is supported by VEP, single-unit, and lesion studies.

Although we are aware of the difficult and unique conceptual and methodological problem in assessing behaviors in immature animals, as

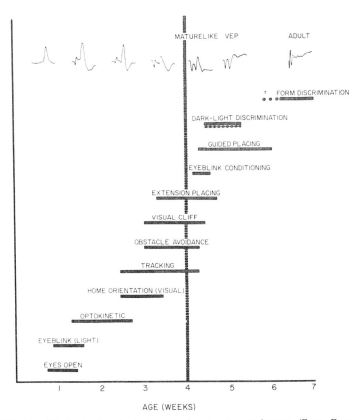

FIGURE 5.5. *Visual behavioral and electrocortical maturation in kittens. (From Rose & Collins, 1975a.)*

discussed elsewhere (Rose, 1975), we chose the overall experimental paradigm shown in Figure 5.6. This consists of a 2 × 2 factorial design, with two levels, each representing a principal area of concern: (*a*) the degree to which initial visual–perceptual abilities do or do not involve early learning proficiencies;

	Nonlearning	Learning
Response independent	Stimulus orientation studies Test: S—ORIENT	Classical conditioning Test: S—CR
Response dependent	Response adjustment procedures (RAP) Test: S_1—R—S	Operant conditioning Test: S—R—S^R

FIGURE 5.6. *Developmental research paradigm.*

and (*b*) the degree to which the immature animal's responses are determinative regarding stimulus change.

That is, we were concerned first of all with separating out those assessment procedures that necessitated a *learning* paradigm, or were actually concerned with learning ability per se, from those in which learning played little or no part in the assessment *(nonlearning)*. We assumed that most (but not all) learning would occur at later ages, in contrast to reflexive-type behavior evident at earlier ages. The nonlearning label does not imply that learning could not be a factor, only that it was not the primary focus. Second, and based primarily on the difference between the classical and operant conditioning paradigms, we made a distinction between *response-independent* (elicited) behaviors, as in classical conditioning, or orientation (orienting responses, reflexive blinking, etc.) in the nonlearning studies in which a reflexive response to a stimulus is part of the procedure, and *response-dependent* (emitted) behaviors, as in operant conditioning, or nonlearning situations in which simple responses to stimuli (reacting to bright light) altered the environmental situation (brightness to darkness). In the latter case, although learning could be a factor, we attempted to concentrate on species-typical behaviors (e.g., bright light avoidance).

Stated otherwise, the difference between the response categories is the degree to which a response is simply elicited (response independent) having no effect on subsequent events and those situations where indeed what occurs depends upon the responses (response dependent). During the presentation of representative studies in each category, the potential relevance to similar research involving the human infant will be briefly noted. As mentioned earlier, a more extensive comment on the relevance of animal as well as human neurophysiological studies will be found in later sections.

Response-Independent Learning

An example of a response-independent learning paradigm is classical eyeblink conditioning. Norman, Collins, and I (Rose, 1975) determined that the onset of stable eyeblink conditioning in kittens, with a shock unconditioned stimulus (UCS), first occurred at a mean age of 29, 31, and 34 days in response to somatic, auditory, and visual conditional stimuli (CS), respectively. That is, independent of when training was initiated, and independent of the number of training trials, conditioned responses to an auditory CS, for example, could not be established until approximately 1 month of age.

However, it was noticed that often when conditioning did appear, responses were seen on the first trials of a session, implying that acquisition had begun initially in earlier sessions, but with an absence of motor expression. This ideas was tested in a subsequent study by training experimental kittens for 7 days beginning at age 21 days, while control littermates received randon presentations of both CS and UCS (see Figure 5.7). After 2 days' rest, both groups

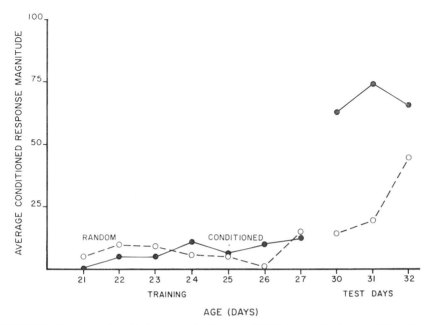

FIGURE 5.7. Conditioned eyeblink magnitude (integrated EMG from orbicularis oculi) in arbitrary units averaged over 100 trials per daily session. Conditioned group received conditioning trials on all days, while the random group received random presentation of CS and US during days 21-27 and were switched to paired presentation on days 30-32. The immediate acquisition of the conditioned group on test days indicates that the response was "learned" during initial training in the absence of motor expression. Solid line shows conditioned group; broken line shows random group. (From Rose, 1975.)

received conditioning trials. The animals that had previous pairings showed immediate conditioning, often on the first trials, while the control animal took 200–300 trials to condition. We tentatively concluded that the prior experience of paired presentation of the CS and UCS was facilitated at some earlier age (21–27 days) but could not be expressed because of some maturational block beyond the associative state in neural processing, principally in effecting a motor response.

In another classical conditioning study with light as the CS, shock as the UCS, and leg flexion as the conditioned response, Dalhouse and I (Rose & Dalhouse, 1974) found that although stable behavioral conditioning was not evident until age 6 weeks, a difference between control and experimental animals with regard to physiological measures (EP and galvanic skin response [GSR]) was seen as early as 2 weeks. The increase and subsequent diminution of autonomic responses prior to somatic expression of conditioning has also been noted by Volokov (1970).

Since the newborn infant is also limited in terms of motor expression, these animal studies suggest that, along with the substitution of nonmotor physiological (e.g., heart rate, GSR, etc.) for overt behavioral responses, a latent learning paradigm with tasks appropriate for the human infant may be very useful.

These studies motivated us to begin a further search for unique ways of establishing the onset of learning abilities that take into account the immaturity of motor expression especially at the younger ages. This is further illustrated in the next two examples of response-dependent learning paradigms.

Response-Dependent Learning

In the first study of operant conditioning (Rose & Collins, 1975a), we devised a system of training young kittens in light–dark discrimination by utilizing a Y water maze, since we discovered that the kittens are capable of swimming by 1 week of age, detest the water, and hence are motivated to escape. Two age groups were studied: one beginning at 35 days, when visual cortical evoked potentials are maturelike; the second beginning at about 3 weeks, when the evoked potentials are still immature. All animals were given 6 daily trials, until a criterion of 12 consecutive correct choices was reached.

The results shown in Figure 5.8 indicate that, whereas the more immature group, A, needed 90 trials (15 days) to reach criterion at 48 days of age, Group B, although begun in training 2 weeks later, reached criterion at 46 days in only 60 trials (10 days). Since both groups were equally adept at swim-

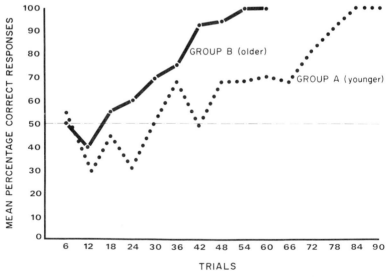

FIGURE 5.8. *Acquisition of light-dark discrimination. Mean percentage correct responses in younger (Group A) versus older (Group B) kittens as a function of training sessions (6 trials/day). Training was initiated at 21-23 days of age for Group A and 35-37 days of age for Group B. Dotted line shows Group A (younger); solid line shows Group B (older). (From Rose & Collins, 1975a.)*

ming, we concluded that a particular level of neural organization, beginning in the fifth postnatal week, was necessary for the acquisition of this particular task.

I would, however, in the light of previous comments, emphasize "this particular task." Although it presents a unique method of early assessment, it is highly artificial, which in itself may produce emotional states in the younger kittens that could interact with early learning potentials or reflect learning abilities under difficult species-atypical circumstances. The same argument might be applied to the classical conditioning studies. Therefore, we emphasize that these kinds of studies, while valid as an initial step in the assessment of learning potential, need additional confirmation, that is, studies sensitive to the issue regarding species-relevant tasks and environments. For example, at what age would kittens in a more natural setting, have chosen the correct arm, not as a function of the presence or absence of light, but rather as a function of the presence or absence of the sight or call of the mother cat? Stated otherwise, at some point the relationship between baseline and normative data needs to be assessed. These concerns become even more important when one attempts to establish neural correlates of early learning, whether in infant animals or humans.

By now convinced that some assessment procedures of early perceptual–learning abilities were hindered primarily by the immaturity of motor response systems, we devised an unorthodox feedback operant technique, in which specified reinforced amplitude changes of a particular component (N_2 wave) of the immature visually evoked potential substituted for a motor operant response (Rose, Norman, Naifeh, & Collins, 1975). That is, kittens as young as 2 weeks were trained to increase or decrease the N_2 component recorded from the visual cortex, using tone as a discriminative stimulus (SD), light flash as the CS, and mild electrical shock as a negative reinforcer in a shock-avoidance paradigm. Specific criterion changes within a specified time-amplitude window were analyzed by an on-line computer, which determined whether to withhold or deliver reinforcement. The animal could use any strategy (e.g., head orientation, pupillary changes) to produce the desired result, since we were interested in learning not in the feedback technique per se.

The results demonstrated that kittens can be trained to both increase (see Figure 5.9) and decrease that amplitude of the N_2 wave as early as 2 weeks of age. Conditioned amplitude shifts in the N_2 wave of 100% to cover 500% were obtained. Yoked controls (e.g., light flash only; noncontingent shock) showed a maximum amplitude increase or decrease of 35% from baseline, depending on age.

These results represent some of the earliest ages at which operant conditioning, utilizing the visual modality, has been demonstrated. What is puzzling is that controls indicate that the results are not due to such trivial factors as eye movement and pupillary changes. We can speculate that the evoked potential

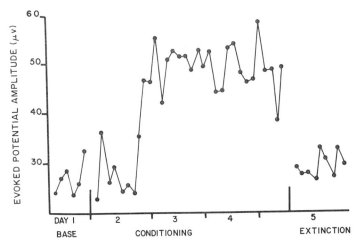

FIGURE 5.9. *The peak amplitude of the N_2 wave is shown for successive blocks of 50 trials during conditioned increases in the flash-evoked potential recorded from the visual cortex in a 20-day-old kitten. The evoked potential remains relatively stable both during initial baseline sessions and following the introduction of shock on early acquisition trials. As the animal learned to increase the prespecified portion of the potential, the criterion level was adjusted upward until maximum performance was reached. (From Rose, Norman, Naifeh, & Collins, 1975.)*

increases or decreases may reflect tonic conditioned behavioral state alterations. That is, a further EEG-behavioral analysis might detect whether in fact general state alterations, as opposed to discrete neural events, have been conditioned.

Various feedback techniques, while extensively investigated in adult humans and applied clinically for epileptic seizures, for example (see review by Schwartz & Beatty, 1977), have yet to be attempted in human infants. Antecdodatal evidence, however, suggests that EEG feedback training (alpha) is much easier for young children than for adults. Although perhaps of limited value with infants near term, such specialized techniques may be indicated when one is faced with unique assessment problems or to establish the age at which an infant is capable of regulating his or her state for positive rewards (milk, attention, etc.) In kittens, this occurs at a surprisingly early age compared to other learning measures.

Response-Dependent Nonlearning

The final two examples of early infant animal assessment procedures attempt to avoid or minimize the use of learning procedures (i.e., *nonlearning* procedures). In the *response-dependent* situation, we devised a method dubbed *response-adjusting procedures* (RAP) to study the infant animal's control over sitmulus preferences. Briefly, instead of measuring a predetermined response to specified stimuli of interest, as in most orientation studies,

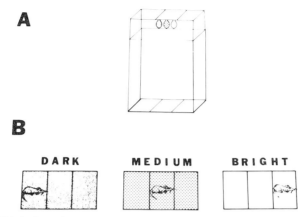

FIGURE 5.10. *(A)* *Light preference test apparatus. (B)* *Animal's position determines light in entire box.*

the animal's developmentally appropriate response or responses (e.g., crawling) are utilized to select preferred stimulation from an array varying in one or more dimensions (e.g., light of different intensities).

In one such study, using infant rats, the animal's position in a box determined lighting conditions in the entire box, as illustrated in Figure 5.10. Infant rats showed a highly reliable preference for dark over dim or bright light (controls for positions, activity, etc.) by 10 days of age, as seen in Figure 5.11.

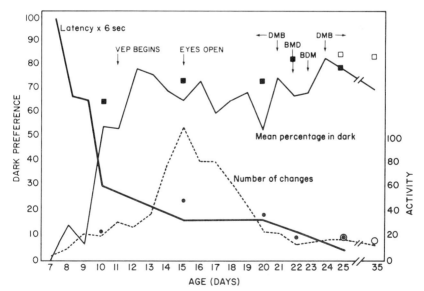

FIGURE 5.11. *Mean percentage time in darkness and activity levels in rats as a function of age. Solid line shows time in darkness; dotted line shows activity levels.*

This is 5–6 days prior to eye opening but coincident with the initial onset of visual evoked potentials in rats at 10 days of age. Furthermore, it is independent of dramatic changes in activity levels (number of lines crossed) shown by the dotted line.

Preliminary data also suggest that prior experience between age 5–7 days, consisting of either handling (H) or handling plus alternating light exposure (HL), produces, in varying degrees, a yet earlier preference for darkness when compared with nonhandled groups (NH), as shown in Figure 5.12.

It needs to be determined, of course, whether the prior experience caused a general increase in the maturational process or whether the effects were more modality specific. Furthermore, as Shapiro's (1971) studies emphasize, early stimulation with resultant early induction of behavioral and/or physiological activities may cause an overload on the age-appropriate systems resulting in deficiencies later in development. The point may be relevant to early stimulation in very young human prematures, particularly while in intensive care.

By utilizing a yet simpler procedure involving activity transducers, the infant rats showed a clear movement reaction to light as early as 5 days of age. This has also been confirmed recently by Routtenberg, Strop, and Jerdan (1978) and shown to involve the superior colliculus.

The activity at 5 days coincides with the earliest onset of significant measurable rhodopsin but precedes by 6–7 days significant synaptic formation, especially in the inner plexiform layer, that is, between bipolar and ganglion cells of the retina (Weidman & Kuwabara, 1968).

We believe that these data make a very significant point for developmental psychobiology. Here is an example in which evidence regarding the behavioral onset of function precedes what is known to date regarding the histology and physiology of this system, necessitating a reevaluation of the latter.

The uniqueness of these results justifies in part early behavioral onset studies, since it forces a more careful analysis of the anatomical–physiological data with regard to the retina or suggests alternative structures meditating

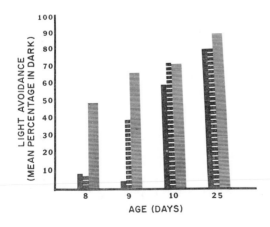

FIGURE 5.12. Mean percentage time in darkness at ages indicated as a function of prior experience Fine stripes = HL, thick stripes = H, and solid line = NH.

early reactions to light, for example, the pineal gland, as suggested by Zweig, Snyder, & Axelrod, (1966), or direct stimulation of the ganglion cells.

As stated earlier, it is also important to repeat these baseline studies utilizing wild strains of rats under field conditions to obtain normative data and determine the generality of these findings. What is the function of light avoidance at 10 days of age? Does it occur as a natural protective device against leaving the dark nest and falling into the mouths of predators? And what are the biological mechanisms that must be available to avoid this disaster? However, we need not lose sight of the fact that it was the artificial situation that provided the behavioral evidence to suggest a reevaluation of the biological data. The kinds of baseline data obtained depend upon the questions of interest; whether or not the data are normative in a species-appropriate ecological sense is an important but separate issue to be faced at some level if the animal data are to have some relevance for the human infant.

There is, however, another point I wish to make about this study. The activity measure (number of lines crossed), although independent of darkness preference, does confirm a trend often reported by Campbell and his associates (Campbell, Lytle, & Fibiger, 1969; Campbell & Mabry, 1972), namely, inhibition of activity in novel environments beginning at approximately 16 days of age. These studies also sought neurochemical correlates of this inhibition.

We have seen clear evidence of earlier behavioral inhibition of a different sort. As early as 9 days, obvious inhibition of forward movement by light onset was clearly evident, as shown in Figure 5.13, which is a RAP sequence taken from a videotape.

The point is, of course, that the concept of behavioral inhibition, and subsequent search for the relevant brain mechanisms, must be related to specific kinds of inhibition that may vary with age and task. This underscores again the need for obtaining the necessary baseline behavioral data. It is most probable that different- or similar-appearing behavioral inhibition is mediated by various neurochemical mechanisms at different stages of development, in different species, under different early experience and testing conditions, etc.

These kinds of studies relate to similar procedures used with human infants in which a change in stimulus conditions (causing an overhead mobile to turn) is brought about by motor activity, such as sucking. The animal studies further seek to establish the developmental sequence of neural mechanisms necessary to begin to initiate responses and to detect changes in stimulus parameters in early infancy.

Response-Independent Nonlearning

Finally, as an example of a response-independent assessment technique, one with obvious human clinical potential, Collins and I (Collins & Rose, 1975) studied the early responsiveness of newborn kittens to light as measured by

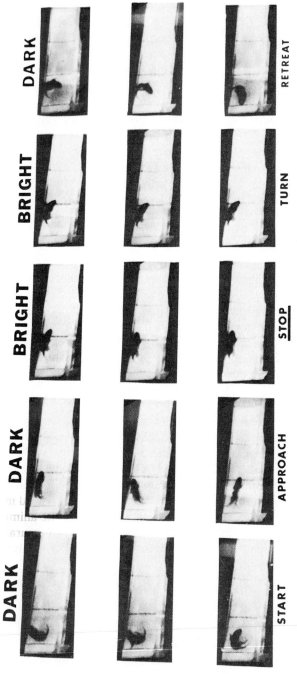

FIGURE 5.13. *Videotaped sequence of movement inhibition in response to light onset (light avoidance) in 10-day-old rat.*

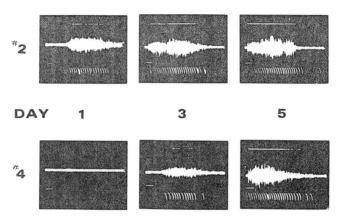

FIGURE 5.14. *EMG responses to light flash at indicated ages; # 2 is a normal kitten; # 4 is runt of the litter.*

behavioral (blink and squint) and electromyographic (EMG) activity (see Figure 5.14) from the eyelid muscles (orbicularis oculi).

At birth, a threshold flash duration of 500 msec evoked a 1200–1500 msec EMG and behavioral responses. A dramatic change in light duration threshold and consequent EMG latency is seen over the next several days, resulting in a 125–150 msec EMG to a single light flash (15 usec) at 6 days of age in normal kittens. The occasional kitten that did not show this pattern usually was the runt of the litter and had later difficulties generally resulting in death.

Furthermore, by determining threshold responses to varying wavelengths of light in the dark-adapted kitten, we have been able to obtain scotopic spectral sensitivity curves using only the EMG as the response measure, as shown in Figure 5.15. The data reflect sensitivity relative to that at 500 nm. Even on the first day of life, there appears a tendency for the curves to peak at 500 nm; this is quite evident by day 2, and by day 4, the curves appear stable. The form of the curves on day 6 describe a very close approximation of the rhodopsin absorbance curves (Wald, 1945) and to the spectral sensitivity curves for the adult cat (Dodt & Walther, 1958). The primary deviation is a tendency for the curves to fall off more sharply at 450 nm than would be predicted based on rhodopsin absorbance. This is possible because the lens and pupil are covered with a vascular tunica during this period (Thorn, Gollender, & Erickson, 1976). The hemoglobin absorption of this network, and that of the closed eyelid itself, would be expected to produce this sharpening effect because of the strong absorbance bands of hemoproteins found between 400 and 450 nm (Crawford & Marc, 1976).

The potential application of the kitten visual blink-response technique in human infant assessment is suggested for the following reasons:

1. This reflex is currently part of the Brazelton newborn infant neurobehavioral examination (Brazelton, 1973). Our method provides for the quantification of both the stimulus and response aspects.

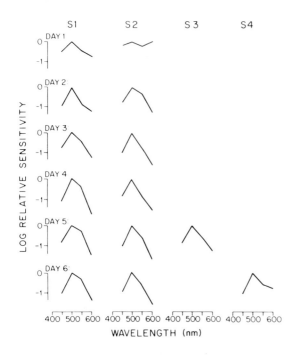

FIGURE 5.15. *Log sensitivity relative to 500 nm standard at different wavelengths during dark adaptation (scotopic curves) in kittens (S_1, S_4) at ages indicated.*

2. Adult animal evidence (Tokunaga, Oka, Muras, Yokoi, Okumura, Hirata, Miyashita, & Yoshitatsu, 1958) indicates that the resultant EMG activity involves two types of reflexive responses; a short latency monosynaptic reflex mediated by the sensory nucleus of the fifth nerve and a longer latency polysynaptic reflex involving thalamic nuclei and possibly the reticular formation. These responses have been differential in the adult animal by lesions and anesthetics, which once again suggests a developmental differentiation in kittens and possibly human infants as well.

3. Finally, the procedure may present a method for obtaining photopic and scotopic spectral sensitivity curves very early in human development.

In summarizing the results to date using the 2 × 2 research strategy outlined in Figure 5.6, several general statements can be made. First, in most of the studies involving immature systems, total reliance on overt responses confounds associative abilities with maturation of motor systems. Substitution of various physiological responses, including evoked potentials for overt responses, while holding constant other variables in a learning paradigm, can result in earlier learning onset age correlations. These, however, may reflect different learning phenomena or strategies. Second, the latent learning paradigm used in conjunction with motor responses may profitably be explored further in animal and human infant studies as an alternative method of establishing associations prior to expressive abilities. Third, there is a need to utilize and quantify early behaviors or physiological responses that avoid or minimize learning in addition to typical reflex measures. These behaviors in animals may, as shown, establish very early abilities for which current biological correlations are found to be inadequate, necessitating a reexamining of the latter as in the RAP studies. Likewise, as illustrated by the EMG studies, simple physiological responses first studied in animals when subsequently quantified in humans may (*a*) reflect activity in different central nervous system (CNS) regions (see also discussion of far-field potentials in the next section); and (*b*) be utilized to assess behavioral (perceptual) capabilities in immature and term human infants. The latter study also illustrates the fact that some physiological responses to light (EMG-squint) precede developmentally the cortical VEP, thus demonstrating the obvious contributions of subcortical processes, so difficult to assess in humans.

The data in the earlier section on animal neurophysiological studies relate to those in the section on animal neurobehavioral studies with regard to the following dimensions:

1. One can establish correlations between developing neurophysiological parameters (latency, amplitude, and waveform) and evolving behaviors.

2. Various manipulations (light intensity, lesions, etc.) may influence both evoked potential characteristics as well as emerging behaviors (e.g. Atwell & Lindsley, 1974), which strengthens biobehavioral correlations and provides evidence of causative neural factors, be they primarily cortical, subcortical, or peripheral.

3. As previously mentioned, such physiological measures as evoked potentials, EMG, and GSR may be profitably substituted for behavioral responses when assessing immature subjects with poor motor control.

4. Specific alterations in physiological responses, such as selective changes in evoked potential components, may correlate with or reflect behavioral processes. For example, an alteration in one component may relate to attentional variables and another to informational properties, within an age-specific (e.g., first postnatal week) research paradigm.

The appropriate analysis of waveform changes (in contrast to latency) in premature infants, as well as postterm infants may undergo some revision based on newer techniques, as discussed in the next section.

Human Neurophysiological Studies

The previous section emphasized the potential relationship between animal neurobehavioral studies and human infant studies. In this section, I wish to briefly provide a sample of current studies of the human evoked potential, or event-related potential (ERP) as it is now called, so that the reader may (*a*) become familiar with the kinds of recent advances made in the recording, analysis, and application of ERPs, especially those involving human infants;

and (b) appreciate the importance and usefulness of further analysis of the various CNS regions and mechanizing involved in EP developmental changes by the use of animal models.

Until fairly recently, most human evoked potential studies, especially those with infants, used simple stimuli, such as a stroboscopic flash, and concentrated on general independent variables, such as attention, treating the whole evoked potential as a global representation of cortical activity. The latency and amplitude of the EP was the dependent variable of interest, with less concern about the often variable individual components.

A careful reexamination of the adult human EP recorded with different time bases and averaging techniques reveal a far more complex situation, as shown in Figure 5.16 (Donchin, 1979). Instead of the previous time base of 500 msec, many new so-called far-field studies analyze the wavelets seen in the first 10 msec following stimulus presentation. The subcortical contributions of these components have been established in animal studies, especially in the auditory system (Buchwald & Huang, 1975). This, of course, has potential application in clinical neurology. The origin of components within the first 50 sec, also shown in Figure 5.16, is far less certain. Alterations seen, however, have found use in human audiometry (Davis, 1976).

It has been suggested by several authors (see Donchin, 1979) that the shorter latency components are *obligatory* or *exogenous* responses, since they are always present under varying conditions and appear to be responsive to exter-

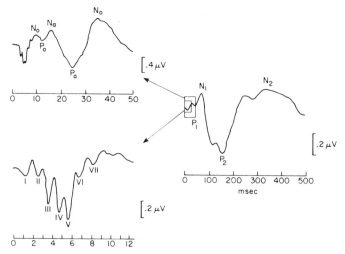

FIGURE 5.16. *A schematic presentation of the configuration of the event-related potential elicited by a click of moderate intensity. Note the different time bases and different callibration signal in each of the three insets. Note also that different peak nomenclatures are used in the three cases and that component labelings for the data shown for the last 500 msec are different from those used in the rest of this chapter. (After Picton, Hillyard, Krausz, & Galambos, 1974.)*

nal stimuli. The longer latency waves, especially beyond 200 msec, appear to be in response to psychological variables. Thus "these *endogenous* components [which are of variable amplitude and not obligatory] appear to represent activities invoked by the system rather than evoked by the stimuli [Donchin, 1979 p. 26]."

The current human evoked potential differentiation is aided in part by more sophistication in measurement of the components as well as in experimental design. Figure 5.17 illustrates a principal-component analysis (PCA) method suggested by Donchin (1966, 1969) by which a grand mean waveform (middle graph) computed from the raw average obtained under varying conditions (bottom graph) can be further partitioned into components, as in the top graph, by the PCA technique. This helps to identify how much of the variance between waveforms is related to different experimental variables, that is, to subject variables, to electrodes, or to random uncontrollable variation. To

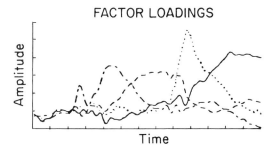

FACTOR LOADINGS

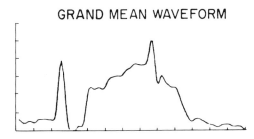

GRAND MEAN WAVEFORM

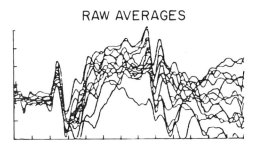

RAW AVERAGES

FIGURE 5.17. *The center graph shows the grand average ERP computed on the basis of the data obtained from all subjects in all experimental conditons from all electrodes in an experiment (McCarthy & Donchin, in press). The bottom panel shows some of the superimposed ERPs obtained for a specific experimental condition in this same experiment. Clearly, most of the ERPs deviate from the grand mean waveform. There are different degrees of variance at different segments of the epoch. The PCA is a technique for determining the extent to which the grand mean can be partitioned into components. As the top panel shows, PCA of these data identified five components. The segment of the epoch over which each component is active is indicated by the magnitude of the factor loading. (From McCarthy & Donchin, in press.)*

quote Donchin (1979): "It has proven, however, far more fruitful to consider the ERP as a sequence of overlapping components, each possibly representing activity of different populations of nerve cells and each standing in a different, often orthogonal, relation to experimental variables [p. 24]."

Such an analysis, which has yet to be used in developmental studies, may, for example, further elucidate the similarities and differences between the human premature infant's cortical components and those obtained at later ages or in animal models (e.g., kittens).

The following is a human adult study, which illustrates the use of the ERP measure in complex adult situations. This will be followed by examples of infant studies that focus on the three different time bases shown in Figure 5.16.

An example (Sutton, Tueting, Zuben, & John, 1967) in which the cortical waveform elicited by identical physical stimuli can be shown to vary as a function of psychological factors is illustrated in Figure 5.18. Event-related potentials were elicited by either single or paired tones that were either loud or soft. That is, in the experimental situation, the subjects were to respond either to the intensity or the frequency dimensions, but never to both. A positive deflection at 300 msec (the P300) was the component of interest. When subjects were told to categorize tones by their intensity, then only one P300 component was recorded to either one or two tones (solid line). In this case, a second of two tones carried redundant information. If, however, the subject was to determine if one or two stimuli (either loud or soft) were presented on a given trial, two large P300 components appeared regardless of whether one or two tones were actively presented. Sutton *et al.* (1967) cite this as evidence of an endogenous event elicited in the absence of (yet expectation of) a physical stimulus.

These kinds of studies and their accompanying analyses have only recently been studied from a developmental perspective in human infants. With respect to far-field potentials, Hecox and Galambos (1974) and Salamy, McKean, and Buda (1975) published the initial cross-sectional age comparisons between infants and adults (see Figure 5.19). Subsequently, Starr, Amlie, Martin, and Sanders (1977) studied the newborn infant in detail. These reports indicate that although far-field auditory evoked potentials are seen in the youngest prematures, the stimuli (clicks) must be of high intensity, above 75 dB, resulting in a long latency potential with components missing or weak until 3–10 months of age, when the adult configuration becomes established.

We now have information, based on adult and infant animal models (Buchwald & Huang, 1975; Shipley, Buchwald, Norman, & Guthrie, 1980), on the possible genesis of the various components of this response. The studies suggest that wave I represents activity in peripheral (eighth nerve) structures, whereas waves II–VII are due to activity in auditory pathway structures, primarily in the brain stem. Furthermore, the evidence indicates a differential development of peripheral and central neural processes that is of

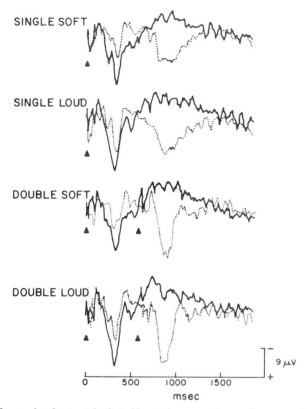

FIGURE 5.18. *Event-related potentials elicited by single or paired tones that were either loud or soft. When a subject is categorizing tones by their intensity, only the first stimulus of a pair elicits a P300 component. When the subject has to determine if one or two stimuli were presented on a given trial, both the presence of a second tone in the pair and the absence of a second tone following a single stimulus elicit a large P300. These data provide strong evidence that P300 is an endogenous component that can be elicited in the absence of a physical stimulus. Solid lines show soft-loud criterion, dotted lines show single-double criterion. (From Sutton, Tueting, Zuben, & John, 1967. Copyright 1967 by the American Association for the Advancement of Science.)*

considerable importance in normal or abnormal neurobehavioral assessment.

Human developmental studies involving the longer duration ERPs are becoming more common. Figure 5.20, taken from a study by Hoffman (Karmel & Maisel, 1975), illustrates changes in potentials evoked by differences in contour density in human infants. The data represent composite ERPs of 6- (dotted line) and 10-week-old children (solid line), taking individual variance into account. Briefly, the shorter latency P_2 amplitude, a wave restricted to the occipital region, showed significant sensitivity to contour density differences in the older but not the younger subjects, whereas the longer latency L–N amplitude corresponded to preferences in the younger but

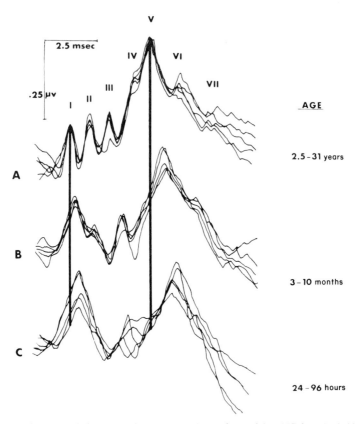

FIGURE 5.19. *Maturational changes in the latency and waveform of the VER from birth (C) to adulthood (A). The vertical lines through waves I and V of the adult record emphasize the age-related shifts (shortening in latency) that occur with increasing age. The multiple tracings superimposed for adults (A), infants (B), and newborns (C) emphasize the consistent changes in VER waveform that take place as a function of age. Each trace represents an average of 1600-2400 responses obtained from a different subject in each age category. The stimulus was presented at a rate of 15 clicks/sec. Positivity at the active (Cz) electrode is indicated by an upward deflection. (From Salamy, McKean, & Buda, 1975.)*

not the older children. This suggests a possible complex maturational interaction of mechanisms mediating contour density preferences and attention, which may relate to Cohen's (1973) distinction between visual attention getting and visual attention holding.

Although in need of considerable further analysis, the kitten studies also suggest a maturational differentiation between mechanisms subserving general attention or arousal initiated by light (early development), those essential for visual feature detection, and those important in complex perception and visual learning (later development).

Finally, a developmental study similar to that of Sutton *et al.'s* original study has been reported (Prichep, Sutton, & Hakerem, 1976). Children (8–11

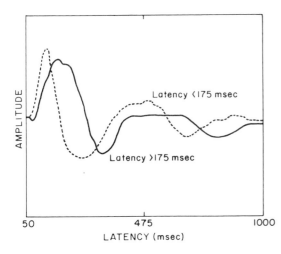

FIGURE 5.20. *Composite event-related potentials across infants and stimuli where infants are grouped on the basis of neurological age based on P₂ latency. Average chronological age was 6 and 10 weeks for the longer and shorter neurological age groups, respectively. Dotted line shows 6-week-old infants, latency <175 msec; solid line shows 10-week-old infants, latency >175 msec. (Adapted from Hoffman, 1973, as shown in Karmel & Maisel, 1975.)*

years old) were either informed in advance (certain condition) or told to guess (uncertain condition) whether single or double clicks would be presented. Under the uncertain condition only, the ERP to the second click of a pair contained larger long latency positive components. Furthermore, the degree of amplitude differentiated these children from a group of hyperactive children. However, the difference in amplitude in the long latency waves as a function of certainty–uncertainty was enhanced—that is, a change in normal direction occurred—by a clinical dose of methylphenidate (Ritaline) in the hyperactive group.

Summary

It would appear then that we are making considerable advances in human ERP studies that may be applicable to assessing possible developmental differences in the human preterm infant, that is the infant with an atypical normative–baseline sequence. These advances also suggest a renewed effort at attempts to elucidate the underlying neural mechanisms and systems of the evoked potentials themselves, by more systematic neurophysiological and anatomical analysis in infant animal models.

To date the premature infant's EP sequence appears to correlate best with the data obtained in species born relatively premature, such as kittens and rats. Such species are appropriate as animal models, not only to analyze neural mechanisms contributing to the evoked potentials, but also to study the influence of unusual environmental events during early development. For example, Rose and Gruenau (1973) demonstrated that kittens reared under constant illumination from birth to 8 months showed a threefold increase in VEP amplitude as well as behavioral defects (diminished reflexes to approaching objects and light). Such stimulation also results in an increase in dendritic spine density in the visual cortex of rats (Parnavelas, Globus, & Kaups, 1973).

Since a premature infant is exposed to an environment that is abnormal in its intensity and complexity, and is also subjected to earlier-than-usual exposure, it would be of interest to analyze the changes in the VEP components in these infants under various experimental conditions.

It is obvious that animal developmental studies of gross electrical phenomena must be accompanied by further electrophysiological, biochemical, and anatomical analysis at the cellular level. My concern is that the former not be abandoned just yet in the current reductionalistic trend, while we are still limited to evoked potential analysis in the preterm human infant. Likewise, continued neurobehavioral studies in animal models are essential for correlation with the physiological activity and to provide useful suggestions for similar human infant research as illustrated by the EMG study cited earlier.

In conclusion, it is via a combined baseline–normative, descriptive–manipulative approach that infant animal psychobiological research may have clinical relevance for the term as well as the preterm human infants. The data furthermore suggest the potential value of a combined animal–human research, as especially illustrated by the far-field studies. Such an approach can provide a foundation for the understanding of aberrant as well as normal systems in various young species, including human infants.

References

Anokhin, P. K. Systemogenesis as a general regulator of brain development. In W. A. Himwich & H. E. Himwich (Eds.), *Progress in brain research*. (Vol. 1). *The developing brain*. Amsterdam: Elsevier, 1964.

Atwell, C. W., & Lindsley, D. B. Development of visually evoked responses and visually guided behavior in kittens: Effects of superior colliculus and lateral geniculate lesions. *Developmental Psychobiology*, 1975, *8*, 465–478.

Brazelton, T. B. *Neonatal behavioral assessment scale*. Philadelphia: Lippincott, 1973.

Bronson, G. W. The postnatal growth of visual capacity. *Child Development*, 1974, *45*, 873–890.

Buchwald, J., & Huang, C. Far field acoustic response: Origins in the cat. *Science*, 1975, *189*, 382–384.

Campbell, B. A., Lytle, L. D., & Fibiger, H. C. Ontogeny of adrenergic arousal and cholinergic inhibitory mechanisms in the rat. *Science*, 1969, *166*, 637–638.

Campbell, B., & Mabry, P. D. Ontogeny of behavioral arousal: A comparative study. *Journal of Comparative Physiological Psychology*, 1972, *81*, 371–379.

Carmichael, L. *Manual of child psychology*. New York: Wiley, 1946.

Coghill, G. E. *Anatomy and the problem of behavior*. Cambridge: University Press, 1929.

Cohen, J. B. A two-process model of infant visual attention. *Merrill-Palmer Quarterly*, 1973, *19*, 157–180.

Collins, J. P., & Rose, G. H. *Behavioral and electromyographic responses to light in newborn kittens*. Paper presented at the meeting of the International Society for Developmental Psychobiology, New York, 1975.

Crawford, M., & Marc, R. Light transmission of cat and monkey eyelids. *Vision Research*, 1976, *16*, 323–324.

Davis, H. Principles of electric response audiometry. *The Annals of Otology, Rhinology, and Laryngology*, 1976, Suppl. 28, *85*, (3, Pt. 3.).

Dodt, E., & Walther, J. Der skotopsiche dominatar der katz im sichbaren und ultravioletten spektralbreich. *J. Pflugers Archi.*, 1958, *266*, 175–186.

Donchin, E. A multivariate approach to the analysis of average evoked potentials. *IEEE Transactions on Bio-Medical Engineering*, 1966, *Bio-Medical Engineering, 13*, 131–139.

Donchin, E. Data analysis techniques in average evoked potential research. In E. Donchin & D. B. Lindsley (Eds.), *Average evoked potentials: Methods, results and evaluations.* (NASA SP-191) Washington, D.C.: U.S. Government Printing Office, 1969.

Donchin, E. Event-related brain potentials: A tool in the study of human information processing. In H. Begleiter (Ed.), *Evoked potentials and behavior.* New York: Plenum, 1979.

Ellingson, R. J. The study of brain electrical activity in infants. In L. P. Lipsitt & C. C. Spiker (Eds.), *Advances in child development and behavior* (Vol. 3). New York: Academic Press, 1967.

Ellis, N. *Aberrant development in infancy: Human and animal studies.* Hillsdale, N.J.: Erlbaum, 1975.

Fox, M. W. Neuronal development and ontogeny of evoked potentials in auditory and visual cortex of the dog. *Electroencephalography and Clinical Neurophysiology*, 1968, *24*, 213–226.

Glass, J. D. Photically evoked potentials from cat neocortex before and after recovery from visual deprivation. *Experimental Neurology, 1973, 39*, 123–139.

Gottlieb, G. *Studies on the development of behavior and the nervous system* (Vol. 1). *Behavioral embryology.* New York: Academic Press, 1973.

Gottlieb, G. *Studies on the development of behavior and the nervous system* (Vol. 2) Aspects of neurogenesis. New York: Academic Press, 1974.

Gottlieb, G. *Studies on the development of behavior and the nervous system* (Vol. 3) *Neural and behavioral specificity.* New York: Academic Press, 1976.

Gottlieb, G. *Studies on the development of behavior and the nervous system* (Vol. 4) *Early influences.* New York: Academic Press, 1978.

Graybiel, A. M. Studies on the anatomical organization of posterior association cortex. In F. O. Schmitt & F. G. Worden (Eds.), *The neurosciences: Third study program.* Cambridge, Mass.: MIT. Press, 1974.

Hebb, D. O. *The organization of behavior.* New York: Wiley, 1949.

Hecox, K., & Galambos, R. Brain stem auditory evoked responses in human infants and adults. *Archives of Otolaryngology*, 1974, *99*, 30–33.

Himwich, W. A. *Developmental neurobiology.* Springfield, Ill.: Thomas, 1970.

Hooker, D. *The prenatal origin of behavior.* Lawrence: Univ. of Kansas Press, 1952.

Humphrey, T. Postnatal repetition of human prenatal activity sequences with some suggestion of the neuroanatomical basis. In R. J. Robinson (Ed.), *The brain and early behavior.* New York: Academic Press, 1969.

Jacobson, M. *Developmental neurobiology* (2nd ed.). New York: Plenum, 1978.

Jones, E. G. The anatomy of extrageniculate visual mechanisms. In F. O. Schmitt & F. G. Worden (Eds.), *The neurosciences: Third study program.* Cambridge, Mass.: MIT. Press, 1974.

Karmel, B. Z., & Maisel, E. B. A neuronal activity model for infant visual attention. In L. B. Cohen & P. Salapatek (Eds.), *Infant perception: From sensation to cognition* (Vol. 1) *Basic visual processes.* New York: Academic Press, 1975.

Marley, E., & Key, B. J. Maturation of the electrocorticogram and behavior in the kitten and guinea pig and the effect of some sympathomimetic amines. *Electroencephalography and Clinical Neurophysiology, 1963, 15*, 620–636.

Marty, R. Développement post-natal des résponses sensorielles du cortex cérébral chez le chat et le lapin. *Arch. Anat. micr. Morph. exp.*, 1962, *51*, 129–264.

Mayers, K. S., Robertson, R. T., Rubel, E. W., & Thompson, R. F. Development of polysensory responses in association cortex of kitten. *Science, 1971, 171*, 1038–1040.

McCleary, R. A. *Genetic and experiential factors in perception.* Glenview, Ill.: Scott, Foresman, 1970.

Myslivecek, J. Electrophysiology of the developing brain—Central and Eastern European contributions. In W. A. Himwich (Ed.), *Developmental neurobiology*. Springfield, Ill.: Thomas, 1970.

Parnavelas, J. P., Globus, A., & Kaups, P. Continuous illumination from birth affects spine density of neurons in the visual cortex of the rat. *Experimental Neurology,* 1973, *40,* 742–747.

Picton, W. W., Hillyard, S. A., Krausz, H. T., & Galambos, R. Human auditory evoked potentials, I: Evaluation of components. *Electroencephalography and Clinical Neurophysiology,* 1974, *36,* 179–190.

Preyer, W. *Die seele des kindes.* Leipzig: Fernau, 1882.

Preyer, W. *Specielle physiologie des embryo untersuchungen über die lebenserscheinungen von der geburt.* Leipzig: Grieben, 1885.

Prichep, L. S., Sutton, S., & Hakerem, G. Evoked potentials in hyperkinetic and normal children under certainty and uncertainty: A placebo and methylphenidate study. *Psychophysiology,* 1976, *13,* 419–428.

Riesen, A. H. *The developmental neuropsychology of sensory deprivation.* New York: Academic Press, 1975.

Rose, G. H. The development of visually evoked electrocortical responses in the rat. *Developmental Psychobiology,* 1968, *1,* 35–40.

Rose, G. H. The relationship of electrophysiological and behavioral indices of visual development in mammals. In M. B. Sterman, D. J. McGinty, & A. M. Adinolfi (Eds.), *Neural ontogeny and behavior.* New York: Academic Press, 1971.

Rose, G. H. CNS maturation and behavioral development. In N. A. Buchwald & M. A. B. Brazier (Eds.), *Brain mechanisms in mental retardation.* New York: Academic Press, 1975.

Rose, G. H. The use of adult and immature ferrets (Mustela Putorius) in biomedical research: Neurophysiological and behavioral studies. *Journal of the Maine Medical Association,* in press.

Rose, G. H., & Collins, J. P. Light-dark discrimination and reversal learning in early postnatal kittens. *Developmental Psychology,* 1975, *8,* 511–518 (a).

Rose, G. H., & Collins, J. P. Assessing early visual-perceptual abilities in animals using *Response Adjusting Procedures (RAP).* Paper presented at the meeting of the International Society for Developmental Phychobiology, New York, 1975. (b)

Rose, G. H., & Dalhouse, A. Neurophysiological correlates of learning in young kittens. *Electroencepholography and Clinical Neurophysiology,* 1974, *37,* 428.

Rose, G. H., & Goodfellow, E. F. *A stereotaxic atlas of the kitten brain: Coordinates of 104 selected structures.* UCLA Brain Information Service, Los Angeles, 1973.

Rose, G. H., & Gruenau, S. P. Alterations in visual evoked responses and behavior in kittens reared under constant illumination. *Developmental Psychobiology,* 1973, *6,* 69–77.

Rose, G. H., Gruenau, S. P., & Spencer, J. W. Maturation of visual electrocortical responses in unanesthetized kittens: Effects of barbituate anesthesia. *Electroencephalography and Clincal Neurophysiology,* 1972, *33,* 141–158.

Rose, G. H., & Lindsley, D. B. Visually evoked electrocortical responses in kittens: Development of specific and nonspecific systems. *Science,* 1965, *148,* 1244–1246.

Rose, G. H., & Lindsley, D. B. Development of visually evoked potentials in kittens: Specific and nonspecific responses. *Journal of Neurophysiology,* 1968, *31,* 601–623.

Rose, G. H., Norman, R. J., Naifeh, K., & Collins, J. P. Plasticity of visual evoked potential in kittens demonstrated by operant conditioning. *Physiology and Behavior,* 1975, *14,* 557–561.

Routtenberg, A., Strop, M. & Jerdan, J. Response of the infant rat to light prior to eyelid opening: Mediation by the superior colliculus. *Developmental Psychobiology,* 1978, *11,* 469–478.

Salamy, A., McKean, C. M., & Buda, F. B. Maturational changes in auditory transmission as reflected in human brain potentials. *Brain Research,* 1975, *96,* 361–366.

Schlag, J. Generation of brain evoked potentials. In R. F. Thompson & M. M. Patterson (Eds.),

Bioelectric recording techniques (Pt. A) *Cellular processes and brain potentials.* New York: Academic Press, 1973.

Schwartz, G. E., & Beatty, J. *Biofeedback: Theory and research.* New York: Academic Press, 1977.

Seligman, M. & Hager, J. *Biological boundaries of learning.* New York: Appleton, 1972.

Shapiro, S. Hormonal and environmental influences on rat brain development and behavior. In M. B. Sterman, D. J. McGinty, & A. A. Adinolfi (Eds.), *Brain development and behavior.* New York: Academic Press, 1971.

Shipley, C. Buchwald, J. S., Norman, R., & Guthrie, D. Brain stem auditory evoked response development in the kitten. *Brain Research,* 1980, *182,* 313–326.

Solomon, R. L., & Lessac, M. S. A control group design for experimental studies of developmental processes. *Psychological Bulletin,* 1968, *70,* 145–150.

Starr, A., Amlie, R. N., Martin, W. H., & Sanders, S. Development of auditory function in newborn infants evaluated by auditory brain stem potentials. *Pediatrics,* 1977, *60,* 831–839.

Sterman, M. B., McGinty, D. J., & Adinolfi, A. M. *Neural ontogeny and behavior.* New York: Academic Press, 1971.

Sutton, S., Tueting, P., Zuben, J., & John, E. R. Information delivery and the sensory evoked potential. *Science,* 1967, *155,* 1436–1439.

Thompson, R. F., Johnson, R. H., & Hoopes, J. J. Organization of auditory, somatic sensory, and visual projection to association fields of cerebral cortex in the cat. *Journal of Neurophysiology,* 1963, *26,* 343–364.

Thorn, F., Gollender, M., & Erickson, P. The development of the kitten's visual optics. *Vision Research,* 1976, *16,* 1145–1149.

Tokunaga, A., Oka, A., Muras, H., Yokoi, X., Okumura, T., Hirata, T., Miyashita, Y., & Yoshitatsu, S. An experimental study on facial reflex by evoked electromyography. *Medical Journal Osaka University,* 1958, *9,* 397–411.

Umezaki, H., & Morrell, F. Developmental study of photic evoked responses in premature infants. *Electroencephalography and Clinical Neurophysiology,* 1970, *28,* 55–63.

Volokhov, A. A. The ontogenetic development of higher nervous activity in animals. In W. A. Himwich (Ed.), *Developmental Neurobiology.* Springfield, Ill.: Thomas, 1970.

Wald, G. *Human vision and the spectrum. Science,* 1945, *101,* 653–658.

Watanabe, K., Iwase, K., & Hara, K. Visual evoked responses during sleep and wakefulness in pre-term infants. *Electroencephalography and Clinical Neurophysiology,* 1973, *34,* 571–577.

Weidman, T. A., & Kuwabara, T. Postnatal development of the rat retina. *Archives of Opthamology,* 1968, *79,* 470–484.

Windle, W. F. Genesis of somatic motor function in mammalian embryos: A synthesizing article. *Physiological Zoology,* 1944, *17,* 247–260.

Zweig, M., Snyder, S. H., & Axelrod, J. Evidence for a nonretinal pathway of light to the pineal gland of newborn rats. *Proceedings of the National Academy of Sciences,* 1966, *56,* 515–520.

6

Development of Vocal Communication in an Experimental Model

JENNIFER S. BUCHWALD

As auditory and vocalization systems become increasingly mature during development, vocal communication gradually emerges. However, the extent to which adult vocal communication is rooted to neonatal audition and vocalization or to their interactions in the neonatal period is poorly understood. Investigation of bird song ontogeny as a function of sensory and motor control systems indicate, for example, quite different degrees of auditory dependence among different bird species; the neonatally deafened ring dove and domestic fowl develop normal vocal repertoires in the absence of auditory feedback, whereas the deafened song sparrow or junco does not. The chaffinch and white-crowned sparrow must hear not only themselves but also conspecific vocalizations within a critical period for normal song development (Nottebohm, Konichi, Hillyard, Marler, 1972).

In mammals, such neonatal interactions between audition and vocalization have not been extensively studied. It would seem essential to establish the ontogenetic role of auditory feedback as a forerunner to investigations of subsequent, more mature vocal forms emerging from the primitive neonatal cries. Existing data indicate that audition is essential for normal speech, so that human vocal behavior clearly does come under auditory control at some point in development. It is not clear, however, whether this control exists at birth, guiding even neonatal vocalizations; whether it gradually emerges in the early postnatal period; or whether it only occurs as infant vocalizations give way to more adults forms.

The deficit in our understanding of the development of human auditory–vocal interactions may in part reflect the emphasis of developmental investigations on auditory acuity rather than on more subtle auditory percep-

PRETERM BIRTH AND
PSYCHOLOGICAL DEVELOPMENT

tual processes (Eisenberg, 1976). Nevertheless, a clearer understanding of early auditory perception and vocal production is of utmost concern given the vulnerability of the auditory system to perinatal complications (Buchwald, 1975) and the importance of audition for language acquisition. The magnitude of this problem is indicated by a study of Friedlander (1970), who found that only 14 of 2312 children in a special-education program had problems of a visual nature, whereas 1050 had problems related to hearing or language.

Technical and theoretical advances now make it possible to assess auditory responsiveness of the mammalian neonate in both primary and nonprimary systems by surface recorded evoked potentials and also to quantify neonatal vocalizations in terms of glottal components and vocal tract resonances. We are presently using these combined techniques to establish a normative developmental data base of vocalization and auditory evoked responses studied concurrently in the same subjects. While we are particularly interested in this problem as it relates to the human, we are currently studying an animal model, the kitten. Use of the kitten affords analytical opportunities not possible in the human. Recording sessions can easily be prolonged, repeated, and controlled. Vocal behavior can be studied under rigidly controlled conditions to optimize quantitation, and auditory evoked responses can be obtained both before and after specific lesions are induced within the auditory system. Technical and interpretive insights gained from the kitten should facilitate the more difficult studies of the human neonate that we hope to carry out in the future.

Role of Auditory Feedback in Neonatal Vocalization

The dependence of human speech development on audition is clearly exemplified by the abnormal vocalizations of the congenitally deaf child. However, there is a lack of data on the nature of the interactions between auditory and vocal processes and on the stage of development during which these interactions begin to occur (Eisenberg, 1976; Strange & Jenkins, 1978). That the onset of such interactions must occur early in development is suggested by the data of Lach, Ling, Ling, & Ship, (1970) showing that the vocalizations of deaf infants are distinguishable from normal phonemic babbling even during the prelinguistic period of 9–12 months. Lenneberg (1967) suggests that deaf infants' utterances differ from those of normal infants even at 6 months of age. Profound disturbances of auditory and vocal channels appear to be coupled in children with Down's syndrome (e.g., Burr & Rohr, 1978; Rohr & Burr, 1978), although causal relations in such complex cases are difficult to infer.

Inherent in the motor regulation of normal neonatal crying is the control of loudness. Insofar as increasing cry loudness provides a means of maximizing information transfer to the caretaker, loudness may be a significant, that is, adaptive—vocal parameter in the neonate. Loudness is a function of both pitch intensity, regulated by the amount of air expelled through the glottis, and resonances, produced by the internal configuration of the vocal tract. In contrast to the expiratory effort needed to maximize pitch intensity, loudness can be increased with relatively little effort by changing the vocal tract contours so as to maximize the resonances of the pitch. In the adult, the shaping of the vocal tract to provide resonances and increase output intensity is a learned skill, exemplified in the singing of professional vocalists, which is typically under auditory control. In the infant, the strategy of optimizing vocal tract resonances would also seem to be an efficient means of enhancing call loudness. We do not presently know to what extent neonates utilize resonances or how important auditory feedback might be to this regulation. However, throughout most of the 28–40 week preterm period, the human auditory system is relatively high in threshold and low in fidelity (Parmelee, this volume). Thus, auditory feedback control of vocalization, as well as central auditory processing of environmental auditory signals, would predictably be less effective in the preterm than in the full-term infant.

The extent to which auditory–vocal interactions occur in animals has unfortunately not been systematically studied in any mammalian model. The vocalization of one squirrel monkey was reported to be unchanged after neonatal deafening (Winter, Handley, Ploog, & Schott, 1973), but these data were not quantified and additional subjects were not reported. Although the auditory system of the cat has been studied extensively, observations of cat vocal behavior are surprisingly scarce. Outside of our own laboratory, we know of only two specific reports on the vocal repertoire of the domestic cat, one a very extensive study utilizing a descriptive phonetic notation (Moelk, 1944) and the other a spectrographic analysis of a relatively restricted variety of vocal responses (Hartel, 1975). Vocal responding in kittens has been investigated (Haskins, 1977; Rosenblatt, 1971), but the development of vocalizations has not been analyzed in detail.

Over the past few years, we have been investigating various aspects of vocal behavior, using cats and kittens as our model systems (Brown, Buchwald, Johnson, & Mikolich, 1978; Buchwald & Brown, 1977; Carterette, Shipley, & Buchwald, 1979; Harrison, Buchwald, Norman & Hinman, 1979). The object of these studies has been to establish a normative data base relative to the structure and behavioral significance of specific classes of cat and kitten vocalizations and then to determine the effects of experimental interventions. Data of particular relevance to the neonatal period will be emphasized in this chapter, although the vocal repertoire of the adult cat will be used as a point of departure.

In our first study of cat vocalizations, vocal responses were classified into several types on the basis of a variety of standardized, response-evoking procedures commonly encountered in a laboratory environment. Vocalizations grouped according to this procedure were then examined for systematic structural or developmental differences. Measurements from sonographic records of call duration, initial and peak values of the fundamental frequency, and changes in these parameters with development indicated that the vocalizations evoked in different behavioral situations showed differences in several quantifiable dimensions (Brown *et al.*, 1978). Moreover, marked qualitative differences between calls that could not be expressed by simple quantitative measures of the sonograms were exemplified by the overall structural patterns of the vocalizations emitted in each behavioral situation (see Figure 6.1). These data indicated that the vocal repertoire of the cat included an array of identifiable, differentiated call types that were selectively emitted under particular circumstances.

Vocalizations of the neonatal kitten were found to be consistently emitted under conditions of stress, for example, removal from mother. From birth to approximately 2 months of age, the rather smooth harmonic structure of the stress call remains relatively constant. Thereafter, this cry gives way to other vocal responses of the adult repertoire. The stress call shows a fundamental frequency beginning at 500–800 Hz, which rises over approximately 100 msec to a steady state of 1250–1500Hz. This steady state segment lasts about 500 msec and is followed by a gradual decline in frequency as the call ends. Typically, several harmonic components are clearly visible (see Figure 6.2; Brown *et al.*, 1978). In general, the form and harmonic structure of the kitten stress call was found to be remarkably similar to that of the human neonatal "stress" cry (Wasz-Höckert, Lind, Vuorenkoski, Partanen, & Valenné, 1968; Zeskind & Lester, 1978).

As we were particularly interested in the role of auditory feedback in the control of infant vocalization, the effects of total deafness were studied in six kittens after the cochlea were bilaterally destroyed at a postnatal age of 4 weeks. Stress calls emitted after deafening indicated a marked disruption of the preoperative formant structure (Figure 6.2; Buchwald & Brown, 1977), although data on fundamental frequency did not indicate significant differences between the normal and deafened kittens. The failure to demonstrate significant pitch differences may reflect the relatively small number of samples obtainable by hand measurement of the sonograms. However, the data suggest that the formant frequencies are relatively more dependent upon intact auditory feedback than is pitch. Taken one step further, these results suggest that some degree of auditory control over vocal behavior, that is, over vocal tract configuration, is present early in development.

Quite different auditory–vocal interactions are suggested by other experiments in which we placed lesions in the central auditory pathway at the upper brain-stem level. The forebrain projection of the inferior colliculus was sectioned bilaterally in kittens 4 weeks of age. In two animals, the inferior colliculus brachium was almost totally destroyed, and in three other animals, incomplete but substantial destruction of this pathway was found histologically

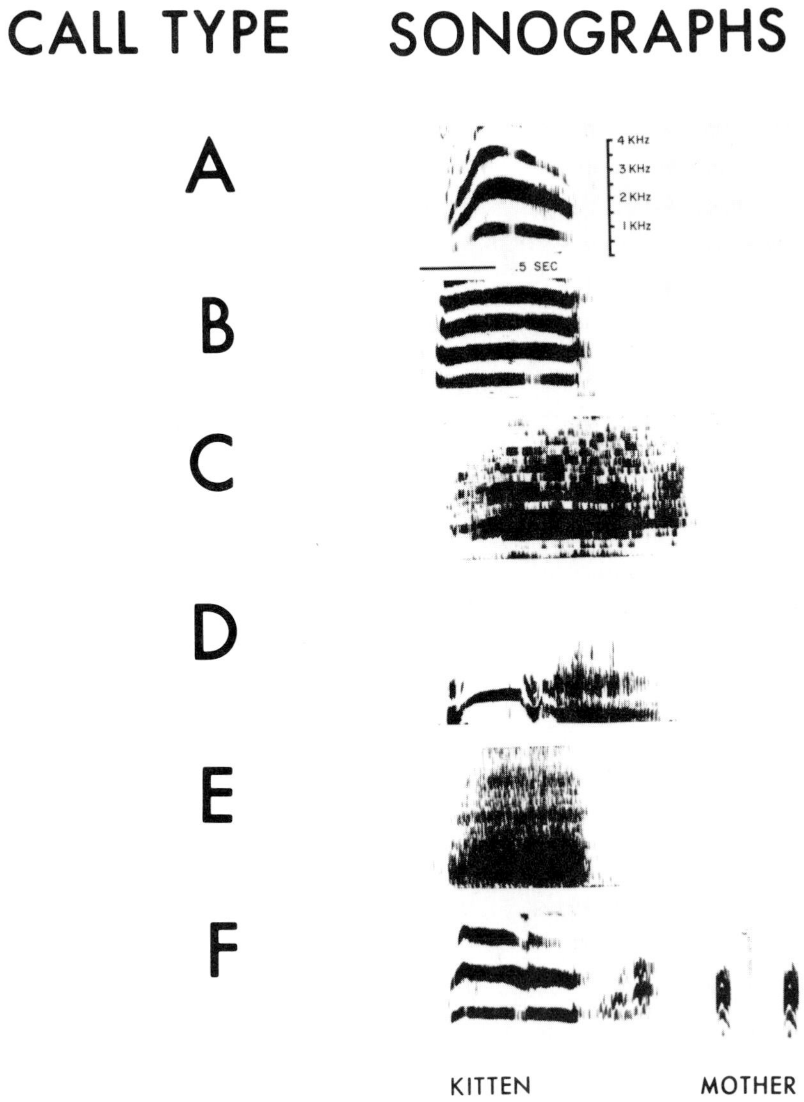

CALL TYPE   SONOGRAPHS

FIGURE 6.1. *Classes of calls in cat vocal repertoire: kitten stress call after isolation from mother; call from adult cats prior to feeding; adult pain call; calls recorded in territorial disputes or in threatening situations; kitten stress call and maternal response.*

(Buchwald & Brown, 1977). Comparisons of the preoperative stress calls with those emitted over the month following surgery indicated no significant differences in fundamental frequency of call structure. However, a significant ($p < .01$) prolongation in call duration was found in all of the lesioned kittens (see Figure 6.3; Brown, Buchwald, Schwafel, Kanegawa, & Johnson, 1976).

Taken together, these studies suggest that auditory feedback plays a role in

PRE-OPERATIVE   POST-OPERATIVE

DAY   6   DAY   32

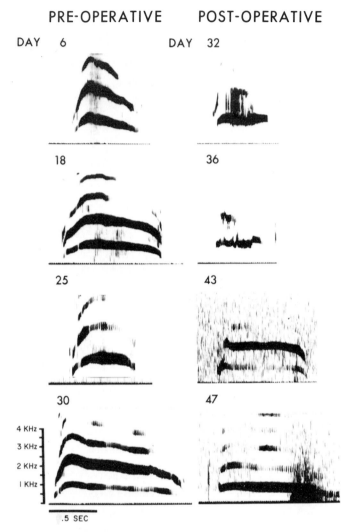

FIGURE 6.2. *Stress calls recorded before and after bilateral cochlear destruction in one kitten. Postnatal age in days indicated in upper left corner of each sonograph. (From Buchwald & Brown, 1977.)*

maintaining normal neonatal vocalization in the kitten. Moreover, the data suggest that more than one kind of auditory control may be important in vocal behavior insofar as total deafness produced loss of formant frequencies and a disintegration of call structure, whereas lesions in the auditory pathway at the upper brain-stem level did not change call structure but significantly elongated call duration.

With the use of a more sophisticated analytical method in our studies (Carterette *et al.*, 1979), we hope to establish normative values for a variety of

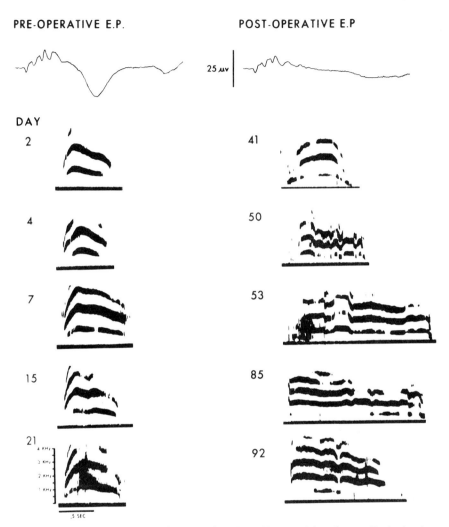

FIGURE 6.3. *Stress calls recorded before and after bilateral lesions of the inferior colliculus brachium in one kitten. Postnatal age indicated on each sonograph. Brain histology indicated almost total bilateral interruption of the brachium. Surface recorded auditory evoked potentials before and after the lesions are indicated by traces above; trace duration is 50 msec.*

stress call parameters so that vocal behavior can be compared along multiple dimensions early and late in development, as well as in normal and experimentally lesioned kittens. We postulate that auditory feedback may have little effect on cry regulation until after the first 1 or 2 postnatal weeks, since this is the period in which the poorly functioning auditory system undergoes a marked decrease in threshold and an increase in transmission fidelity.

In the human neonate, auditory functions progress through a similar developmental sequence in the preterm period between 28 and 40 weeks gestational age (Parmelee, this volume). Thus, we might infer that auditory control of vocal behavior in the preterm infant would be poor, whereas in the full-term infant this mechanism would be more mature and possibly of considerable functional utility.

Significant Elements in Neonatal Vocalizations

In response to a crying infant, increases in diastolic blood pressure and skin conductance have been shown to occur in both male and female parents, whereas a smiling and cooing infant elicits negligible autonomic changes (Frodi, Lamb, Leavitt, & Donovan, 1978). Clearly, information is provided by these two situations but, since both the sight and sound of the infant were available as cues, the relative significance of the two kinds of auditory signals cannot be inferred.

In developing an experimental model to define behaviorally significant components of a vocalization, we have again utilized the kitten stress call (Harrison et al., 1979). Then the kitten is isolated from its mother, it repeatedly cries, and, in response to the cry, the mother retrieves the kitten and carries it back to the nest. In parallel with the studies described in the preceding section on the role of auditory feedback in shaping call structure, we have been investigating the kitten stress call for its behavioral significance. The objective of these studies is to determine which components within the call, for example, those that depend upon auditory feedback, provide salient auditory cues to the mother.

Maternal retrieval in response to kitten vocalizations was investigated by placing the test subject in a cylindrical chamber in which there was a nest box opposite two wall apertures of approximately 6 × 6 cm covered by opaque curtains (see Figure 6.4). Behind each aperture a 6 × 6 × 8 cm box was mounted with a speaker at the back. After several days of habituation within

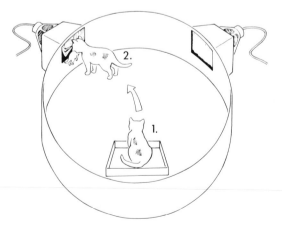

FIGURE 6.4. *Test situation for assaying retrieval responses to stress calls. The test subject was unable to see whether or not a kitten was placed in one or the other box on any particular trial.*

the chamber, the test subject predictably went to the nest box and curled up for the duration of the observation period. Experimental sessions consisted of 12 2-min trials separated by intertrial intervals of 5 min, with no more than two sessions per week per subject. During each 2-min trial, one of five test stimuli was continuously delivered: stress calls from a vocalizing kitten within one of the wall-mounted boxes, tape-recorded stress calls from one of the two boxes, tape-recorded square waves, triangular waves, or sine waves from one of the boxes with frequency modulation and duration and fundamental frequency appropriate to the stress call. These stimuli were delivered pseudorandomly so that presentations of the vocalizing kitten always occurred throughout the session to mitigate against habituation effects.

Fourteen adult females were tested with the same stimuli during the month immediately before and after parturition. "Retrieval" responses were scored when the test subject's head contacted the curtain of the box from which the call originated. None of the animals was observed to retrieve in the absence of a call stimulus.

The graphs in Figure 6.5 summarize for all cats the response level induced by each call type as a percentage of all presentations of that call within a session. As indicated by these data, the highest levels of retrieval occured postnatally and to the vocalizing kitten. In general, whether or not the kittens were of the mother's litter, she retrieved them. A response gradient from retrieval in response to the kitten to retrieval in reponse to the taped kitten call to retrieval in response to the three different kinds of synthesized calls (frequency-modulated sine wave, square wave, or triangular wave at the fundamental frequency of the call) was consistently seen in all animals in the postnatal period. A similar response gradient occured during the prenatal period, although prenatally all retrieval levels were lower.

Within the postnatal test month, some litters were permanently removed from their mothers. When tested subsequent to kitten deprivation, these mothers continued to retrieve but at lower levels than those of mothers in contact with their litters. Three nonlactating, nonpregnant resting mothers were primed sequentially over an 8-week period with appropriate amounts of

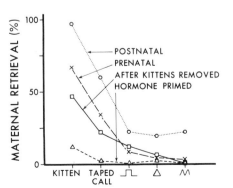

FIGURE 6.5. *Retrieval responses of female cats in four different conditions to stress call vocalizations emitted by kitten, a tape recorded stress call or a square wave, triangular wave, or sine wave synthesized stress call. Each point is the mean retrieval level to a particular call type, expressed as a percentage of all calls of that type delivered per session.*

estrogen, progesterone, and prolactin so as to approximate hormonal changes prior to and immediately after parturition (Verhage, Beamen, & Brenner, 1976; Zarrow, Gandleman, & Dennenberg, 1971). As indicated in Figure 6.5, the hormone-primed animals showed almost no retrievals and generally evinced little interest in kittens. Although hormones in these animals may not have replicated the natural pre- and postpartum levels, this result emphasizes the specificity of the retrieval response as one extremely vigorous in the pregnant and lactating female but not easily induced artificially.

These experimental data suggest that the strong autonomic responses induced by human infant cries in parents (Frodi et al., 1978) may not be elicitable in nonparents. It would be of interest to determine whether the prolonged exposure of caretakers, such as pediatric intensive care nurses, to crying infants results in the acquisition of the same autonomic responses as those shown by parents. Similarly, it would be important to know whether extremely pathological or deviant cries, for example, the cries of Down's syndrome infants (Lind, Vuoroenkosin, Rosberg, Partanen, Wasz-Höckert, 1970) or infants at risk (Michelsson, 1971; Zeskind & Lester, 1978), might be less likely than a normal cry to induce a caretaker response.

We are interested in further defining basic components of the stress call that are important in triggering high levels of retrieval responding; presumably, these would be the most significant elements of this vocalization. Through an analysis program now in use, vocalizations in the normal behavioral repertoire of the cat can be synthesized and displayed as three-dimensional sonographs (see Figure 6.6) with numerical values available for specific call components, for example, onset frequency modulation (Carterette et al., 1979). Such specific call components are presently being used as acoustic stimuli in the maternal retrieval test. Ultimately, the elements of the normal stress call found to be most significant to maternal retrieval will be compared

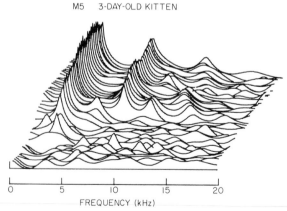

M5   3-DAY-OLD KITTEN

FREQUENCY (kHz)

FIGURE 6.6. *Three-dimensional plot of kitten stress call with amplitude on the vertical axis, time on the oblique axis.*

with those elements in the human infant's stress call which induce parental reponses. One aim of this work is to develop generic indices of behaviorally significant neonatal call components as a basis for quantitating normal and abnormal vocalization changes during development.

Development of Central Auditory Functions

Plasticity in mammalian auditory development as a function of acoustic inflow has been demonstrated anatomically in studies of congenitally deaf humans (Fisch, 1959), cats (Brouwer, 1912), and mice (Ross, 1962). In all of these subjects deprived of acoustic stimulation from birth, the cochlear nuclei were abnormal or missing. More recent studies of mice raised in a sound-deprived environment have further demonstrated abnormally small neurons in the cochlear nucleus as well as in the nucleus of the trapezoid body (Webster & Webster, 1977). Functional abnormalities in the sensitivity of inferior colliculus neurons were found in rats raised in an abnormal sound environment (Clopton & Winfield, 1976) or with asymmetrical auditory inflow as a result of blocking one ear (Clopton & Silverman, 1977; Silverman & Clopton, 1977). Furthermore, rats deprived of auditory stimulation during early development were behaviorally unable to integrate tone sequences as adults (Tees, 1967a, 1967b). These data suggest that an early structural and functional plasticity exists in the auditory system akin to that which has been extensively demonstrated for the mammalian visual system (Blakemore, 1974; Pettigrew, 1974; Wiesel & Hubel, 1965).

The significance of vocalization to early auditory development is suggested by the apparent tuning of the infant auditory system to conspecific vocalizations. Behavioral and electrophysiological studies in the human neonate show much greater responsivity to frequencies in the speech range than to high-pitched tones and much more responsiveness to speech and other complex stimuli than to simple tones or noise (Eisenberg, 1970a, 1970b, 1976). There is also growing evidence that infants as young as 1–2 months can make very fine discriminations along speech-related dimensions (e.g., Elimas, Siqueland, Juscyzk, & Viqouto, 1971; Morse, 1972; Trehub, 1973; Trehub & Rabinovitch, 1972). Behavioral studies of kittens also indicate earlier and more marked orientating responses to conspecific vocalizations than to other types of auditory stimuli (Villablanca & Olmstead, 1978). Electrophysiological studies indicate that the 500–2500 Hz frequency range, encompassed by the kitten cry and other conspecific vocalizations (Brown et al., 1978), elicits the first cochlear microphonic response (Pujol & Hilding, 1973; Romand, 1971), as well as the earliest response from the acoustic nerve (Pujol & Hilding, 1973; Romand, 1971),cochlear nucleus (Pujol, 1972; Romand & Marty, 1975), inferior colliculus (Pujol, 1972), and primary auditory cortex (Pujol, 1972).

There is a growing literature demonstrating that qualitatively different auditory-processing functions are reflected by surface recorded auditory evoked potentials ranging from 1 to 1000 msec in latency (e.g., Picton, Hillyard, Krauz, & Galambos, 1974). To the extent that the generator of any particular potential can be identified, that potential provides a noninvasive functional probe of a particular brain region. Thus, the use of the entire sequence of auditory evoked potentials is particularly attractive for developmental studies of auditory information processing; functional and structural development at multiple brain levels can be concurrently monitored by recordings that can be carried out longitudinally in the same subject.

In our laboratory, we have been investigating neural substrates of both short- and long-latency auditory evoked responses in the adult cat (Buchwald, Hinman, Norman, Huang, & Brown, in press; Buchwald & Huang, 1975; Huang & Buchwald, 1977) as well as the development of these responses in the kitten. As indices of early auditory function, maturation of the auditory evoked response components will be compared with vocalization development in the same animal. Although the correlative auditory response–vocal response data have not yet been collected, work to date on the development of the auditory brain-stem response in the kitten (Shipley, Buchwald, Norman, & Guthrie, 1980) will be briefly summarized.

Short-latency, volume-conducted auditory evoked responses have been recorded from surface electrodes in cat (Buchwald & Huang, 1975; Huang & Buchwald, 1977; Jewett, 1970; Lev & Sohmer, 1972; Plantz, Williston, & Jewett, 1974) and human subjects (Jewett & Williston, 1971; Lev & Sohmer, 1972; Picton et al., 1974; Starr & Achor, 1975). The first five waves recorded under these conditions have been termed autitory brain-stem responses (ABRs) because both experimental (Achor, 1976; Buchwald & Huang, 1975; Huang & Buchwald 1977; Jewett, 1970; Jones et al., 1977; Plantz et al., 1974) and clinical (Lev & Sohmer, 1972; Starr & Achor, 1975; Starr & Hamilton, 1976; Stockard & Rossiter, 1977) studies indicate that these waves originate from generators in the brain-stem. In the adult cat, the five ABR peaks occur at extremely constant latencies within 7 msec and show interpeak intervals of approximately 1 msec (see Figure 6.7). Evidence from lesion experiments (Buchwald & Huang, 1975) and depth evoked potential recordings (Achor, 1976; Jewett, 1970; Lev & Sohmer, 1972) in the cat indicate that the major, although not necessarily sole, generator of wave 1 is the acoustic nerve; of wave 2, the cochlear nucleus; of wave 3, the region of the superior olivary complex; of wave 4, the preolivary region and lateral leminiscus; and of wave 5, the region of the inferior colliculus (see Figure 6.7). Furthermore, the invariance in peak latency of the ABR waves has been correlated with subpopulations of cells in each of the brain-stem relay nuclei that also show constant response latencies, for example, less than .1 msec standard deviation (Huang & Buchwald, 1977). Such "high synaptic security" cells would appear to be likely neuronal generators of the ABRs.

Since the ABRs reflect activation of the brain-stem auditory pathway, they

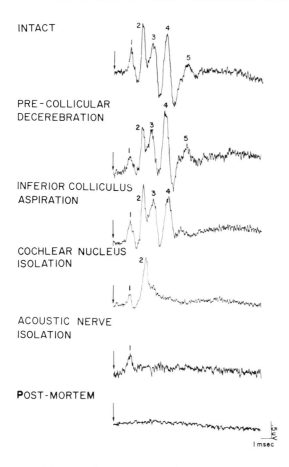

INTACT

PRE-COLLICULAR
DECEREBRATION

INFERIOR COLLICULUS
ASPIRATION

COCHLEAR NUCLEUS
ISOLATION

ACOUSTIC NERVE
ISOLATION

POST-MORTEM

FIGURE 6.7. *ABRs after a series of lesions. The potential sequence recorded from the intact cat in response to binaural click presentations was unaltered following precollicular decerebration. Subsequent bilateral aspiration of the inferior colliculi largely eliminated wave 5. Following surgical isolation of the cochlear nuclei from the brain stem, waves 3 and 4 disappeared. Isolation of the acoustic nerve from the cochlear nucleus resulted in the loss of potential 2. No potential remained in the postmortem recording. Positivity is above the baseline. (From Buchwald & Huang, 1975.)*

provide a unique opportunity to study development from the level of the acoustic nerve to inferior colliculus in the same subject from birth to maturity. Jewett and Romano (1972) noted the first appearance of ABRs in the kitten at 12–14 days after birth. In contrast to these observations, local evoked potentials and single-unit responses to loud sound stimuli have been recorded throughout the auditory system of the kitten as early as 1–4 days postnatally (Pujol, 1969; Pujol, 1972; Pujol & Hilding, 1973; Romand, 1971; Romand, Granier, & Marty, 1973; Romand & Marty, 1975).

In a series of 28 kittens over a postnatal period ranging from birth to 60 days, we have carried out repeated, longitudinal observations of ABR development (Shipley *et al.,* 1980). The position of the animal and sound source within the recording chamber were held constant across recording sessions, as was click intensity except during recordings in which intensity effects were specifically studied. Click rates of 1,10, 50, and 100 per sec were routinely presented. Reference electrodes at the tongue, pinna, and neck showed volume conducted responses to the click stimuli and resulted in considerable distortion of the activity recorded by the vertex electrode; the forepaw, in contrast, showed no activity and a vertex–forepaw electrode configuration provided good resolution of ABRs across development.

A number of new observations were made. ABRs were first observed at 4 days, approximately the same age at which depth evoked potentials are first recorded in brain-stem auditory nuclei. Initially, the ABRs were diffuse, showed high threshold, and fatigued rapidly, characteristics shared with depth evoked potentials in the early postnatal period (see Figure 6.8). Over the first 3 weeks, the potentials showed marked decrease in threshold, increased resistance to fast click rates, and better definition of wave forms (see Figure 6.9). All ABR components showed exponential decreases in latency. Because all of the brain-stem potentials could be recorded concurrently and longitudinally in the same subject, a number of developmental comparisons were possible among the ABR components. Wave 1, related to the acoustic nerve in the adult cat, showed a marked developmental time course and adult latency similar to that reported for N_1 (Romand, 1971). Wave 2, related to the cochlear nucleus in the adult, showed a marked bimodality over the first month; wave 2a was a large amplitude wave that gradually fused as an inconspicuous leading shoulder on wave 2b. Wave 2b developed with a time course and adult latency similar to that reported for ventral cochlear nucleus (Pujol, 1972; Romand & Marty, 1975). Wave 3, related to the region of the superior olivary complex in the adult, showed a clear but transient bimodality during the third week of development. Wave 5, related to the region of the inferior colliculus in the adult, appeared later than waves 1–4 and showed a significantly slower rate of development than these waves. The preceding data indicate that differential developmental changes occur within the brain-stem auditory pathway and that the ABRs provide a probe of these concurrent maturational interactions.

Human developmental studies indicate that ABRs can be recorded in preterm infants as early as 28 weeks gestational age and responses to high-intensity stimuli at even earlier gestational ages (Starr, Amlie, Martin, & Sanders, 1977). Peripheral transmission (latency to wave I) reaches adult latency by 6 weeks after full-term birth, while the morphology of wave I matures only at 3–6 months, and the central conduction time (wave V minus wave I latency) continues to decrease until at least 1 year of age (Hecox & Galambos, 1974; Starr et al., 1977). Increased stimulation rates have a greater effect on wave latencies in the infant than in the adult (Fujikawa & Weber, 1977). There are reports that infants showing absence of the brain-stem potentials may later be identified as deaf (Starr et al., 1977), although these click-induced responses do not constitute an audiological examination in the common sense. The brain-stem potentials have also been useful in identifying neurological disorders in the neonate (Starr et al., 1977) as well as in children (Sohmer & Student, 1978).

In general, the kitten and infant evoked potential data show similar trends

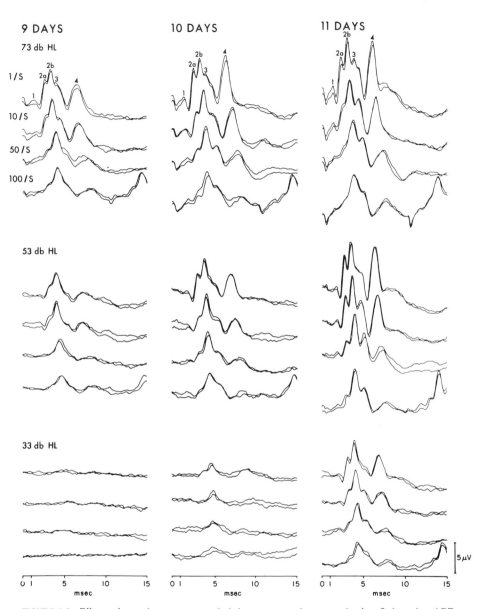

FIGURE 6.8. *Effects of stimulus intensity and click rate in one kitten on the first 3 days that ABRs were evoked by a 73 dB HL stimulus. (From Shipley, Buchwald, Norman, & Guthrie 1980.)*

of decreasing stimulus intensity threshold, decreasing sensitivity to rapid rates of stimulation, and a caudal to rostral brain-stem maturation gradient. Because of the greater ease with which these studies can be carried out in the kitten, the ABR waves are clearer than in the human and the data indicate a

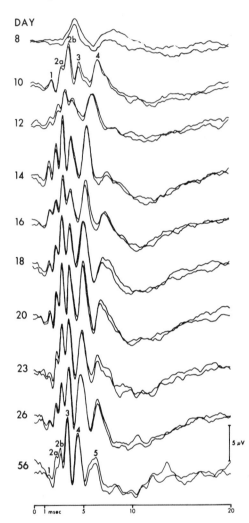

FIGURE 6.9. *ABR developmental sequence from one kitten across the first 2 months of life. The stimulus (46 dB HL, 10/sec clicks) occurs at trace onset. (From Shipley, Buchwald, Norman, & Guthrie, 1980.)*

complex and differential development of particular waves that the human developmental work has not reported. However, the kitten studies suggest that the brain-stem potentials may provide a probe for discrete developmental events, for example, the appearance and disappearance of bimodality in wave 3, in addition to reflecting the more general functional maturation of the brain-stem auditory pathway.

For the future, we plan to continue experimental studies of auditory and vocal behavior in the developing kitten and ultimately to extend this work to the human neonate. As our data base increases, the extent to which specific auditory and vocal functions interact in the neonatal period should become increasingly clear. We hope that the kitten model will provide insights relevant to the human and to the many unresolved general questions concerning the otogeny of mammalian vocal communication.

Acknowledgments

The material presented in this chapter reflects work with a number of collaborators: K. Brown, J. Harrison, C. Hinman, C.-M. Huang, R. Norman, C. Shipley, and N. Squires.

References

Achor, L. J. Field analysis of auditory brainstem responses. *Neuroscience Abstract,* 1976, *2,* 12.

Blakemore, C. Developmental factors in the formation of feature extracting neurons. In F. O. Schmitt & F. G. Worden (Eds.), *The neurosciences: Third study program.* Cambridge, Mass.: MIT Press, 1974.

Brouwer, B. Das Gehrin einer congenital tauben Katze. *Folia Neuro-Biologica* 1912, *6,* 197–208.

Brown, K. A., Buchwald, J. S., Johnson, J. R. & Mikolich, D. J. Vocalization in the cat and kitten. *Developmental Psychobiology,* 1978, *11* 559–570.

Brown, K. A., Buchwald, J. S., Schwafel, J. A., Kanegawa, K. & Johnson, J. R. Behavioral effects on damage to auditory pathways in kittens. *Neuroscience Abstract,* 1976, *2,* 207.

Buchwald, J. S. Brainstem substrates of sensory information processing and adaptive behavior. In N. A. Buchwald and M. A. B. Brazier (Eds.), *Brain mechanisms in mental retardation.* New York: Academic Press, 1975.

Buchwald, J. S., & Brown, K. A. The role of acoustic inflow in the development of adaptive behavior. *Annals of the New York Academy of Sciences,* 1977 *290,* 270–284.

Buchwald, J. S., Hinman, C., Norman, R. J., Huang, C. M., & Brown, K. A. Middle- and long-latency auditory evoked responses recorded from the vertex of normal and chronically lesioned cats. *Brain Research,* in press.

Buchwald, J. S., & Huang, C. M. Origins of the far-field acoustic response in the cat. *Science,* 1975, *189,* 382–384.

Burr, D. B., & Rohr, A. Patterns of psycholinguistic development in the severely mentally retarded: A hypothesis. *Social Biology,* 1978, *25,* 15–22.

Carterette, E., Shipley, C. & Buchwald, J. S. Linear prediction theory of vocalization in cat and kitten. In B. Lindholm & S. Ohman (Eds.), *Frontiers of speech communication research.* London: Academic Press, 1979.

Clopton, B. M. & Silverman, M. S. Plasticity of binaural interaction. II. Critical period and changes in midline responses. *Journal of Neurophysiology,* 1977, *40,* 1275–1280.

Clopton, B. M., & Winfield, J. A. Effect of early exposure to patterned sound on unit activity in rat inferior colliculus. *Journal of Neurophysiology,* 1976, *39,* 1081–1089.

Elimas, P. D., Siqueland, E. R., Juscyzk, P., & Viqouto, J. Speech perception in infants. *Science,* 1971, *171,* 303–306.

Eisenberg, R. B. The development of hearing in man: An assessment of current status. *Journal of the American Speech and Hearing Association,* 1970, *12,* 199–223. (a)

Eisenberg, R. B. The organization of auditory behavior. *Journal of Speech and Hearing Research,* 1970, *13,* 454–471. (b)

Eisenberg, R. B. *Auditory competence in early life.* Baltimore: University Park Press, 1976.

Fisch, L. Deafness as part of an hereditary syndrome. *Journal of Larynogology and Otology,* 1959, *73,* 355–382.

Friedlander, B. Z. Receptive language development in infancy: Issues and problems. *Merrill-Palmer Quarterly,* 1970, *16,* 7–51.

Frodi, A. M., Lamb, M. E., Leavitt, L. A., & Donovan, W. L. Fathers' and mothers' responses to infant smiles and cries. *Infant Behavior and Development*, 1978, *1* 187-198.

Fujikawa, S. M., & Weber, B. A. Effects of increased stimulus rate on brainstem electric response (BER) audiometry as a function of age. *Journal of the American Audiological Society*, 1977, *3*, 147-150.

Harrison, J. B., Buchwald, J. S., Norman, R. J. & Hinman, C. Acoustic analysis of maternal retrieval to kitten stress call. *Neuroscience Abstracts*, 1979, *5*, 22.

Hartel, R. Zur struktur und funktion akustischer signale im pflegesystem der hauskatze (Felis catus L.). *Biologisches Zentralblatt*, 1975, *94*, 187-204.

Haskins, R. Effect of kitten vocalizations on maternal behavior. *Journal of Comparative Physiology and Psychology*, 1977, *91*, 830-838.

Hecox, K., & Galambos, R. Brainstem auditory evoked responses in human infants and adults. *Archives of Otolaryngology*, 1974, *99*, 30-33.

Huang, C. M., & Buchwald, J. S. Interpretation of the vertex short-latency acoustic response: A study of single neurons in the brainstem. *Brain Research*, 1977, *137*, 291-303.

Jewett, D. L. Volume-conducted potentials in response to auditory stimuli as detected by averaging in the cat. *Electroencephalography and Clinical Neurophysiology*, 1970, *28*, 609-618.

Jewett, D. L., & Romano, M. N. Neonatal development of auditory system potentials averaged from the scalp of rat and cat. *Brain Research*, 1972, *36*, 101-115.

Jewett, D. L., & Williston, J. S. Auditory evoked far-fields averaged from the scalp of humans. *Brain*, 1971, *94*, 681-696.

Jones, T. A., Schorn, V., Siu, G., Stockard, J. J., Rossiter, V. S., Bickford, R. J., & Sharbrough, F. W. Effects of local and system cooling on brainstem auditory responses. *Electroencephalography and Clinical Neurophysiology*, 1977, *43*, 469-470.

Lach, R., Ling, D., Ling, A., & Ship, N. Early speech development in deaf infants. *American Annals of the Deaf*, 1970, *115*, 522-526.

Lenneberg, E. H. *Biological foundations of language*. New York: Wiley, 1967.

Lev, A., & Sohmer, H. Sources of averaged neural responses recorded in animal and human subjects during cochlear audiometry (electrocochleogram). *Archiv Fuer Klinische und Experimentelle Ohren-Nasan-und Kehlkopfheilkunde*, 1972, *201*, 79-90.

Lind, J. Vuorenkoski, V., Rosberg, G., Partanen, T. J., & Wasz-Höckert, O. Spectrographic analysis of vocal response to pain stimuli in infants with Down's Syndrome. *Developmental Medicine and Child Neurology*, 1970, *12*, 478-486.

Michelsson, K. Cry analysis of symptomless low birth weight neonates and of asphyxiated newborn infants. *Acta Paed Scandinavica Supplement* AC 8196, 1971, *1*, 1-45.

Moelk, M. Vocalizing in the house-cat. A phonetic and functional study. *American Journal of Psychology*, 1944, *57*, 184-204.

Morse, P. A. The discrimination of speech and nonspeech stimuli in early infancy. *Journal of Experimental Child Psychology*, 1972, *14*, 477-492.

Nottebohm, F., Konichi, M., Hillyard, S., & Marler, P. Auditory templates and the ontogeny of birdsong. In F. G. Worden & R. Galambos (Eds.), *Auditory processing of biologically significant sounds*. *Neuroscience Research Program Bulletin*, 1972, *10*, 34-39.

Pettigrew, J. D. The effect of visual experience on the development of stimulus specificity by kitten cortical neurons. *Journal of Physiology* (London), 1974, *237*, 49-74.

Picton, T. W., Hillyard, S. A., Krausz, H. K., & Galambos, R. Human auditory evoked potentials. I. Evaluation of components. *Electroencephalography and Clinical Neurophysiology*, 1974, *36*, 179-190.

Plantz, R. G., Williston, J. S., & Jewett, D. L. Spatio-temporal distribution of auditory evoked far field potentials in rat and cat. *Brain Research*, 1974, *68*, 55-71.

Pujol, R. Développement des résponses à la stimulation sonore dans le colliculus inférieur chez le Chat. *Journal de Physiologie* (Paris), 1969, *61*, 411-421.

Pujol, R. Development of tone-burst responses along the auditory pathway in the cast. *Acta Oto-Laryngologica*, 1972, *74*, 383-391.

Pujol, R., & Hilding, D. Anatomy and physiology of the onset of auditory function. *Acta Oto-Laryngologica*, 1973, *76,* 1-10.

Rohr, A., & Burr I. G. Etiological differences in patterns of psycholinguistic development of children of IQ 30 to 60. *American Journal of Mental Deficiency*, 1978, *82,* 549-553.

Romand, R. Maturation des potentiels cochléaires dans la période périnatale chez le Chat et chez le Cobaye. *Journal de Physiologie* (Paris), 1971, *63,* 763-782.

Romand, R., Granier, M. R., & Marty, R. Développement postnatal de l'activité provoquée dans l'olive supérieure latérale chez le chat par la stimulation sonore. *Journal de Physiologie* (Paris), 1973, *66,* 303-315.

Romand, R., & Marty, R. Postnatal maturation of the cochlear nuclei in the cat: A neurophysiological study. *Brain Research*, 1975. *83,* 225-233.

Rosenblatt, J. S. Suckling and home orientation in the kitten: A comparative developmental study. In E. Tobach, L. R. Aranson, & E. Shaw (Eds.), *The biopsychology of development*. New York: Academic Press, 1971.

Ross, M. D. Auditory pathway of the epileptic waltzing mouse. I. A comparison of the acoustic pathways of the normal mouse with those of the totally deaf epileptic waltzer. *Journal of Comparative Neurology*, 1962, *119,* 317-339.

Shipley, C. Buchwald, J. S., Norman, R., & Guthrie, D. Brainstem auditory evoked response development in the kitten. *Brain Research*, 1980, *182,* 313-326.

Silverman, M. S., & Clopton, B. M. Plasticity of bianural interaction. I. Effect of early auditory deprivation. *Journal of Neurophysiology*, 1977, *40,* 1266-1274.

Sohmer, H., & Student, M. Auditory nerve and brainstem evoked responses in normal, autistic, minimal brain dysfunction and psychomotor retarded children. *Electroencephalography and Clinical Neurophysiology*, 1978, *44,* 380-388.

Starr, A., & Achor, L. J. Auditory brain stem responses in neurological disease. *Archives of Neurology*, 1975, *32,* 761-768.

Starr, A., Amlie, R. N., Martin, W. H., & Sanders, S. Development of auditory function in newborn infants revealed by auditory brainstem potentials. *Pediatrics*, 1977, *60,* 831-839.

Starr, A., & Hamilton, A. Correlation between confirmed sites of neurological lesions and abnormalities of far-field auditory brainstem response. *Electroencephalography and Clinical Neurophysiology*, 1976, *41,* 595-608.

Stockard, J. J., & Rossiter, V. S. Clinical and pathologic correlates of brain stem auditory response abnormalities. *Neurology*, 1977, *27,* 316-325.

Strange, W., & Jenkins, J. J. Role of linguistic experience in the perception of speech. In R. D. Walk & H. L. Pick, Jr. (Eds.), *Perception and experience*. New York: Plenum, 1978.

Tees, R. C. Effects of early auditory restriction in the rat on adult pattern discrimination. *Journal of Comparative Physiology and Psychology*, 1967, *63,* 389-393. (a)

Tees, R. C. The effects of early auditory restriction in the rat on adult duration discrimination. *Journal of Auditory Research*, 1976, *7,* 195-207. (b)

Trehub, S. E. Infant's sensitivity to vowel and tonal contrasts. *Developmental Psychobiology*, 1973, *9,* 91-96.

Trehub, S., & Rabinovitch, S. Auditory-linguistic sensitivity in early infancy. *Developmental Psychobiology*, 1972, *6,* 74-77.

Verhage, H. G., Beamen, N. B., & Brenner, R. M. Plasma levels of estradiol and progesterone in the cat during polyestrus, pregnancy and pseudopregnancy. *Biology of Reproduction*, 1976, *14,* 579-585.

Villablanca, J. R., & Olmstead, C. E. Neurological development of kittens. *Developmental Psychobiology*, 1978, *12,* 101-127.

Wasz-Höckert, O., Lind, J. Vuorenkoski, V., Partanen, T., & Valnné, E. *The infant cry. A spectrographic and auditory analysis.* Suffolk, England: Lavenham, 1968.

Webster, D. B., & Webster, M. Neonatal sound deprivation affects brain stem auditory-nuclei. *Archives of Otolaryngology*, 1977, *103,* 392-396.

Wiesel, T. N., & Hubel, D. H. Comparison of the effects of unilateral and bilateral eye closures on cortical unit responses in kittens. *Journal of Neurophysiology,* 1965, *28,* 1029–1046.

Winter, P., Handley, P., Ploog, D., & Schott, D. Ontogeny of squirrel monkey calls under normal conditions and under acoustic isolation. *Behavior,* 1973, *47,* 230–239.

Zarrow, M. X., Gandelman, R., & Dennenberg, V. H. Prolacten: Is it an essential hormone for maternal behavior in the mammal? *Hormones and Behavior,* 1971, *2,* 343–354.

Zeskind, P. S., & Lester, B. M. Acoustic features and auditory perceptions of the cries of newborns with prenatal and perinatal complications. *Child Development,* 1978, 49, 580–589.

7

Auditory Function and Neurological Maturation in Preterm Infants[1]

ARTHUR H. PARMELEE, JR.

Infants born many weeks before their expected date of birth are now able to survive despite the extreme immaturity of all their organs, including the nervous system. Of particular interest to us is the degree to which the maturation of the immature nervous system can be influenced by the nursery environment. Most neuronanatomical and neurophysiological studies have demonstrated a surprising number of similarities between the preterm infant at the time of his expected date of birth and the infant born at term. Almost all studies, however, have also mentioned some differences that have generally been less striking than the similarities. These differences have not been consistently in the direction of advancing or retarding nervous system maturation in the preterm at term. Different parameters in an individual infant may be both advanced and delayed in development. Furthermore, most of the neurophysiological differences between preterm and term infants disappear in the first months after term. Similarly, it has been difficult to demonstrate persisting behavioral differences between preterm and term infants in the first months of life when compared at comparable conceptional ages (i.e., age calculated from onset of mother's last menses to time of observation. [Parmelee, 1975]).

Perhaps with more infant observations and assessments, we will find more persisting effects of the exposure of the immature nervous system to the

[1] This research is supported by National Institutes of Health—National Institute of Child Health and Human Development Contract No. 1-HD-3-2776, "Diagnostic and Intervention Studies of High-Risk Infants," and National Institute of Child Health Development Grant No. HD-04612, Mental Retardation Research Center, University of California at Los Angeles.

nursery environment. On the other hand, the extreme immaturity of the nervous system may provide a form of protection by its limited capacity to respond to all the stimuli presented.

At present, we have very limited neuroanatomical information about the nervous system of preterm infants of various gestational and conceptional ages and even more limited neurophysiological information. For many practical and ethical reasons, there will always remain many gaps in our knowledge. It is important therefore to look for animal models to attempt to resolve the issue of the responsive capacity of the nervous system at various levels of maturity. There are several animals whose newborns are very immature. Among these, the kitten seems to be the best comparative model for the preterm human infant. In terms of state organization, electrocortical activity, evoked potential latencies, and nerve conduction velocities, the kitten at birth is like a preterm infant born about 15 weeks before term (25 weeks gestation and barely viable). The kitten then matures about five times as rapidly as the infant. Thus the kitten of 3 weeks is like the full-term infant or preterm infant at his expected birth date (Parmelee & Sigman, 1976; Verley, 1974). The rat and mouse are also very immature at birth but mature so rapidly that comparative studies are difficult. Fortunately, there have been many excellent neuroanatomical, neurophysiological, and behavioral studies in kittens.

A comparative review of the anatomical and physiological development of the auditory system in kittens and infants and their responses to auditory stimuli will be presented. This will illustrate in one system the limitations in stimulus processing imposed by the level of maturity of the anatomy and physiology of that particular system and the nervous system in general.

The auditory system provides a good model for discussion of the influences of sensory stimulation on neurological development in the preterm infant. There is, possibly, some auditory functioning even in the smallest and youngest viable infants, and the auditory environment in the nursery to which the infant is exposed before its expected date of birth has been studied to some degree.

Infants born preterm, if not exposed to more sounds than *in utero,* are probably exposed to different sounds. Among these are noises within incubators, due to air circulation motors, etc., that may be at a 70–80 dB level in the frequency range of 63–250 Hz, with the peak at 125 Hz. This is continuous and without patterning. Additional and more varied increases in sound level come from the clatter of doors, handling of equipment, and nursery staff conversation (Svenningsen, & Almquist, 1974; Committee Academy of Pediatrics, 1974; Lawson, Daum, & Turkewitz, 1977; Selency & Streczyn, 1969).

The effects of this noise pollution on the later auditory perception of preterm infants has been difficult to determine. Other factors that can cause hearing losses confound follow-up studies. These include hypoxia, infections, drugs, and hyperbilirubinemia, all potentially ototoxic and not uncommon complications for preterm infants.

Schulte and Stennart (1978) in a follow-up study of preterm infants found 12.4% with some neurosensory loss compared with a generally reported .5% incidence for all children. There was no correlation of the neurosensory hearing loss in the preterm infants with gestational age or length of stay in the incubator. There was, however, a correlation with a perinatal nonoptimal risk score. This suggests that the hearing losses were more related to illnesses during pregnancy, delivery, and immediate postnatal problems than to nursery noise pollution. As will be discussed later, longitudinal studies of auditory evoked potentials in the neonatal period are also not altered in their development by the nursery environment.

Preterm infants have been reported to have language difficulties in childhood with somewhat greater frequency than full-term infants (DeHirsch, Jansky, & Langford, 1964; Neligan, Kolvin, Scott, & Garside, 1976). Variables other than preterm birth have been difficult to control in analyses. We are increasingly aware of the importance of demographic variables and parent–infant interactions. Beckwith, Cohen, Kopp, Parmelee, and Marcy (1976) reported the influence of caregiver–infant interactions and the general level of competence of preterm infants. Cohen and Beckwith (1977) further observed that the ordinal position of the preterm infants influenced early cognitive development. Cohen, Beckwith, and Parmelee (1978) also found specific influences of parental caregiving on the receptive language competence of a 2-year-old preterm infants. Neligan *et al.* (1976) also found a strong environmental influence on language competence of preterm infants at 5 and 7 years of age.

O'Connor (1980) studied 30 preterm and 20 full-term infants at 4 months of age using a variable trials habituation–dishabituation procedure in an auditory discrimination task with heart rate as a response measure. The preterm and full-term infants were indistinguishable on the habituation parameters even though many infants who were in incubators for prolonged periods were included in the preterm group since the mean gestational for the group was 32 weeks with a range of 26–37 weeks.

Beckwith, Sigman, Cohen, and Parmelee (1977) reported that the vocal output of preterm and full-term infants at 1 and 8 months was similar. The full-term infants, however, increased the amount of their vocalization more rapidly from 1 to 3 months than the preterm infants and then did not change as much from 3 to 8 months.

The potential for auditory and language difficulties in preterm infants seems to be present. It is still unclear, however, that the unusual auditory environment of the preterm has a significant impact on the immature but rapidly developing auditory system.

Fetal and Preterm Infant Responses to Auditory Stimulation

How early in life the fetus responds to auditory stimulation has not been definitely established. Stirnimann (1940) reports that one mother told him that she stopped attending concerts at the sixth month of pregnancy because she experienced violent child movements during these concerts. Fleischer (1955), in a systematic study of 78 subjects, did not find movement reactions of the fetus to auditory stimulation before the seventh month of gestation, and these were inconsistent until the eighth month. There have been many other observations of this nature. In all of them, there remains the possibility of the influence of the sound on the mother, who in turn influences the fetus to movement via some nonauditory mechanism. Thus, they have not provided clear evidence for the development of auditory function in the fetus.

Heart rate acceleration in the fetus *in utero* to 500 and 4000 Hz sine wave tone stimulation at 100 dB was observed in one subject at 30 weeks gestation by Murphy and Smyth (1962), and by Johansson, Wedenberg, and Westin (1964) in a fetus of 33 weeks to 3000 Hz tone at 110 dB. Bench and Vass (1970), however, were unable to get fetal heart rate responses to 500 and 4000 Hz tone at 100 dB in 20 subjects at even later gestational ages. Sontag, Steele, and Lewin (1969) obtained fetal heart rate acceleration when music was played at 75 dB while the mother rested. They concluded that this effect on the fetus was more likely through indirect influences from the mother than direct auditory perception by the fetus. From these studies, we are still not sure whether the fetus *in utero* before 34 weeks gestation respond to auditory stimulation through the maternal abdominal wall.

There are a few descriptions of the behavioral responses of preterm infants to sound. Gesell and Amatruda (1945) state that infants of 28–32 weeks conceptional age respond to sound by "a slight frown, a 'squinch' with a blink followed by a short wave of activity which soon subsides. On repeated stimulation the fetal–infant rapidly becomes impervious to sound [p. 112]." Monod and Garma (1971) made repeated detailed observations of seven preterm infants with birthweights of 980–1510 gm from birth to term. Videotape recordings were made during 2-hour polygraphic sleep recordings. Clicks with components of 600–900 Hz at 103 dB were the stimuli. These were presented randomly with 70–120 clicks each session. Motor responses were obtained 29% of the time in the infants of 30–31 weeks conceptional age and blinks only 5%. With maturation, the motor responses remained at the same level at all conceptional ages in active sleep, but dropped to 6% in quiet sleep. Blinks, on the other hand, increased with maturation in active sleep from 5–25% at 37–39 weeks conceptional age. There was no increase in blinks in quiet sleep.

Bench and Parker (1971) determined that preterm infants of 30–38 weeks gestation had a greater reaction to broad-spectrum noise band sounds presented at 85 dB in light sleep (active sleep) than full-term infants, but the preterm infants also had a higher level of spontaneous activity. On the other hand, the full-term infants responded more frequently to this sound level. They concluded that the hyperreaction of the preterm infants was evidence of hyperresponsivity rather than hypersensitivity to sound.

Als, Lester, and Brazelton (1979) have described in detail the responses to auditory stimulation of a preterm infant of 34 weeks conceptional age. This infant responded in sleep to a rattle with gradual response decrement and did not awaken. Later, while awake, he turned a soft noise with visual fixation but startled to a loud sound.

From the various reports, we may conclude that the preterm infant responds behaviorally to loud sounds but inconsistently before 36 weeks conceptional age. Als *et al.* (1979) suggest that more careful observation of behavior of preterm infants to a greater variety of sounds, including the human voice, and at a lower level may reveal more responsiveness that has so far been reported.

Cortical auditory evoked potentials have been obtained from the youngest viable preterm infants of 25 weeks gestation. The evoked potentials of these infants is a single negative wave (N_1) with a latency of 180–270 msec, sometimes followed by a positive wave (P_2) at 600–900 msec. By 35 weeks conceptional age, the latencies of these waves decrease to 150–200 for N_1 and 250–350 for P_2 and an N_2 wave of 500–600 msec latency forms at term, 40 weeks conceptional age. At term, about 20% of the infants also have a P_1 component with a latency of 50–120 msec. These P_1, N_1, P_2, N_2 components are those usually seen in older children and adults but have longer latencies at term, (see Figures 7.1 and 7.2) (Akiyama, Schulte, Schultz, & Parmelee, 1969, Barnet, Ohlrich, Weiss, & Shanks, 1975; Engel, 1967; Weitzman & Graziani, 1968).

In recent years, auditory brain-stem evoked potentials have been studied in preterm infants, (see Figure 7.3). As with cortical evoked responses, there is a rapid decrease in latency for all wave components between 28 and 36 weeks conceptional age, with a smaller decrease from 36 to 44 weeks (Hecox & Galambos, 1974; Schulman-Galambos & Galambos, 1975; Starr, Amlie, Martin & Sanders, 1977). These changes in latency are the same for the infants born at 28–30 weeks gestation and followed longitudinally to 44 weeks conceptional age and newly born preterm infants at comparable conceptional ages (see Figure 7.4). This indicates that these latency changes are not enhanced or delayed by environmental experiences. Higher decibel levels were needed to obtain any responses at all in two preterm infants born before 28 weeks (Starr *et al.,* 1977).

Schulte, Stennert, Wulbrand, and Eichorn (1977) studied the ontogeny of cortical auditory evoked potentials in preterm infants followed longitudinally and compared these with newly born preterm infants of comparable conceptional age. No consistent differences in waveform or latency could be found between the two groups.

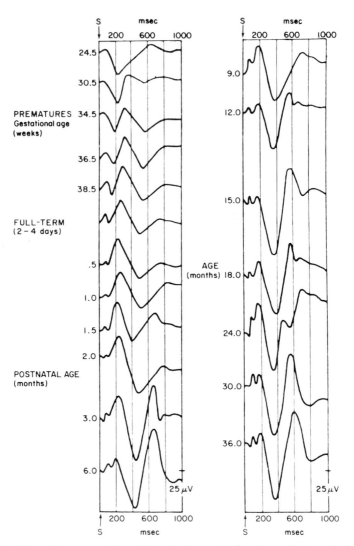

FIGURE 7.1. *Schematic representation of the development of vertex auditory evoked potentials from pre-term 24.5 weeks conceptional age to 3 years. Upward deflection is positive at vertex electrode and downward negative. (From Barnet, Ohlrich, Weiss, & Shanks, 1975.)*

Schulman (1969) obtained heart rate responses to auditory stimulation of 80 dB in three of four infants as early as 29–32 weeks conceptional age but not until 35 weeks for one infant. All responses were acceleratory during sleep at all ages, but some infants responded with decelerations of heart rate during wakefulness by 36 weeks gestation. This latter observation was not confirmed by Berkson, Wasserman, and Behrman (1974).

Lennard, Schulte, Eichorn, Meyer, and Busse (1977) studied heart rate re-

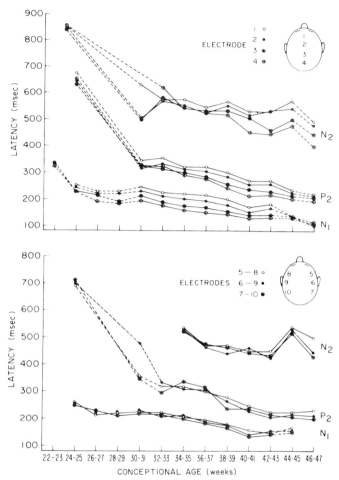

FIGURE 7.2. *Change in peak latencies in msec for three cortical auditory evoked potential waves* N_1, P_2, N_2. *(From Weitzman & Graziani, 1968.)*

sponses to auditory stimuli in preterm infants followed longitudinally and observed less heart rate response as the infants matured when compared with newly born preterm infants of comparable conceptional ages. They interpreted this difference to be the result of environmental experiences in the longitudinal group. At least in this parameter, there may be some evidence for environmental influences on auditory responses in preterm infants.

Infants after term, 40 weeks conceptional age, have rapidly growing auditory competence that is far greater than that of the fetus *in utero* or of preterm infants. Young infants in the first weeks past term respond consistently and with a greater variety of behavioral responses. They show some selectivity for the frequency range and patterning of human speech sounds.

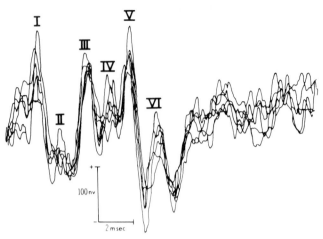

FIGURE 7.3. *Auditory brain-stem potential from a normal term infant at 40 weeks gestation measured six times in 2 hours. Six distinct components designated I-VI can be identified. Click rate 10/sec; click intensity 65 dB sensation level. Positivity at vertex electrode. (From Starr, Amlie, Martin, & Sanders, 1977. Copyright American Academy of Pediatrics 1977.)*

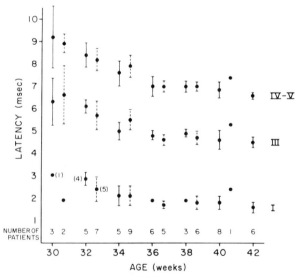

FIGURE 7.4. *Comparison of mean latencies at 65 dB sensation level of major waves between gestational age group tested at birth and conceptional age group tested several weeks after birth at comparable ages. Solid lines show gestational age group; broken lines show conceptional age group. One standard deviation of the mean is indicated by bars; numbers in parentheses indicate number of infants, with clearly defined components of total group tested indicated at lower part of graph. (From Starr, Amlie, Martin, & Sanders, 1977. Copyright American Academy of Pediatrics 1977.)*

134

Within a few months after term, infants can habituate rapidly to repeated sounds and discriminate fine differences in speech sounds. They also show marked maturational changes in electroencephalographic characteristics, auditory evoked potentials, and heart rate responses. At this level of auditory and general competence, it is possible to demonstrate more clearly persisting influences from environment inputs (Berg & Berg, 1979; Butterfield & Cairns, 1976; Eisenberg, 1976; Graziani, Korberly, & D'Amato, 1977; Morse, 1974).

The fetus or preterm infant of 25–26 weeks conceptional age may show some response to sound behaviorally and in heart rate, but these responses are inconsistent. Cortical and brain-stem evoked potentials are also present but have long latencies and incomplete forms. There is, however, rapid improvement in all these characteristics to 36 weeks conceptional age, with more gradual changes thereafter to term and beyond. Studies comparing preterm infants followed longitudinally from 28 to 30 weeks gestation with later born preterms and term infants at comparable conceptional ages have not yet demonstrated environmental influences on the ontogenetic changes at least to 36 weeks conceptional age. This is surprising considering the apparently noise-polluted environment of the preterm nursery.

It is, of course, possible that our measures are still inadequate to detect changes that may be occurring. Certainly, studies with preterm infants have not paid close attention to the characteristics of the auditory stimuli that have been recognized as critical in studies of older infants.

It is also possible that the nervous system of the very immature preterm infant does not respond sufficiently to be readily influenced by the environment. This possibility will be elaborated in the following sections.

Anatomical Development of the Human Auditory System

There is limited information concerning the development of the human auditory system. The earliest studies were concerned with the development of the bony structures of the inner and middle ear and the general contour of the cochlea. These develop rapidly in fetal life to nearly adult proportions (Bast & Anson 1949). The statoacoustic system in the brain stem, including the vestibular and cochlear system, tectospinal tract, and inferior colliculi, myelinate early, starting about the fifth fetal month, with complete myelination by the middle of the ninth month (Yakovlev & Lecours, 1967). These two observations have stimulated considerable speculation concerning the early and complete functioning of the auditory system.

On the other hand, the cochlea is slow to develop microscopic structures considered important to auditory function (Selnes & Whitaker, 1976), and auditory radiation paths to the cortex have protracted myelination well beyond the end of the first year after birth (Yakovlev & Lecours, 1967).

Light microscopy of the human cochlea was done by Bredberg (1967) in fetuses of 2½, 3, 4, and 6 months gestation and in term infants. At 6 months, the microscopic structure is still in evolution but is considered complete at term. Illustrated by Tuchman–Duplessis, David, and Haegel (1972) in Figure 7.5 are the cochlear ducts of a 5 month embryo and a term infant. Nakai (1970) provided electron microscopic studies of the cochleas from 5–6-month-old human fetuses. He concludes that "the organ of corti in the 6 month fetus has not begun to carry out its auditory function yet because auditory function does not begin before the pillars separate to form the tunnel of corti and the arrival of the efferent nerve endings [p. 264]." Selnes and Whitaker (1976) indicate the organ of corti is fully developed at about 8 months with respect to the pattern of sensory and supporting cells and fluid spaces. They state "the question of the onset of functional maturity of the organ of corti is not clear [p. 131]." They cite the delay until 3–5 weeks after birth in detachment of the tectorial membrane at its outer edge to the long microvilli of Deiter's cells in the kitten cochlea and point out that there is no available information concerning the time at which the tectorial membrane in the human fetus and infant becomes detached. There is also very little information concerning the structural maturation of the cells and their synaptic connections to the various nuclei of the human auditory pathway.

Hecox (1975) in his review states "the gross structural features of the inner ear are attained by the sixth month of intrauterine life. While certain structural details such as the formation of spaces within the organ of corti are known to change up to the time of birth [p. 162]." He also states that additional information is needed concerning hair cell maturation and the geometry between hair cells, tectorial membrane, and basilar membrane to determine the role played by the immaturity of cochlear structure in the reduced responsivity of infants to auditory stimuli.

The middle ear ossicular chain reaches adult proportions by 6–8 months gestation, and transfer efficiency of the ossicles may be mature. On the other hand, adult dimensions of the middle ear cavity, tympanic membrane, and external auditory canal are not found until 1 year or more after birth. These changes produce some shifts in resonance and transfer function of the middle ear and impedance matching properties of the middle ear.

While myelination studies of the auditory nerve describe it as well myelinated at term birth, detailed studies of the components of the nerve are not sufficiently known to explain function. It does appear that peripheral transducers lag behind neural elements in development in humans as well as in kittens.

The long latencies of auditory evoked potentials and the high threshold sensitivity of the preterm infant can be explained by limited function at all levels from the transducers to the cortex.

The limited information we have of the development of the human auditory system is confusing. Some portions develop rapidly in fetal life, particularly

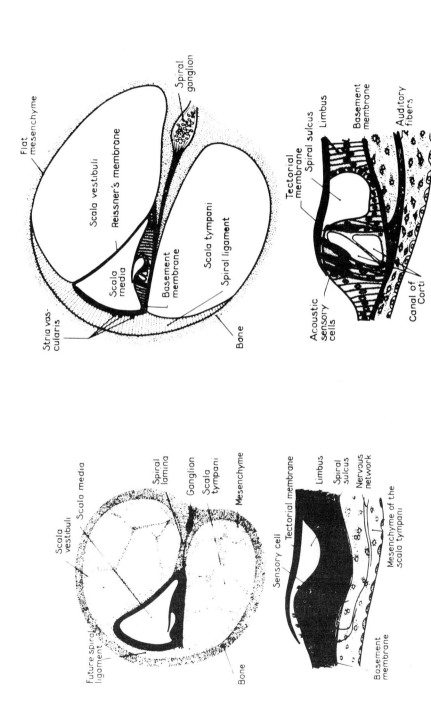

FIGURE 7.5. Differentiation of cochlear duct. Left: embryo of 5 months. Right: at term. (From Tuchmann-Duplessis, David, & Haegel, 1972.)

the bone structure for the cochlea and middle ear. Portions of the auditory nerve and brain-stem pathways myelinate early. On the other hand, the microphonic tranducer components of the organ of corti develop slowly and may be incomplete until term or later. Also the auditory radiation pathway to the cortex slowly myelinates long after term birth.

We have practically no details concerning the neurophysiological development of the system except for brain-stem and cortical auditory evoked potentials. These have long latencies and high stimulation thresholds in preterm infants. We need to turn to animal models to try to gain further insight to maturational changes in function. The kitten is a good model and is being actively studied. Some of these studies will be discussed in the next section.

Development of the Auditory System in the Kitten

According to Pujol and Marty (1970), at birth the otic capsule of the kitten has reached its final size, but only the first coil of the lamina spiralis is ossified (see Figure 7.6). Histologically, most of the components of the adult organ can be identified in an immature state. The cochlea matures from the base at birth. There the hair cells are present, but few features differentiate internal from external hair cells with no visible intercellular space. The tunnel of the corti is not yet differentiated. Near the apex, the hair cells can barely be distinguished from the mass of pseudostratified cells, and the basilar membrane is still very thick.

About 12 days after birth, the base of the cochlea is mature. The external hair cells are clearly separated by intercellular spaces, and the internal hair cells have matured. The tunnel of corti shows its adult form (see Figure 7.7). By 15 days, the apex of the cochlea is mature in appearance.

At birth, the neural components of the cochlea have a myelin sheath, but the neurons appear immature in arrangement and contour. Nevertheless, they are more mature in development than the epithelial elements of the cochlea and continue to mature more rapidly.

Pujol and Marty (1970) state that the cochlea becomes responsive to auditory stimulation about 3 days after birth. Marty (1967) observed that cortical evoked potentials can be obtained in the kitten at birth by stimulation of the auditory nerve. Thus, the central nervous system is responsive to stimulation befor the transducer, the cochlea. Pujol and Marty (1970) state that the important changes in the cochlea in the first 3 days are the differentiation of the tunnel of corti and the space of Nuel, lengthening of the external hair cells, and freeing of the internal spiral sulcus.

Neurophysiological studies demonstrate a rapid decrease during the first 15 days in latencies of cochlear nerve and cochlear nucleus evoked responses to auditory stimuli (see Figures 7.8 and 7.9). There are also marked changes in the response characteristics during this period. At 3 days, the responses

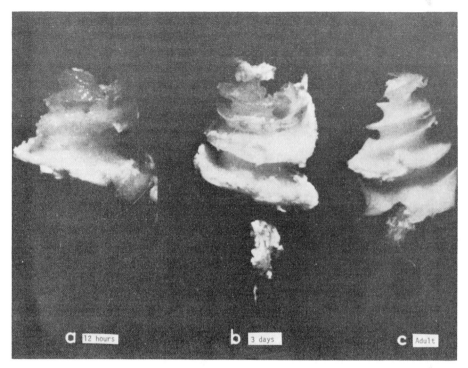

FIGURE 7.6. *Development of the modiolus and lamina spiralis of the cochlea in the cat. (a) Age 12 hours. (b) Age 3 days. (c) Adult. (From Marty, 1967.)*

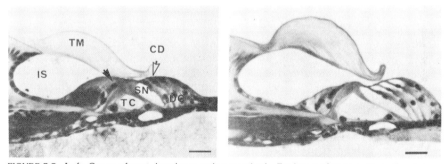

FIGURE 7.7. *Left: Organ of corti, basal turn in kitten at birth. Evidence of immaturity in the absence of spaces around the outer hair cells and the relative squatness of Deiter's cells and the primitive cells still associated with the inner hair cells. Right: Organ of corti, middle turn in a kitten of 15 days. Complete anatomical differentiation has just been attained. CD, cochlear duct; DC, Deiter's cells; IS, internal nucleus; SN, space of Nuel; TC, tunnel of corti; TM, tectorial membrane; solid arrow, inner hair cell; open arrow, outer hair cells. Marker, 40 μm. (From Bosher, 1975.)*

139

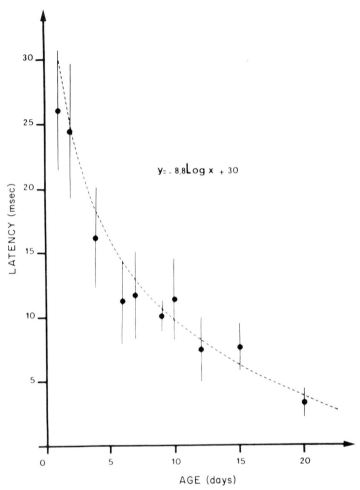

FIGURE 7.8. *Latencies of unit activity in the cochlear nerve to auditory stimulation in the kitten from 1 to 20 days. (Carlier, Abonnenc, & Pujol, 1975.)*

recorded to a 500 msec stimulus are weak, brief, and only at the onset. By 10 days, the responses persist during the stimulus period but in periodic bursts, and the spike intervals are variable. At 15–20 days, the responses are sustained during the stimulus period, and the spike intervals are short and uniform (see Figure 7.10). (Carlier, Abonnenc, & Pujol, 1975; Pujol, 1976; Romand & Marty, 1975). In a study of the tonotopic organization of the inferior colliculus of the kitten, Aitkin and Moore (1975) observed a sharp drop in threshold sensitivity to auditory stimulation between 11 and 22 days and an increasing range of the frequency responses, particularly for the higher frequencies (see Figure 7.11).

Buchwald (this volume) has described similar maturational changes in the

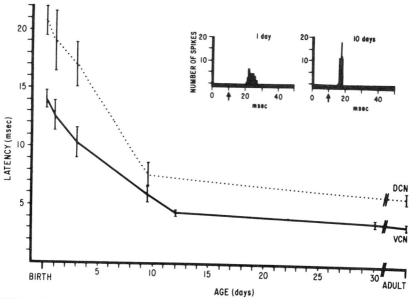

FIGURE 7.9. *Development in the latency of the first spike recorded in the ventral cochlear nucleus (VCN) and the Dorsal Cochlear Nucleus (DCN) in the cat from birth to adult. In upper right corner are two examples of latency histograms showing the variation in latency between two cells of kittens of 1 and 10 days. Each histogram corresponds to 50 stimulations and arrow indicates onset of stimulation. (From Romand & Marty, 1975.)*

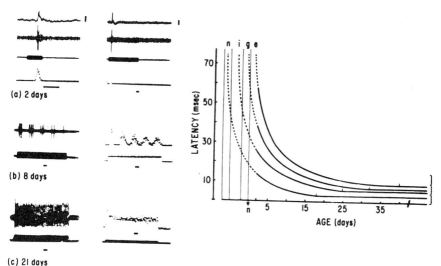

(a) 2 days

(b) 8 days

(c) 21 days

FIGURE 7.10. *Two physiological criteria for evaluation of the maturation of the auditory system in the kitten. Left: Maturation of unit responses in the cochlear nerve. The response to a sound of long duration is (a) only an "on" response at 2 days with wide distribution of spikes; (b) an intermittent rhythmic response at 8 days; (c) continuous response at 21 days. Sound duration in (a) is 500 msec and in (b) and (c) 800 msec. Right: Decrease in latencies to auditory evoked potentials in different places in the auditory path in the kitten. (n) Cochlear nucleus. (i) Inferior colliculus. (g) Medial geniculate. (e) Cerebral cortex. (From Pujol, 1970.)*

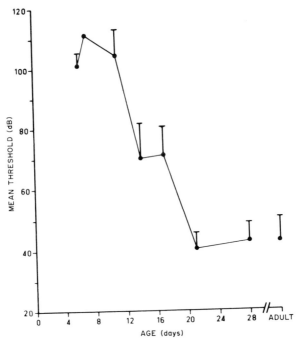

Figure 7.11. *Mean threshold in decibels sound pressure level and standard deviations required to elicit unit responses for best frequencies in cells in the inferior colliculus of kittens from 5 to 28 days. (From Aitkin & Moore, 1975.)*

latencies and response charateristics of brain-stem evoked potentials in the kitten from birth to 28 days. Studies of the auditory cortical evoked potentials in kittens have also demonstrated the long latencies of all the components in the 4–8 day-old kitten. These decrease rapidly to about 21 days of age (see Figure 7.12). The form of the waves is immature at birth, in that it is predominantly negative. There are progressive changes to term, with development of several positive and negative components (see Figure 7.13) (Ellingson & Wilcott, 1960; Marty, 1967).

The maturation of these characteristics of cortical evoked potentials of the kitten in the first 21 days is similar in the preterm infant from 25 weeks gestation to term, 40 weeks conceptional age.

In the kitten, the auditory transducer, the cochlea, places major limits on the early reception of sound. At birth, no responses can be obtained central to the cochlea. When the responses first appear at 1–2 days, loud stimuli are required, and the unit responses in the cochlear nucleus have a long latency, are brief, and occur only at the onset of sound. With maturation, the latencies and thresholds decrease and the responses become more prolonged though at first variable. These changes take place in the first 2–3 weeks. Similarly, there are maturational changes in the brain-stem and cortical evoked responses to

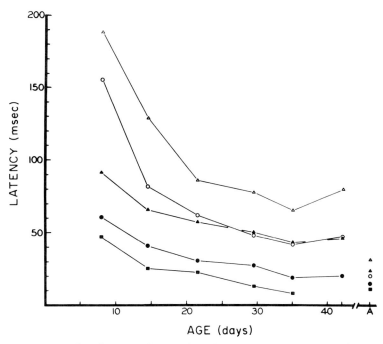

FIGURE 7.12. *Relationship of age to auditory and visual evoked response latencies in kittens. Closed symbols, auditory; open symbols, visual. (From Ellingson & Wilcott, 1960.)*

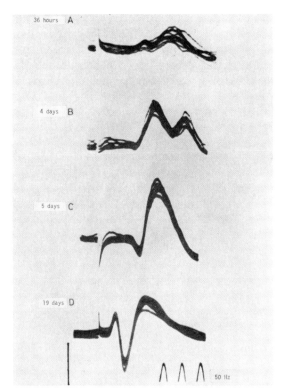

FIGURE 7.13. *Postnatal development of the cortical response to electrical stimulation of the auditory nerve in the kitten. (A) 36 hours; (B) 4 days; (C) 5 days; (D) 19 days. Upward deflection negative and downward positive. Time marker 50 Hz; amplitude marker 200 μv. (From Marty, 1967.)*

143

auditory stimuli. These consist of decreases in stimulus thresholds, latencies of responses, and "fatiguability," to repeated stimulation. This maturation occurs somewhat more slowly than the cochlear changes over the first 3–4 weeks.

The changes described during the first 3 weeks of the kitten's life parallel the developmental changes in the auditory system of the human preterm infant from 25 weeks gestation to term. This may explain the delay in behavioral responsiveness of the very early preterm infants to auditory stimulation.

Neurophysiological Organization and Behavioral Development in Kittens and Infants

Similar neurophysiological and behavioral maturational changes take place in several systems in the kitten in the first 3 postnatal weeks and in the preterm infant during 12–15 weeks before term. The visual system in both kittens and preterm infants is more immature than the auditory system initially but matures more rapidly. Other systems have not been studied sufficiently for comparison, though there is some information on the somesthetic system in the kitten. It is the most mature system at birth in the kitten and matures slowly. Scherrer (1974) has compared the latencies of cortical evoked potentials for auditory, visual, and somesthetic systems in kittens and finds they converge to equivalent ratios of adult levels around the third week (see Figure 7.14). He feels that the slow spleed of central processing of all input limits the information content and behavioral significance of environmental stimuli.

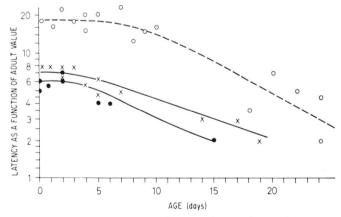

FIGURE 7.14. *Latencies of afferent signals as a function of age in the cat. Age is expressed as days along the abscissa and latency as multiples of the adult value along the ordinate. Electrical stimulation to the optic nerve, open circle; to the auditory nerve, x; to the somesthetic nerve, closed circle. (From Scherrer, 1974.)*

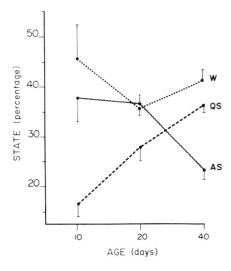

FIGURE 7.15. *Sleep-waking state distribution during kitten development. Mean state percentage and standard error in 10, 20, and 40 day kittens. W, wake; QS, quiet sleep; AS, active sleep. (From McGinty, Stevenson, Hoppenbrowers, Harper, Sterman, & Hodgman, 1977.)*

Of interest to me is the parallel organization of states of arousal and sleep in kittens from birth to 3 weeks and in preterm infants from 25–28 weeks gestation to term. For both, there is no recognizable state organization at birth. Two weeks postnatally in the kitten and at 35–37 weeks conceptional age in the human infant, state organization begins to be recognizable, and by 3 weeks in the kitten and term in the infant, sleep states are fairly well organized and stable (see Figures 7.15 and 7.16). (McGintly, Stevenson, Hoppenbrowers, Harper, Sterman, & Hodgman, 1977; Parmelee & Stern 1972;

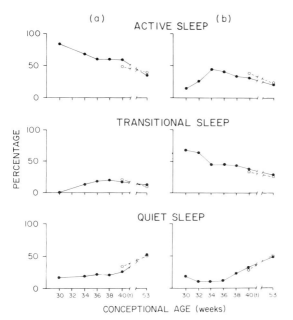

FIGURE 7.16. *Development of distribution of sleep states in preterm and term infants in 3-hour interfeeding polygraphic recordings— 40 (t) week conceptional age is term and 53 weeks is 3 months past term. Solid line shows preterm infants; broken line shows term infants. (From Parmelee, Wenner, Akiyama, Schultz, & Stern, 1967.)*

Parmelee, Wenner, Akiyama, Schultz, & Stern, 1967) At these ages, both kittens and preterm infants also become more responsive to visual and auditory stimuli, neurophysiologically and behaviorally.

Organization of states of sleep and arousal is not necessarily causally related to the responsiveness of kittens or infants to their environment. It may well be, however, a reasonable index of the level of central nervous system cybernetic networks necessary for significant interaction of the kitten or infant with the environment (Parmelee & Sigman, 1976).

General Discussion

From the standpoint of a long-term impact of auditory stimulation on neurophysiological and behavioral development, it may be important to distinguish between the initial simplest form of response of the auditory system to intense stimulation and some later stage in development when responsiveness is more complex and more easily obtained.

In the kitten, auditory responses can be obtained at some levels of the auditory system at birth or soon after. However, these initial responses are only at the onset of an intense stimulus, and the latencies at all levels of the system are long. There is also an inability to respond to rapidly repeated stimulation. Within the first 2–3 weeks, these inadequacies of the system rapidly change. The unit responses in the cochlear nucleus and inferior colliculus become more regular and sustained to a continuous stimulus and are responsive to rapidly repeated stimuli and at lower thresholds of intensity of stimulation. Latencies of responses recorded at all levels from cochlear nerve to cortex rapidly decrease to near-adult levels. These changes in the auditory system are coincidental with similar changes in the visual system (Parmelee & Sigman, 1976). Scherrer (1974) has indicated that the slow responsiveness of the neonatal kitten's central nervous system to stimulation markedly limits the impact and significance of the stimulus.

Further, as has been pointed out, there is a coincidental development of sleep state organization in the kitten during the first 2–3 weeks that probably reflects the development of feedback systems at all levels of the nervous system. It is at least concurrent with rapid dendritic development at all levels of the nervous system as well as with the development of interconnecting short axon neurons, particularly in the cortex (see Figure 7.17).

There is much less information concerning the neurophysiological development of the auditory system in the infant. The information we have from preterm infants from 25 weeks gestation to term demonstrates changes parallel to those in the kitten in the first 3 postnatal weeks. This is particularly evident in the decrease in brain-stem and cortical evoked potentials and the drop in stimulus threshold. The organization of sleep states in preterm infants also parallels that in the kitten in the same time period. In addition,

Inferior Colliculus   Auditory Cortex

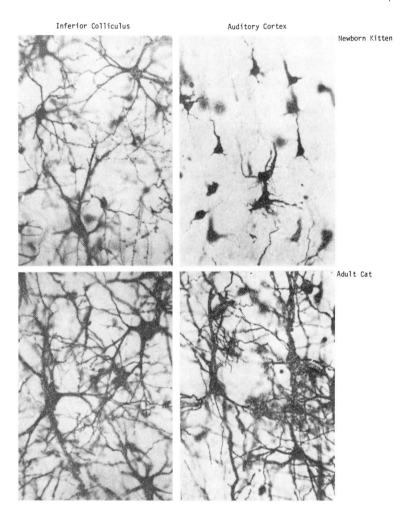

FIGURE 7.17. *Maturational changes in the inferior colliculus and auditory cerebral cortex in the cat. Note the development of dendritic branching and short axon neurons. Left: inferior colliculus. Right: auditory cerebral cortex; top, newborn kitten; bottom; adult cat. (From Pujol, 1976.)*

neuroanatomical studies of dentritic and short axon neuron development in the cortex are similar in preterm infants and kittens in this period (Parmelee & Sigman, 1976).

These similarities of the auditory system and other neurophysiological parameters between the kitten from birth to 3 weeks postnatally and the preterm infant from 25 to 40 weeks conceptional age may allow us to use the more detailed information from the kitten to attempt to explain some of our observations in preterm infants. In particular, they may explain in part why we can find so little impact of the noise-polluted environment of the nursery on the neurophysiological and behavioral development of the preterm infant. This is especially true from 25 to 35 weeks conceptional age. At the latter age, sleep states begin to become organized in the preterm infants and they might become more vulnerable to the noise pollution of the nursery. However, most preterm infants are currently sent home from the nursery at about this age.

Future studies that provide us with many of the details now missing are likely to alter the sequence of some of the development and the behavioral outcomes as described. Still it may remain useful to consider the possibility that some level of neurophysiological functioning more complex than that at the onset of response is necessary before significant impact of the environment on development can be expected.

References

Aitkin, L. M., & Moore, D. R. Inferior colliculus. II. Development of tuning characteristics and tonotopic organization in central nucleus of the neonatal cat. *Journal of Neurophysiology,* 1975, *38,* 1208–1216.

Akiyama, Y., Schulte, F. J., Schultz, M. A., & Parmelee, A. H., Jr. Acoustically evoked responses in premature and full term newborn infants. *Electroencephalography and Clinical Neurophysiology,* 1969, *26,* 371–380.

Als, H., Lester, M. B., & Brazelton, T. B. Dynamics of the behavioral organization of the premature infant: A theoretical perspective. In T. Field, S. Goldberg, A. Sostek, & H. H. Shuman (Eds.), *The high risk newborn.* New York: Spectrum, 1979.

Barnet, A. B., Ohlrich, E. S., Weiss, I. P., & Shanks, B. Auditory evoked potentials during sleep in normal children from ten days to three years of age. *Electroencephalography Clinical Neurophsiology,* 1975, *39,* 29–41.

Bast, C. H., & Anson, B. J. *The temporal bone and the ear.* Springfield, Ill.: Thomas, 1949.

Beckwith, L., Cohen, S. E., Kopp, C. B., Parmelee, A. H., & Marcy, T. G. Caregiver–infant interaction and early cognitive development in pre-term infants. *Child Development,* 1976, *47,* 579.

Beckwith, L., Sigman, M., Cohen, S. E., & Parmelee, A. H. Vocal output in pre-term infants. *Developmental Psychobiology,* 1977, *10,* 543–554.

Bench, J., & Parker, A. Hyper-responsivity to sounds in the short-gestation baby. *Developmental Medicine Child Neurology,* 1971, *13,* 15–19.

Bench, R. J., & Vass, A. Fetal audiometry. *The Lancet,* 1970, *1,* 91–92.

Berg, W. K., & Berg, K. M. Psychophysiological development in infancy: State, sensory function and attention. In J. Osofsky (Ed.), *Handbook of infant development.* New York: Wiley, 1979.

Berkson, G., Wasserman, G. A., & Behrman, R. Heart rate response to an auditory stimulus in premature infants. *Developmental Psychobiology,* 1974, *11,* 244–246.

Blennow, G., Svenningsen, N. W., & Almquist, B. Noise levels in infant incubators (Adverse effects?). *Pediatrics,* 1974, *53,* 29–32.

Bosher, S. K. Morphological and functional changes in the cochlea associated with the inception of hearing. In R. J. Bench, A. Pye, & J. D. Pye (Eds.), *Sound reception in mammals.* Symposia of the Zoological Society of London, No. 37. London: Academic Press, 1975.

Bredberg, G. The human cochlea during development and aging. *Journal of Laryngology and Otology,* 1967, *81,* 739–758.

Butterfield, E. C., & Cairns, G. G., The infant's auditory environment. In T. D. Tjossem (Ed.),

Intervention strategies for high risk infants and young children. Baltimore: University Park 1976.

Carlier, E., Abonnenc, M., & Pujol, R. Maturation des réponses unitaires à la stimulation tonale dans le nerf cochléaire du chaton. *Journal de Physiologie.* (Paris), 1975, *70*, 129-138.

Cohen, S. E., & Beckwith, L. Caregiver behaviors and early cognitive development as related to ordinal position in pre-term infants. *Child Development,* 1977, *48,* 152-157.

Cohen, S. E., Beckwith, L., & Parmelee, A. H. Receptive language development in pre-term infants as related to caregiver–child interaction. *Pediatrics,* 1978, *61,* 1620.

Committee on Environmental Hazards of the American Academy of Pediatrics. Noise pollution: Neonatal aspects. *Pediatrics,* 1974, *54,* 476-479.

DeHirsch, K., Jansky, J. J., & Langford, W. S. The oral language performance of prematurely born children and controls. *Journal of Speech and Hearing Disorders,* 1964, *29,* 60-69.

Eisenberg, R. B. *Auditory competency in early life: The roots of communicative behavior.* Baltimore: University Park, 1976.

Ellingson, R. J., & Wilcott, R. C. Development of evoked responses in the visual and auditory cortices of kittens. *Journal of Neurophysiology,* 1960, *23,* 363-375.

Engel, R. Electroencephalographic responses to sounds and light in premature and full term neonates. *The Journal-Lancet,* 1967, *87,* 181-186.

Fleischer, J. Utersuchungen zur Entwiklung der Innenohr funktion: Intrauterine Kindesbewegungen nach Schallreizen. *Zeitschrift fur Laryngologie, Rhinologie, Otologie,* 1955, *34,* 733-740.

Gessell, A., & Amatruda, C. S. *The embryology of behavior.* New York: Harper, 1945.

Graziani, L. J., Korberly, B., & D'Amato, G. Brain and behavior in the neonatal period. In M. E. Blaw, I. Ropin, & M. Kinsbourne (Eds.), *Topics in child neurology.* New York: Spectrum, 1977.

Hecox, K. Electrophysiological correlates of human auditory development. In L. B. Cohen & P. Salapatek (Eds.), *Infant perception: From sensation to cognition* (Vol. 2), *Perception of space, speech, and sound.* New York: Academic Press, 1975.

Hecox, K., & Galambos, R. Brain stem auditory evoked responses in human infants and adults. *Archives of Orolaryngology,* 1974, *99,* 30-33.

Johansson, B., Wedenberg, E., & Westin, B. Measurement of tone response by the human fetus. *Acta oto-laryngology,* 1964, *57,* 188-192.

Lawson, K., Daum, C., & Turkewitz, G. Environmental characteristics of a neonatal intensive care unit. *Child Development,* 1977, *48,* 1633-1639.

Lenard, H. G., Schulte, F. J., Eichorn, W., Meyer, S., & Busse, C. Die Entwicklung sensorischer Funktionen bei Fruhgeborenen in den ersten Lebens wachen. *Mschr. Kinderheilkunde,* 1977, *125,* 383-385.

McGinty, D. J., Stevenson, M., Hoppenbrowers, T., Harper, R. M., Sterman, M. B., & Hodgman, J. Polygraphic studies of kitten development: Sleep state patterns. *Developmental Psychobiology,* 1977, *10,* 455-469.

Marty, R. Maturation post-natale du système auditif. In A. Minkowski (Ed.), *Regional development of the brain in early life.* Oxford: Blackwell, 1967.

Monod, N., & Garma, L. Auditory responsivity in the human premature. *Biology of the Neonate,* 1971, *17,* 292-316.

Morse, P. A. Infant speech perception: A preliminary model and review of the literature. In R. L. Schiefebusch & L. L. Lloyd. (Eds.), *Language perspectives—acquisition, retardation and intervention.* Baltimore: University Park, 1974.

Murphy, K. P., & Smyth, C. N. Response of foetus to auditory stimulation. *The Lancet,* 1962, *1* (pt. 2) 972-973.

Nakai, Y. An electron microscopic study of the human fetus cochlea. *Practice oto-rhino-laryngology,* 1970, *32,* 257-267.

Neligan, G. A., Kolvin, I., Scott, D. McL., & Garside, R. F. *Born Too Soon or Born Too Small.* Philadelphia: Lippincott, 1976.

O'Connor, M. J. A comparison of preterm and full-term infants on parameters of habituation at 4 months and performance on the Bayley Scales of Infant Development at 18 Months. *Child Development,* 1980, in press.

Parmelee, A. H., Neurophysiological and behavioral organization of premature infants in the first months of life. *Biological Psychiatry,* 1975, *10,* 501–512.

Parmelee, A. H., & Sigman, M. Development of visual behavior and neurological organization in pre-term and full-term infants. In A. D. Pick (Ed.), *Minnesota symposia on child psychology* (Vol. 10). Minneapolis: Univ. of Minnesota Press, 1976.

Parmelee, A. H., & Stern, E. Development of states in infants. In C. Clemente, D. Purpura, & F. Meyer (Eds.), *Sleep and the maturing nervous system.* New York: Academic Press, 1972.

Parmelee, A. H., Jr., Wenner, W. H., Akiyama, Y., Schultz, M., & Stern, E. Sleep states in premature infants. *Developmental Medicine and Child Neurology,* 1967, *9,* 70–77.

Pujol, R. Maturation du système auditif. *Revue de Laryngologie,* 1976. *97* (Suppl 1976), 551–562.

Pujol, R., & Marty, R. Postnatal maturation in the cochlea of the cat. *Journal of Comparative Neurology,* 1970, *139,* 115–126.

Romand, R., & Marty, R. Postnatal maturation of the cochlear nuclei in the cat: A neurophysiological study. *Brain Research,* 1975, *83,* 225–233.

Scherrer, J. Electrophysiologie et ontogenèse du système nerveux. In S. R. Berenberg, M. Caniaris, & N. P. Masse (Eds.), *Pre- and postnatal development of the human brain.* Basel: Karger, 1974.

Schulman, C. Effects of auditory stimulation on heart rate in premature infants as a function of level of arousal, probability of CNS damage, and conceptional age. *Developmental Psychobiology,* 1969, *2,* 172–183.

Schulman-Galambos, C., & Galambos, R. Brain stem auditory evoked responses in premature infants. *Journal of Speech and Hearing Research,* 1975, *18,* 456–465.

Schulte, F. J., & Stennart, E. Hearing defects in pre-term infants. *Archives of Disease in Childhood,* 1978, *53,* 269–270.

Schulte, F. J., Stennert, E., Wulbrand, H., Eichorn, W., & Lenard, H. G. The ontogeny of sensory perception in pre-term infants. *European Journal of Pediatrics,* 1977, *126,* 211–224.

Seleny, F. L., & Streczyn, M. Noise characteristics in the baby compartment of incubators. *American Journal of Diseases of Children,* 1969, *117,* 445–450.

Selnes, O. A., & Whitaker, H. A. Morphological and functional development of the auditory system. In R. W. Rieber (Ed.), *The neurophysiology of language: Essays in honor of Eric Lennenberg.* New York: Plenum, 1976.

Sontag, L. W., Steele, W. G., & Lewis, M. The fetal and maternal cardiac response to environmental stress. *Human Development,* 1969, *12,* 1–9.

Starr, A., Amlie, R. N., Martin, W. H., & Sanders, S. Development of auditory function in newborn infants revealed by auditory brain stem potentials. *Pediatrics,* 1977, *60,* 831–839.

Stirnimann, E. *Psychologies des Neugeborenen Kindes.* Zurich: Rascher, 1940.

Tuchmann-Duplessis, H., David, G., & Haegel, P. *Illustrated human embryology* (Vol. 3), *Nervous system and endocrine glands.* New York: Springer Verlag, 1972.

Verley, R. Essai sur les critères électrophysiologiques qui permettraient de comparer entre elles les évolutions de diverses espèces, en particulier de l'homme. In S. R. Berenberg, M. Caniaris, & N. P. Masse (Eds.), *Pre- and postnatal development of the human brain.* Basel: Karger, 1974.

Weitzman, E. D., & Graziani, L. J. Maturation and topography of the auditory evoked response of the prematurely born infant. *Developmental Psychobiology,* 1968, *1,* 79–89.

Yakovlev, P., & Lecours, A. The myelogenetic cycles of regional maturation of the brain. In A Minkowski (Ed.), *Regional development of the brain in early life.* Oxford: Blackwell, 1967.

8

Comparative Development of Feline and Human Cerebral Cortex: A Review of Chapters 5-7

DOMINICK P. PURPURA

The central dogma of developmental neurobiology may be summarized in the view: "Neurons make synapses and synapses make behavior." Developmental psychobiologists might add the corollary phrase, "and behavior modifies neurons." Whichever ideology is espoused, what really counts is what one believes to be the relationship between neurons and the emergence of complex behaviors in higher organisms such as mammals. Most developmental neuropsychobiologists would ascribe to the belief that it is simply a matter of time, and considerably more effort, before the development and elaboration of behavior is understood in terms of the distributed properties of neuronal aggregates. Until then, one has little choice but to collect and validate new data, which can be used to formulate new and hopefully testable hypotheses. There is much to be said for this approach, particularly since it rejects dualism and other hazardous detours to progress.

Many developmental data have been collected and summarized in the preceding chapters by Rose, Buchwald, and Parmelee. Their concern with the morphological and physiological basis of sensory processing in the immature nervous systems of the cat and the human infant emphasizes the need for normative data in these species. As noted by several contributors to this volume, a vast literature has accumulated on developmental processes in laboratory animals, but there is a paucity of data on similar studies in the human preterm and full-term infant. Since considerable attention has been focused on developmental events in the kitten by Buchwald and Rose and in view of the concern of Parmelee and Friedman for information on the developmental status of the brain of the preterm human infant, it would seem appropriate to utilize this opportunity to summarize our studies on the comparative develop-

PRETERM BIRTH AND
PSYCHOLOGICAL DEVELOPMENT

ment of the cerebral cortex in the postnatal kitten and preterm human infant. The emphasis here will be on the extent to which structural features of immature cortex in these two mammalian species provide clues to the nature and origin of evoked potential waveforms, considered in detail by Rose, Buchwald, and Parmelee in the preceding chapters.

Our interest in the morphological substrate of evoked potential waveforms in the immature brain may be traced to earlier studies that suggested a predominant role of axodendritic excitatory and inhibitory synaptic activities in the genesis of spontaneous and evoked electrocortical potentials (Purpura, 1959). Because of the extraordinary complexity of the mature feline cerebral cortex, we turned to the immature brain for a preparation that would permit correlations of developmental alterations in evoked potentials with specific morphogenetic events in neurons.

One of the most interesting observations from these early ontogenetic studies was the finding that cortical pyramidal neurons in newborn kittens exhibit prominent apical dendrites but sparse basilar dendrites. Electron microscopy revealed the presence of axodendritic synapses on apical dendritic shafts, whereas direct cortical surface stimulation resulted in well-developed superficial negative responses. A conclusion derived from these morphophysiological studies in neonatal kittens was that superficial neocortical elements (axodendritic synaptic pathways related to apical dendritic shafts of deep-lying pyramidal neurons) were well developed at birth in the kitten and constituted the morphological substrate for surface-negative components of simple evoked potentials (Purpura, 1961). Progressive alterations in somatosensory evoked potentials in young kittens from long-latency cortical surface negativity (at birth) to a diphasic configuration (positive–negative) typical of the 2–3 week-old kitten correlated with elaboration of basilar dendrites of pyramidal cells, axospinodendritic synapse development, and further development of axosomatic synapses (Purpura, Shofer, Housepian, & Noback, 1964). This sequence of cortical synaptogenesis beginning with axodendritic (shaft) synapses then axospinodendritic and axosomatic synapses was suggested as a general principle of synaptogenesis in the mammalian brain.

A number of nagging problems persisted in our attempts to understand the functional properties of evoked potentials in the immature kitten brain. Several of the contributors to the preceding chapters have noted the low-frequency following of evoked potentials in the neonatal kitten, and others have described relatively long functional recovery cycles of evoked responses to repetitive stimulation in young laboratory animals and in the human infant. To explore the basis for these response properties of immature neurons, we undertook an extensive intracellular study of the physiological activities of immature feline neocortical and hippocampal pyramidal neurons (Purpura, Shofer, & Scarff, 1965; Purpura, Prelevic, & Santini, 1968). In these studies, low-frequency discharge characteristics of immature cortical neurons to intracellular and afferent stimulation were observed as well as large amplitude excitatory postsynaptic potentials. These findings taken together with observations of prominent and prolonged inhibitory postsynaptic potentials in cortical neurons of neonatal kittens provided important clues to the fundamental differences in the response properties of evoked potentials in early and late postnatal development in the kitten. Of greater significance, as it turned out, was the finding that dendrites of immature cortical neurons differed from mature cortical neurons in their capacity to generate partial and all-or-none spike potentials. These studies revealed a heterogeneity of membrane properties of dendrites and permitted analysis of the data in terms of a comparative electrogenesis of dendrites of different classes of neurons in different species (Purpura, 1967, 1972).

The ontogenetic studies summarized above provided a framework for our more recent morphophysiological studies of the visual cortex of the human preterm infant. In effect, we attempted to replicate the developmental sequences observed in the kitten in studies of human preterm infants. This required a major collaborative effort on the part of neuroscientists and neonatologists at the Rose F. Kennedy Center for Research in Mental Retardation and Human Development of the Albert Einstein College of Medicine in New York City.

The questions we sought to answer were precisely those raised in our earlier kitten studies. What is the maturational status of visual cortical neurons of the human preterm infant at the earliest stages in which visual evoked potentials (VEPs) are recordable? What is the time course of development of visual cortex neurons in the preterm infant, and how does this relate to evoked potential changes? What morphogenetic events in human immature cortex correlate with the early maturation of VEPs? Finally, a question that is of more than casual interest: Are alterations in VEPs observed in high-risk conditions related to morphological changes in underlying neuronal substrate?

Golgi studies of neurons in the primary visual cortex of the 25-week-old preterm infant may be summarized as follows: Well-developed apical dendrites are present on most pyramidal cells, particularly those of layers V and VI. Basilar dendrites are absent, and no dendritic spines are detectable. Nonpyramidal cells have poorly developed dendrites. With the exception of a few cells migrating along radial glial fibers and presumably destined for layer VI, virtually all the neurons the visual cortex will ever possess are present in the preterm infant at 25–26 weeks post-conceptional age (Purpura, 1975). The morphological picture observed at this developmental stage in the human infant is comparable to that of the neonatal kitten, as Parmelee (Chapter 7, this volume) has indicated. Indeed, the similarities also extend to the electrographic characteristics of flash-evoked VEPs. For at the time when apical dendrites and axonal elements in superficial cortex are identifiable in Golgi material, VEPs consist of an early cortical surface negativity, as is the case for the neonatal kitten.

Morphological maturation of cortical neurons and synapses in the kitten is complete by 30 days. Studies of visual cortex in the human preterm infant reveal a rather narrow temporal span for initial elaboration of cortical dendritic growth and synaptogenesis. Our studies indicate that the period of about 28–34 weeks conceptional age is a phase of rapid dendritic differentiation and synaptogenesis. All the features of the columnar organization of different cell types comprising a cortical "module" are present by 34 weeks, at which time spines are well developed on apical and basilar dendrites of pyramidal neurons and "spiny" stellate cells. During this period, the early component of the VEP is detectable as a surface positivity, and several electrographic features of VEPs acquire mature characteristics (Purpura, 1976).

The extent to which VEP alterations and morphogenetic events are causally related has been examined in several instances involving high-risk preterm infants with stormy postnatal courses and fatal outcomes. In these conditions, ranging from respiratory distress syndrome to overwhelming sepsis, VEPs exhibit either pronounced maturational delays or frankly bizarre electrographic configurations. Dramatic morphological alterations have been observed in visual cortex neurons under these varying high-risk conditions (Purpura, 1976). Despite the apparent relationship between the maturational status of cortical neurons and evoked potential waveforms generated by these elements, it is not possible to extrapolate from conditions with a fatal outcome to more subtle developmental perturbations of the perinatal period. Are there consistent identifiable changes in morphological events in the visual or auditory cortex of the preterm infant that are related to extrauterine environmental influences? Obviously, this question cannot be answered, since any condition that results in postmortem Golgi studies will surely obscure subtle morphological alterations attributable to extrauterine environmental factors per se.

What many developmental neurobiologists really want to know, one can imagine, is whether there is good reason to expect that aberrant behavioral development will be definable in terms of morphophysiological and biochemical parameters of brain operations and processes. The studies on structure–dysfunction relations in the visual cortex of preterm infants are tentative steps in this direction. However, we are on somewhat firmer ground with the possibility of identifying developmental abnormalities in cortical neurons that correlate to the onset and progression of profound neurobehavioral deterioration in the infant and young child.

The use of the Golgi method combined with electron microscopic studies of cortical biopsy tissue has provided new insights into the nature of developmental disorders affecting the immature human brain. Thus, in recent years attention has been focused on developmental alterations in dendritic growth and differentiation and dendritic spine formation in subjects with progressive neurobehavioral deterioration (Purpura, 1974). Morphological studies of cortical neurons in several lipid-storage disorders (gangliosidoses) have yielded new clues to the pathophysiology of neuron-storage diseases and have also pointed to the possible role of gangliosidoses in the growth and differentiation of cortical neuronal and synaptic organizations (Purpura, 1979).

Advances in developmental neurobiology at the cellular level and in developmental psychobiology at the level of the behaving animal are rapidly moving along convergent paths. The focal point of these lines of inquiry will surely illuminate problems of normal and aberrant behavioral development in the human infant.

References

Purpura, D. P. Nature of electrocortical potentials and synaptic organizations in cerebral and cerebellar cortex. In C.C. Pfeiffer & J. R. Smythies (Eds.), *International review of neurobiology* (Vol. 1.) New York, Academic Press, 1959.

Purpura, D. P. Analysis of axodendritic synaptic organizations in immature cerebral cortex. *Annals of the New York Academy of Science, 1961, 94, 606–654.*

Purpura, D. P. Comparative physiology of dendrites. In G.C. Quarton, T. Melnechuck, & F. O. Schmitt (Eds.), *The neurosciences. A study program.* New York: Rockefeller Univ. Press, 1967.

Purpura, D. P. Intracellular studies of synaptic organizations in the mammalian brain. In G.D. Pappas and D.P. Purpura (Eds.), *Structure and function of synapses.* New York: Raven Press, 1972.

Purpura, D. P. Dendritic spine 'dysgenesis' and mental retardation. *Science, 1974, 186,* 1126–1128.

Purpura, D. P. Morphogenesis of visual cortex in the preterm infant. In M. A. B. Brazier, (Ed.), *Growth and development of the brain.* New York: Raven, 1975.

Purpura, D. P. Structure-dysfunction relations in the visual cortex of preterm infants. In M. A. B. Brazier & F. Cocceani (Eds.), *Brain dysfunction in infantile febrile convulsions.* New York: Raven, 1976.

Purpura, D. P. Pathobiology of cortical neurons in metabolic and unclassified amentias. In R. Katzman (Ed.), *Congenital and acquired cognitive disorders.* New York: Raven, 1979.

Purpura, D. P., Prelevic, S., & Santini, M. Postsynaptic potentials and spike variations in the feline hippocampus during postnatal ontogenesis. *Experimental Neurology, 1968, 22,* 408–422.

Purpura, D. P., Shofer, R. J., Housepian, E. M., & Noback, C. R. Comparative ontogenesis of structure-function relations in cerebral and cerebellar cortex. In D.P. Purpura & J. P. Schade (Eds.), *Progress in brain research. Growth and maturation of the brain* (Vol. 4). Amsterdam: Elsevier, 1964.

Purpura, D. P., Shofer, R. J., & Scarff, T. Properties of synaptic activities and spike potentials of neurons in immature neocortex. *Journal of Neurophysiology, 1965, 28,* 925–942.

III

Behavioral Patterns in the Neonatal Period

9

Sensory Processing in Pre- and Full-Term Infants in the Neonatal Period

SARAH L. FRIEDMAN
BLANCHE S. JACOBS
MILTON W. WERTHMANN, JR.

Psychologists have developed and refined measures of sensory processing in young infants (for reviews, see Fitzgerald & Brackbill, 1976; Jeffrey & Cohen, 1971) and some of these measures have been applied to the study of preterms, yielding some evidence for sensory deficits in these infants. The finding of deficits in the sensory processing of preterm infants is not surprising. Preterm infants are exposed to the extrauterine environment before some of their sensory systems have completed maturation (Bradley & Mistretta, 1975), a fact that may interfere with their ability to take advantage of the environmental stimulation to which they are exposed. Moreover, it is possible that the stimulation provided by the extrauterine environment might be damaging to sensory systems that have not completed maturation. The findings of sensory processing deficits in preterm infants mesh nicely with the available information regarding intellective deficits in preterm children and young adolescents (e.g., Caputo & Mandell, 1970; Eames, 1955; Field, Hallock, Ting, Dempsey, Dabiri, & Shuman, 1978; Knobloch, Rider, Harper, & Pasamanick, 1956; Wiener, 1968).

The belief that such intellective deficits as those suffered by preterms originate in infancy and the assumption that early intervention is superior to late intervention have led to intervention programs and studies with preterm infants (Cornell & Gottfried, 1976; Schaefer, Hatcher, & Barglow, 1980). The scarcity of data about sensory processing in very young preterms, however, has precluded the design of scientifically based intervention programs, the effects of which could be predicted and tested. The research described in this chapter was aimed at generating data to guide planners of intervention programs in their decisions concerning tactile, auditory, and visual stimulation of young preterm infants.

PRETERM BIRTH AND
PSYCHOLOGICAL DEVELOPMENT

ISBN 0-12-267880-X

The available information on sensory processing in preterm infants will be reviewed first. We will then describe our study of tactile, auditory, and visual processing in 45 relatively low-risk preterm and 23 healthy full-term infants. Our findings show that at expected date of birth the sensory processing of low-risk preterms is not uniformly different from that of full-term neonates and that the differences between preterm and term infants are not evenly distributed across the tactile, auditory, and visual sensory modalities. Consequently, we will hypothesize that there might be an inverse relationship between the maturity of a sensory system at preterm birth and the damage it suffers due to preterm exposure to the extrauterine environment.

Previous Research

When reviewing studies of sensory processing in preterm infants, one has to keep in mind that preterm infants vary in the amount of medical complications they suffer and that medical technology keeps improving. Consequently, differences in the findings of different studies may be the result of differences in the medical risk (e.g., Berkson, Wasserman, & Behrman, 1974; Schulman, 1969; Sigman, Kopp, Littman, & Parmelee, 1977; Werner & Siqueland, 1978) or medical technology associated with the early life of the infants involved (Teberg, Hodgman, Wu, & Spears, 1977). Differences in findings of different studies may have to do with the fact that the control groups of the various studies are not the same. In some studies, the full-term control subjects are of the same chronological age as the preterms (Fantz & Fagan, 1975), whereas in others, they are of the same conceptional age (Sigman *et al.,* 1977). Discrepant findings may also be attributed to variations in experimental parameters. Usually different laboratories use different experimental procedures, different stimulation procedures, and different observational methods.

The review that follows includes only studies that compare preterm with full-term infants. It excludes studies that do not have a control group. Most of the studies compare processing in a single sensory modality. Consequently, the review is organized around tactile sensory processing, auditory sensory processing, and visual sensory processing.

Tactile Processing

Rose, Schmidt, and Bridger (1976) compared full-term neonates (presumably, of mean conceptional age of 40.0 weeks) with preterms who were biologically somewhat younger (mean conceptional age of 38.5 weeks). They stroked the infants' abdomens with nylon filaments and found that, whereas the full-term group showed both behavioral and heart rate responsiveness, the preterms showed only behavioral responsiveness and that this responsiveness was somewhat lesser than that of the term infants. Field, Dempsey, Hatch,

Ting, and Clifton (1979) compared full-term neonates with preterms (of mean conceptional age of 37.4 weeks). They poked their subjects' abdomens with a filament and found no group differences in cardiac or behavioral responsiveness. However, whereas the behavioral and cardiac responsiveness of term infants decreased over trials, only the behavioral responsiveness decreased in the preterms. These two studies show that preterm infants' processing of tactile stimulation is somewhat deficient and that this deficiency manifests itself primarily in the cardiac system.

Auditory Processing

Katona and Berenyi (1974) found deficits in newborn preterms' behavioral responsiveness to sound only when the gestational age of the infants was less than 29 weeks. Eisenberg, Coursin, and Rupp (1966) found that eight full-term neonates were quicker to habituate to a repeatedly presented modulated tone than were two preterms. (The conceptional age of the preterms was not given.) Bench and Parker (1971) report that term infants can be better sound detectors than preterms. They compared the behavioral responses given by preterm infants and full-term neonates of the same conceptional age (40 weeks) to a repeated sound stimulus. They found that preterm and full-term infants detect sound equally well when they are in quiet sleep but that full-term infants are better sound detectors in active sleep. A fourth study (Field *et al.*, 1979) did not find deficits in the behavioral responsiveness of preterm infants of 37.4 weeks conceptional age but did find that the cardiac responsiveness of the preterms did not significantly decrease when the infants were presented repeatedly with rattle or buzzer noises. The above studies suggest that preterms who are of younger conceptional ages than full-term neonates are less responsive to auditory stimulation than the full-term neonates. They also suggest that in active sleep preterms at expected date of birth are less responsive than full-term neonates.

Visual Processing

Katona and Berenyi (1974) presented neonates with rhythmical visual stimuli and found that preterm neonates of less than 29 weeks gestational age gave fewer motor responses (startles) than full-term neonates. Fantz and Fagan (1975) compared visual preferences in full-term and preterm infants who were tested at 5 and 10 weeks after birth. There was a 5-week difference between the conceptional age of the full-term and preterm subjects at the time of testing. Preterms' duration of attention was shorter than that of full-terms. In a study of blinking in response to an approaching object, Petterson, Yonas, and Fisch (1980) found that 10-week-old preterms blinked on significantly fewer trials than 10-week-old full-terms, thereby suggesting greater immaturity. Differences in visual processing were also found by Sigman and her colleagues (1977), who compared preterms at expected date of birth with full-term neonates. The preterm infants looked for significantly longer periods than the control subjects did. Sigman and Parmelee (1974), who compared preterms and full-terms at 4 months (following expected or real term), found that full-terms but not preterms preferred a novel over a familiar stimulus.

Rose, Gottfried, and Bridger (1979) tested mostly lower socioeconomic class preterm and full-term infants on a visual recognition memory task. The term infants were tested at 6 and 12 months of age. The preterms were tested at 6 and 12 months corrected age (i.e., following expected date of birth). Whereas the term infants discriminated between a familiar and a novel visual stimulus at both ages, preterms did so only at 12 months of corrected age. At 12 months, the preterms' performance was similar to the full-term infants' performance at 6 months, indicating a developmental lag in the visual discrimination abilities of preterm infants.

The differences between the visual processing of preterm and full-term infants did not appear on all visual measures or at all the ages studied: In the study by Fantz and Fagan (1975) described earlier, 15-, 20-, and 25-week-old preterms attended to the visual stimuli for longer periods than did full-terms. The differences, however, disappeared when the preterm and term infants were matched on conceptional age. In their study of 4-month-olds (real age for full-term infants or corrected age for preterm infants), Sigman and Parmelee (1974) found no differences in the preferences shown for specific visual stimuli by full-term and preterm infants. Rose, Gottfried, and Bridger (1978) found that year-old term infants (mean age approximately 54 weeks) and preterms of the same corrected age discriminated between familiar and novel visual stimuli. In summary, in the first year following real or expected date of birth, preterms are likely to respond less maturely than term infants. This developmental deficit, however, does not appear consistently in all the studies comparing visual perception of preterm and term infants.

Our Study

Subjects

Between July 1977 and January 1979, we studied 45 preterm and 23 full-term infants of 40 weeks conceptional age who were born to black mothers at the Washington Hospital Center in Washington, D.C. Our preterm and full-term groups were similar on variables that have been shown in the past to be associated with some of the differences between the behavioral outcome of full-term and preterm children.

1. Our subjects were all of the same conceptional age. Hunt and Rhodes (1977), Parmelee and Schulte (1970), and Tilford (1976), as well as others, have shown the importance of matching preterms and full-terms on this variable in studies of preterms' behavior.

2. Our subjects were all born with weight adequate for gestational age. Drillien (1970), Fitzhardinge and Stevens (1972), Lubchenco, Delivoria-Papadopoulos, and Searls (1972), and Neligan, Kolvin, Scott, and Garside (1976) have shown that being small for date is associated with poorer outcome.

3. Our gestation groups were similar on two indicators of socioeconomic background, mothers' education and prenatal care. In life, prematurity is often confounded with an economically and culturally poor environment; preterm birth occurs more frequently in economically depressed populations (Garn, Shaw, & McCabe, 1977) and the deprived background of preterm children at least partly accounts for their poorer intellective and/or academic performance (Douglas, 1960; Drillien, 1964, 1969).

The full-term infants were all healthy; none was delivered by cesarean section or under general anesthesia. No full-term neonate was circumcised before testing. Using need for intensive care and cost of hospital care as indices, we judged our preterms to be of relatively low medical risk. Neonatal medical risk has been shown to relate to psychological short- and long-term outcome (e.g., Sostek, Quinn, & Davitt, 1979; Wiener, Rider, Oppel & Harper, 1968). Parmelee and Haber (1973) have argued that theoretically it is possible that preterm birth may not be a predictor of later risk if dissociated from the poor medical history and inadequate rearing conditions associated with preterm birth. The preterm subjects of our study may approximate the hypothetical healthy, riskless preterms Parmelee and Haber wrote about. Assuming this to be the case, a comparison of this relatively risk-free group of preterms at expected date of delivery with a control group of healthy neonates of similar background would be expected to reveal few sensory-processing differences between the groups. Some details describing our preterm and full-term infants are given in Table 9.1.

Procedures

We attempted to test the tactile, auditory, and visual processing of each subject. We were successful in completing all procedures with 33 preterms and 16 full-terms. Three preterms and one full-term infant completed one procedure only. The data of all the subjects who participated in each procedure—regardless of whether they participated or did not participate in other procedures—were analyzed.

For 53 out of 68 of the subjects, the tactile experimental procedure was administered first, the auditory second, and the visual third. All subjects were fed and changed immediately following their arrival at the test room. They were then observed for their spontaneous behavior. (Mean length of the procedure for full-terms was 19.0 min and for preterms 15.0 min. Standard deviations were 4.1 and 6.5, respectively). The sensory-processing procedures followed the spontaneous procedure. Before the administration of the auditory procedure all infants were fed, changed, and allowed to rest for 30

TABLE 9.1

Neonatal, Day-of-Test, and Maternal Variables for Full- and Preterm Infants

	Full-term $(N = 23)$	Preterm $(N = 45)$
Gestational age at birth		
Mean	40.2	33.7
SD	(1.2)	(2.2)
Weight at birth		
Mean	3272.1	1819.5
SD	(357.9)	(387.8)
Most intensive care (days)		
Mean	n.a.[b]	2.9
SD	n.a.[b]	(6.2)
Cost of hospital care (dollars)		
Mean	n.a.[b]	5953.2
SD	n.a.[b]	(6315.4)
Conceptional age at test		
Mean	40.2	40.1
SD	(1.2)	(1.2)
Weight at test		
Mean	3272.1	2936.9
SD	(357.9)	(447.3)
Mother's age (years)		
Mean	26.3	24.8
SD	(4.5)	(4.8)
Mother's education (years)		
Mean	13.0	12.5
SD	(2.2)	(2.3)
Prenatal care[a]		
Mean	3.9	3.7
SD	(.4)	(.8)

[a] 1 = none; 2 = first half pregnancy; 3 = second half pregnancy; 4 = throughout pregnancy.

[b] n.a. = not applicable.

min. For the 53 subjects who were administered the visual procedure last, a neurological exam preceded the visual procedure. For the other 15 subjects, the neurological exam was administered last. Within each procedure, and for each gestation × sex group, two psychologists alternated the roles of coder and experimenter. No infant had all three procedures administered by the same experimenter.

The value of having tactile, auditory, and visual sensory data from the same subjects lies in the possibility of identifying strengths and deficits in sensory processing that are not artifacts of using different samples of subjects. As will be shown later, the tactile and auditory procedures were identical except for the nature of the stimuli. The responses coded in each procedure included face, head, and body movements, and vocalizations. The visual procedure differed from the tactile and auditory procedures in the infants' initial state (awake rather than asleep), in the duration of stimulus presentation, in interstimulus intervals, and in the coding of visual attention to the stimulus rather than face and body movements. We tried to compensate for these differences by analyzing the data in terms of conceptually equivalent response measures (latency, initial responsiveness, response decrement, and time to response decrement).

TACTILE STIMULATION

The experimental procedures of this study were carried out in a private patient room that was turned into a laboratory and in which experimental conditions could be carefully controlled. For the tactile procedure, the infant was swaddled snugly and placed supine in a bassinet, with his or her head supported in the midline position (see Figure 9.1). Stimulation started after the baby had spent 60 sec in quiet sleep. No attempt was made to control state after the procedure began. Stimulation consisted of repeated strokes to the infant's left cheek with a Semmes-Weinstein filament #5.46. Each stimulus presentation was applied manually for approximately 2 sec, with a randomly computer-determined interstimulus interval of between 19.75 and 29.75 sec. Stroking was applied either downward from the outer corner of the eye to the outer corner of the mouth or upward from the mouth to the eye. The direction of stroking was counterbalanced across subjects within each gestation $\times$ sex group. Stroking continued in the same manner until either the infant reached

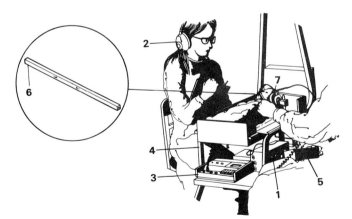

FIGURE 9.1. *The tactile procedure. (1) A specially constructed electronic device controlling the type and duration of stimuli presentations. (2) A pair of Realistic Nova-30 stereo earphones. (3) Superscope tape deck. (4) Air-Shields Infant Warmer Model DR, used as a warmer when the room temperature was below 78°F, otherwise used as a bassinet. (5) A specially constructed box with buttons to activate pens on an event recorder. (6) Filament #5.46 from the Semmes-Weinstein aesthesiometer. (7) Adjustable foam-cushioned silent earphones specially designed to limit ambient noise at infant's ears.*

a predetermined response decrement criterion, or 127 stimulus presentations were applied (this meant an hour of exposure to the procedure), or the infant cried for more than 15 sec. Response decrement criterion was reached either (a) when on six consecutive trials the infant emitted the same degree of activity in the 5 sec prior to and in the 7 sec following the initiation of stimulus presentation; or (b) when equivalent pre- and poststimulation activity level was emitted on five consecutive trials and was resumed for three consecutive trials after a break in this pattern for one trial. Infants' behaviors were tallied on a special form following an observation period of 12 sec, as defined above under (a). The behaviors coded were state (Brazelton, 1973), startles, body movement (the swaddled "bundle" was writhing), head movement, facial movement, tremors, vocalization, or protest.

AUDITORY STIMULATION

The auditory procedure was identical to the tactile procedure except for the stimulus, which was one of two pure tones, a 500 Hz and a 1500 Hz tone, each played at 80 dB for exactly 2 sec, with randomly determined interstimulus intervals of between 19.75 and 29.75 sec. The tone was administered automatically and heard through a pair of adjustable Grason–Stadler TDH–49 earphones placed at each infant's ears (see Figure 9.2). The choice of tone to be presented was counterbalanced across subjects within each gestation × sex group.

VISUAL STIMULATION

The awake infant was swaddled, placed in a bassinet especially modified to serve as a testing apparatus (see Figure 9.3), given a pacifier, and presented with one of two visual stimuli at a distance of 19 cm from his or her eyes. The stimuli consisted of one red and one green three-dimensional lighted, translucent, plastic $2\frac{1}{2}$ in. × $2\frac{1}{2}$ in. × 1 in. box. The stimulus was presented for 30 sec, starting with the beginning of the first fixation, with interstimulus intervals of not less than 10 sec but with maximum limit determined by the infant's directing his or her visual attention to the next presentation of the stimulus. The stimulus was presented until the infant either (a) reached a predetermined response decrement criterion; (b) avoided a stimulus presentation for three times the sum of the latencies on the first three trials; (c) avoided the stimulus for 60 sec; or (d) cried for more than 15 sec. Response decrement criterion was reached when the sum of the latencies to the last three stimulus presentations equaled 1.5 times the sum of the latencies to the first three stimulus presentations. (This criterion was based on pilot data showing that term infants fell asleep shortly after reaching such a criterion.) The choice of stimulus (red or green) was counterbalanced across subjects within each gestation × sex group. The visual responses recorded were the latency to the first response on each trial and the duration of each fixation. The latency was measured with a stopwatch, and the duration of fixation was read off an event recorder.

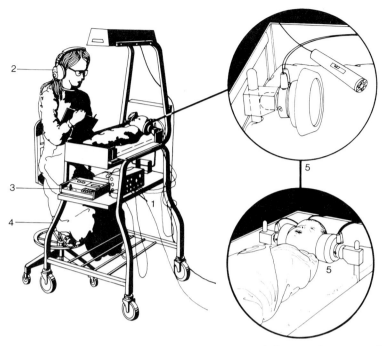

FIGURE 9.2. *The auditory procedure. (1) A specially constructed electronic device controlling the type and duration of stimuli presentations. (2) A pair of Realistic Nova-30 stereo earphones. (3) Superscope tape deck. (4) Air-Shields Infant Warmer Model DR, used as a warmer when the room temperature was below 78°F, otherwise used as a bassinet. (5) A pair of Grason-Stadler TDH-49 earphones padded with foam cushions and mounted on rods that allow the earphones' adjustment against each infant's ears.*

Response Measures

One source of difficulty in assessing the data from different studies is that they use different response measures. In this study, we were interested in comparing tactile, auditory, and visual processing. To maximize the meaning of our comparisons, we analyzed our tactile, auditory, and visual data in terms of conceptually equivalent measures. These were (*a*) quickness of response (latency); (*b*) degree of responsiveness to initial stimulation (three trials); (*c*) presence of response decrement (significant decrement from initial to final trials); and (*d*) duration of time to reaching a response decrement criterion.

QUICKNESS OF RESPONSE (LATENCY)

In the tactile and auditory data, we counted the number of times the stimulus presentations were applied before the infants gave their first response. In the visual data, we noted information as to the number of seconds elapsed between the moment the stimulus was presented above an in-

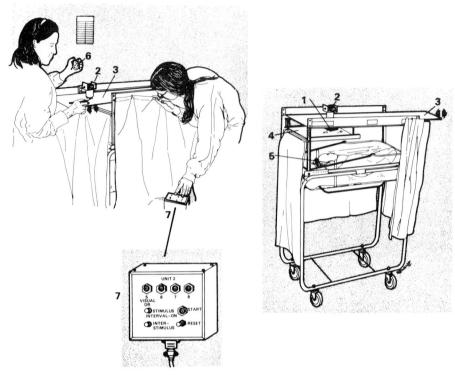

FIGURE 9.3. *The visual procedure. (1) A lighted three-dimensional stimulus that completes two 360° revolutions every 45 sec. (2) A small motor powered by a 15V battery that rotates the stimulus. (3) A sheet of opaque white Plexiglas that can be moved horizontally on a track. (4) A sheet of clear Plexiglas. (5) Adjustable foam-cushioned silent earphones designed to hold the infant's head in mid-line. (6) A stopwatch. (7) A specially constructed experimental box with buttons to activate pens on an event recorder. The box has timing devices with light signals.*

fant's head and the moment the stimulus was reflected on the pupil of at least one of the infant's eyes.

DEGREE OF INITIAL RESPONSIVENESS

In the tactile and auditory data, we identified the trial on which each infant first responded to the stimulus. This trial and the following two trials were considered the "initial" three trials of responding. The responses given preceding and following stimulation on each of these trials (5 sec prior to stimulation; 7 sec following the initiation of stimulation) were weighted and summed. The weighting was done according to the size of the response (tremor = 1; face = 1; head = 2; body = 3; startle = 4; cry = 7). A responsiveness score on each trial was calculated by subtracting the weighted activity preceding stimulation from the weighted activity preceding stimulation from the weighted activity following stimulation. The responsiveness scores on the "initial" three trials were summed and constituted the responsiveness data.

In the visual data, our measure of initial responsiveness was the total atten-tiveness (in seconds) given during the first three presentations of the stimuli.

PRESENCE OF RESPONSE DECREMENT

For the tactile and for the auditory data, the responsiveness on the "initial" three trials was compared (repeated measures ANOVA, Winer, 1971) with that on the last three trials. For the visual data, the duration of attention on the first trial was compared with the duration of attention on the last trial.

TIME TO REACHING DECREMENT CRITERION

In the tactile, auditory, and visual data, we measured the time from the beginning of stimulation to the reaching of response decrement criterion only for those individuals who reached criterion. (Translating number of trials to a duration measure was possible, since the exact time of stimulus presentation was recorded on an event recorder for all procedures.)

RELATIONSHIPS AMONG RESPONSE MEASURES

A review of the experimental literature shows that shorter latencies of re-sponding are associated with more mature and better organized central nervous systems (Barnet, Friedman, Weiss, Ohlrich, Shanks, & Lodge, 1980; Barnet, Ohlrich, Weiss, & Shanks, 1975; Barnet, Weiss, Sotillo, Ohlrich, Shkurovich, & Cravioto, 1978; Bellis, 1932–1933; Gilbert, 1894; Goodenough, 1935; Jones, 1937; Luria, 1932; Miles, 1931; Philip, 1934). Shorter initial respon-siveness is considered an index of better organization (Parmelee & Sigman, 1976). The ability to habituate to repeated stimulation is considered an index of memory and learning, and the quickness of doing so, a measure of matur-ity and central nervous system (CNS) status (Lewis, 1971; Lipsitt, 1979). Reaching a response decrement in this study could be the result of sensory or motor fatigue rather than the result of true habituation (Thompson & Spencer, 1966). Sensory fatigue in response to sensory stimulation is known to decrease with increased maturation (Ellingson, 1964). Because of this uncertainty regarding our response decrement measure and the meager literature regarding the meaningfulness of responsiveness as a maturity and CNS integrity index, we decided to place the most confidence in the latency measure. Consequently, we looked at the correlations between latency of responding and the performance on the other measures.

Our own data show that for full-term infants longer latencies were nega-tively associated with greater responsiveness on initial trials in the three sensory modalities studied ($r = -.22; -.40; -.25$ for tactile, auditory, and visual data, respectively). In the tactile and auditory data, we found that quick-to-respond full-term neonates tended to take longer to reach the response decre-ment criterion than slow-to-respond full-terms ($r = -.20; -.20$). The visual data revealed that full-terms who were quicker to respond were also quicker to shut off their responsiveness ($r = +.33$). The preterm data showed that longer latencies were negatively associated with greater responsiveness ($r = -.26$; $-.60$; and $-.14$ for the tactile, auditory, and visual data, respectively). Latencies were not associated with time to response decrement in the preterms' tactile data ($r = +.06$); they were negatively related in the auditory data ($r = -.24$) and positively related in the visual data ($r = +.58$).

On the basis of the above trends in our data and on the basis of the confidence we had in previous findings that latency is negatively related to maturation, we expected group differences to show longer latencies and less initial responsiveness in the data of the group comprising less well-organized infants. We expected that poor tactile and auditory organization would be manifested by quicker response decrement and that poor visual organization would manifest itself in longer times to response decrement.

RELIABILITY OF CODING RESPONSES

For each of the procedures, two psychologists alternated as coders of infant behaviors. Measures of reliability were calculated using intraclass correlations (Bartko & Carpenter, 1976). These were based on 10 taped tactile sessions, 10 taped auditory sessions, and 4 live visual sessions. The tactile and auditory scores were weighted activity scores on each trial. The visual scores were duration of fixation on each trial. The tactile reliability of average rating was .96 and of single rating .93. The respective scores for auditory reliability were .84 and .73. The respective visual ratings were .94 and .89. All these were significantly different from zero correlations ($p < .001$).

Results

STATE CHANGE

Because the state the infants are in while being stimulated affects their responsiveness (Clifton & Nelson, 1976; Hutt & Hutt, 1970), we first assured ourselves that there were no group differences in terms of the infants' states. No infant was in other than quiet sleep at the first administration of the tactile or auditory stimulus. Consequently, the tactile and auditory latency data is based on responsiveness in quiet sleep. Three preterms changed their state to active sleep during the "initial" tactile trials, and three other preterms changed their state during the "initial" auditory trials. Two full-terms changed state during the "initial" tactile trials. No full-term infant changed state during the "initial" auditory trials. The total number, minus one, of tactile or auditory trials that an infant attended to gave the number of opportunities for state change. The percentage of state change during the tactile procedure had means of .81 and .91 and standard deviations of 1.54 and 1.91 for full-term and preterm infants, respectively (differences are not statistically significant). The mean percentages of state change during the auditory procedure were 1.11 and 1.02 and the standard deviations were 1.88 and 1.57 for term and preterm infants, respectively (differences are not statistically significant). Consequently, it is unlikely that tactile or auditory responsiveness differences between preterm and full-term infants could be explained by differences in state organization. During the visual procedure, all infants were awake, precluding an interaction between state and visual behaviors.

GROUP DIFFERENCES

We compared the full-term and preterm infants on their tactile (see Table 9.2), auditory (see Table 9.3), and visual (see Table 9.4) responsiveness. Comparisons were made on four measures in each sensory modality: quickness of

TABLE 9.2

Tactile Responsiveness to Stimulation: Full-Term versus Preterm Infants of 40 Weeks Conceptional Age

	Quickness of response (trials)	Amount of initial responsiveness	Amount of response decrement	Time to response decrement (sec)
Full-term				
Mean	1.04	9.57	9.38	983.8
SD	.22	4.87	4.72	952.5
N	(21)	(21)	(21)	(18)
Preterm				
Mean	1.20	7.78	5.94	927.2
SD	.67	5.14	8.59	861.3
N	(44)	(43)	(42)	(33)
Comparison (ANOVA)	n.s.[a]	n.s.[a]	n.s.[a]	n.s.[a]

[a] n.s. = nonsignificant.

TABLE 9.3

Auditory Responsiveness to Stimulation: Full-term versus Preterm Infants of 40 Weeks Conceptional Age

	Quickness of response (trials)	Amount of initial responsiveness	Amount of response decrement	Time to response decrement (sec)
Full-term				
Mean	1.78	6.14	5.44	1183.1
SD	1.70	5.36	5.76	1089.9
N	(18)	(18)	(18)	(11)
Preterm				
Mean	2.97	3.88	2.92	558.1
SD	2.48	3.84	4.10	450.5
N	(39)	(39)	(39)	(20)
Comparison (ANOVA)	$p < .09$	$p < .06$	n.s.[a]	$p < .04$

[a] n.s. = nonsignificant.

TABLE 9.4

Visual Responsiveness to Stimulation: Full-Term versus Preterm Infants of 40 Weeks Conceptional Age

	Quickness of response (sec)	Amount of initial responsiveness	Amount of response decrement	Time to response decrement (sec)
Full-term				
Mean	2.00	74.43	8.17	152.0
SD	1.48	14.74	12.93	47.4
n	(23)	(21)	(21)	(15)
Preterm				
Mean	4.74	69.93	7.51	235.0
SD	6.68	20.69	9.49	131.3
n	(44)	(41)	(40)	(36)
Comparison (ANOVA)	$p < .04$	n.s.[a]	n.s.[a]	$p < .01$

[a] n.s. = nonsignificant.

response, amount of initial responsiveness, amount of response decrement, and time to response decrement. Comparisons were done by analyses of variance (Winer, 1971). No group differences were found in the tactile data. The auditory data showed that full-terms were slightly quicker and more responsive than preterms ($p < .10$) and that they took significantly longer to reach the response decrement criterion ($p < .04$). No group differences were found in the auditory presence of response decrement.

The visual data showed that the full-term group was quicker to respond ($p < .04$) and took less time to reach the response decrement criterion ($p < .01$) than did the preterm group. No group differences were found in the visual responsiveness on the initial trials or on the presence of response decrement.

Discussion

We compared the tactile, auditory, and visual processing of preterms at expected date of birth with the sensory processing of healthy full-term neonates. Sensory processing was evaluated by quickness of response (latency), initial responsiveness, amount of response decrement, and time to response decrement. Twelve group comparisons were thus carried out, and only three statistically significant ($p < .05$) group differences were found. Two other comparisons tended toward significance ($p < .10$). We found no differences in the tactile processing of the preterm and full-term infants. The full-term infants were somewhat more responsive to the auditory stimulus and took longer to reach the auditory response decrement criterion. The full-terms were quicker to respond to the visual stimulus and took less time to reach the visual response decrement criterion. Developmental literature clearly shows that short latencies are positively related to developmental status. In order to evaluate the meaning of the responsiveness measure and the response decrement data in our study, we correlated the performance of our subjects on these measures with their latency data. These intercorrelations suggest that the greater auditory responsiveness of full-terms and the longer time it took them to reach the response decrement criterion indicate greater maturity on the part of these infants. The shorter visual latencies in the full-terms' data and these subjects' relative quickness in reaching the visual decrement criterion also indicate greater maturity. These group differences cannot be explained by differences in state while responding or by background (race, socioeconomic) differences between subjects.

Our failure to find group differences in tactile processing is in line with the results of Rose *et al.* (1976) and of Field *et al.* (1979), who did not find statistically significant differences between the behavioral responsiveness of their preterm and full-term subjects. Our finding that preterm infants were quicker to reach the auditory response decrement criterion is neither supported nor contradicted by the available literature. The slight ($p < .10$) tendency of full-terms to be more responsive to the auditory stimulus parallels the finding of Bench and Parker (1971), who showed that full-terms can be better sound detectors than preterms. Our finding that preterms were slower to respond to the first presentation of the visual stimulus is in line with findings of Sigman and Parmelee (1974) and of Rose *et al.* (1979). These authors found that full-term infants but not preterm infants preferred to attend to a novel over a familiar visual stimulus. If latencies to responding can be taken as indexes of interest in novel stimulation (short latencies indicating greater interest than long latencies), one can conclude that the full-term neonates in our study showed more interest in novelty than did the preterms. By not finding differences between the full-terms' and preterms' visual responsiveness on the first three trials, our study fails to support Sigman *et al.*'s (1977) findings. These authors found that preterms at expected date of birth spent more time looking at visual stimuli than did full-term neonates. The differences in the results of the two studies may be quite superficial. In both studies the preterms were found to be slower than term infants in their ability to decrease their responsiveness to visual stimulation. In the Sigman *et al.* (1977) study this slowness manifested itself in the measure of total fixation time; in our study the slowness was picked up by the measure of time to reaching the response decrement criterion. The fact that in our study fixation time during the first three trials was equivalent for both gestation groups may be related to the fact that our stimuli were very attractive (three-dimensional, colored, lighted, revolving) and might have been better attention-holders than the two-dimensional stimuli used by Sigman *et al.* (1977).

The small number of differences between the preterm and full-term groups can be explained in different ways and may in fact be due to a combination of factors: At equivalent conceptional (or maturational) ages the number of differences between preterm and full-term infants is at its minimum (e.g., Fantz & Fagan, 1975; Hunt & Rhodes, 1977; Tilford, 1976). Our preterm and full-term subjects were matched on their estimated conceptional age, thereby minimizing the chance of finding group differences. As indicated in the description of the subjects, our subjects were of the same socioeconomic background and were all born with weight adequate for gestational age. Group differences on these variables have been shown to be associated with differences in the behavioral outcome of full-term and preterm children (e.g., Douglas, 1960; Drillien, 1964, 1969, 1970). Various studies show that low medical risk is associated with low levels of risk in sensory processing (Schulman, 1969; Sigman *et al.* 1977; Werner & Siqueland, 1978). Most of our preterm subjects were of low medical risk and consequently at low risk for deficits in sensory processing. The nature of our sample and our results (indicating a small number of group differences) lend partial support to the hypothesis of Parmelee and Haber (1973) that preterm birth may not be predictor of later risk if disassociated from the poor medical history and inadequate rearing conditions frequently associated with such birth. The differences in the sensory processing abilities of our full-term and preterm subjects could have been more numerous and more pronounced had our subjects been unswaddled during the administration of the stimuli. Swaddling has been shown to have a calming effect on full-term neonates and young infants (Brackbill, 1971; Lipton, Steinschneider, & Richmond, 1960, 1965), and it makes sense to believe that it has a similar effect on preterm infants. By swaddling our subjects, we might have helped the preterms to attend to the stimuli in a way that would not have been possible had they been unswaddled. Observations we made while our subjects were not swaddled (not reported here) showed that when not swaddled the preterms were significantly more irritable than the term infants.

We find the distribution of the group differences across sensory modalities of special interest. We found no statistically significant differences in tactile processing, one significant difference in auditory processing, two almost significant auditory differences, and two significant differences in visual processing. The three sensory modalities we chose to study are not equally developed at the time of preterm birth (Bredberg, 1968; Gottlieb, 1971; Hooker, 1952; Mann, 1969). The fetal tactile sensory modality is the earliest to develop and is functional by the fourth month of gestation (Hooker, 1952). The fetal auditory sensory system is probably not functional before the eighth month of gestation (for a review, see Parmelee, this volume). The visual system continues to develop throughout pregnancy, and structural changes occur even as late as the ninth month of gestation (Mann, 1969). The normal environment for the development of the fetal sensory systems is the intrauterine environment. The extrauterine environment is probably not optimally appropriate for supporting the normal development of fetal sensory structures and functions. Therefore, we would expect the visual system, which is not mature at the time of preterm birth, to suffer by preterm exposure to the extrauterine environment. We would not expect the tactile sensory system, which is mature at the time of preterm birth, to be negatively affected by exposure to tactile extrauterine stimulation. Following the same logic, we would expect the auditory sensory system to be somewhat less negatively affected by preterm birth than we would expect the visual system to be. As already indicated, our results follow the predicted pattern, showing no full-term versus preterm differences on tactile measures, one statistically significant difference in the auditory data, and two such differences in the visual data. The fact that the statistically significant group differences occurred in the visual and auditory data and not in the tactile data could be explained by the infants' state at testing (the infants were asleep in the tactile and auditory procedures and awake in the visual procedure); by the intensity of the stimuli (which could not be equated across procedures); or by other experimental conditions (e.g., length of trials). Nevertheless, the possibility that there is a negative relationship between the maturity of a sensory system at the time of preterm birth and the amount of insult that that system may suffer by virtue of extrauterine experience is an intriguing alternate explanation of the results and calls for further investigation.

If replicated, our study would suggest that planners of intervention programs would do well to study ways of facilitating the optimal auditory and visual development of preterms in the period between birth and expected date of birth. In this short period, even low-risk preterms already accumulate auditory and visual deficits that are likely to affect their later intellective development negatively.

Acknowledgments

We would like to thank Anne Mayfield for her valuable contributions to and dedicated involvement in all aspects of this study. We are also grateful to Marilyn Pickett for her invaluable help in data reduction and analysis and to Rita Dettmers for her patience and help in the preparation of this manuscript. We also thank John Bartko for his help in monitoring our choice of statistical methods. Without the cooperation and help of Alice Thorner and the nursing and administrative staff of the Washington Hospital Center, we would not have been able to carry out the project. Finally, we thank T. M. Field, A. Hollenbeck, B. Lester, A. H. Parmelee, S. Rose, and M. Sigman, whose critical evaluation of this chapter influenced significantly the presentation of the material.

References

Barnet, A. B., Friedman, S. L., Weiss, I. P., Ohlrich, E. S., Shanks, B., & Lodge, A. VEP development in infancy and early childhood: A longitudinal study. *Electroencephalography and Clinical Neurophysiology,* 1980, *49,* 476–489.

Barnet, A. B., Ohlrich, B. S., Weiss, I. P., & Shanks, B. Auditory evoked potentials during sleep in normal children from ten days to three years of age. *Electroencephalography and Clinical Neurophysiology,* 1975, *39,* 29–41.

Barnet, A. B., Weiss, I. P., Sotillo, M. V., Ohlrich, B. S., Shkurovich, M., & Cravioto, J. Abnormal auditory evoked potentials in early infancy malnutrition. *Science,* 1978, *201,* 450–452.

Bartko, J. J., & Carpenter, W. T. On the methods and theory of reliability. *The Journal of Nervous and Mental Disease,* 1976, *163,* 307–317.

Bellis, C. J. Reaction time and chronological age. *Proceedings of the Society for Experimental Biology and Medicine, 1932-1933, 30,* 801–803.

Bench, J., & Parker, A. Hypersensitivity to sounds in the short gestation baby. *Developmental Medicine and Child Neurology,* 1971, *13,* 15–19.

Berkson, G., Wasserman, G. A., & Behrman, R. E. Heart rate response to an auditory stimulus in premature infants. *Psychophysiology,* 1974, *11,* 244–246.

Brackbill, Y. Cumulative effects of continuous stimulation on arousal in infants. *Child Development,* 1971, *42,* 17–26.

Bradley, R. M., & Mistretta, C. M. Fetal sensory receptors. *Physiological Reviews,* 1975, *55,* 352–382.

Brazelton, T. B. *Neonatal behavioral assessment scale.* Philadelphia: Lippincott, 1973.

Bredberg, G. Cellular pattern and nerve supply of the human organ of corti. *Acta Oto-Laryngologica,* 1968, *236,* 1–135.

Caputo, D. V., & Mandell, W. Consequences of low birth weight. *Developmental Psychology,* 1970, *3,* 363–383.

Clifton, R. K., & Nelson, M. N. Developmental study of habituation in infants: The importance of paradigm, response systems and state. In T. J. Tighe & R. N. Leaton (Eds.), *Habituation.* Hillsdale, N.J.: Erlbaum, 1976.

Cornell, E. H., & Gottfried, A. W. Intervention with premature human infants. *Child Development,* 1976, *47,* 32–39.

Douglas, J. W. B. Premature children at primary schools. *British Medical Journal,* 1960, *1,* 1008–1013.

Drillien, C. M. *The growth and development of the prematurely born infant.* Edinburgh: Livingstone, 1964.

Drillien, C. M. School disposal and performance for children of different birth weight born 1953-1960. *Archives of Diseases in Childhood,* 1969, *44,* 562–570.

Drillien, C. M. The small-for-date infant: Etiology and prognosis. *Pediatric Clinics of North America,* 1970, *17,* 9–24.

Eames, T. H. The relationship of birth weight, the speed of object and word perception and visual acuity. *Journal of Pediatrics,* 1955, *47,* 603–606.

Eisenberg, R. B., Coursin, D. B., & Rupp, N. R. Habituation to an acoustic pattern as an index of differences among human neonates. *The Journal of Auditory Research,* 1966, *6,* 239–248.

Ellingson, R. J. Cerebral electrical responses to auditory and visual stimuli in the infant (human and subhuman studies). In P. Kellaway & I. Petersen (Eds.), *Neurological and electroencephalographic correlative studies in infancy.* New York: Grune & Stratton, 1964.

Fantz, R. L., & Fagan, J. F., III. Visual attention to size and number of pattern details by term and preterm infants during the first six months. *Child Development,* 1975, *46,* 3–18.

Field, T. M., Dempsey, J. R., Hatch, J., Ting, G., & Clifton, R. K. Cardiac and behavioral responses to repeated tactile and auditory stimulation by preterm and term neonates. *Developmental Psychology,* 1979, *15,* 406–416.

Field, T. M., Hallock, N., Ting, G., Dempsey, J., Dabiri, C., & Shuman, H. H. A first-year follow-up of high-risk infants: Formulating a cumulative risk index. *Child Development,* 1978, *49,* 119–131.

Fitzgerald, H. E., & Brackbill, Y. Classical conditioning in infancy: Development and constraints. *Psychological Bulletin,* 1976, *83,* 353–376.

Fitzhardinge, P. M., & Steven, E. M. The small-for-date infant. II. Neurological and intellectual sequelae. *Pediatrics,* 1972, *50,* 50–57.

Garn, S. M., Shaw, H. A., & McCabe, K. D. Effects of socioeconomic status (SES) and race on weight defined and gestational prematurity in the U.S.A. In D. M. Reed & F. J. Stanley (Eds.), *The epidemiology of prematurity.* Baltimore-Munich: Urban & Schwarzenberg, 1977.

Gilbert, J. A. Researches on the mental and physical development of school children. *Yale University Psychological Lab Studies* (Superseded by Yale Psychological Studies), 1894, *2,* 40–100.

Goodenough, F. L. The development of the reactive process from early childhood to maturity. *Journal of Experimental Psychology,* 1935, *18,* 431–450.

Gottlieb, G. Ontogenesis of sensory function in birds and mammals. In E. Tobach, I. R. Aronson, & E. Shaw (Eds.), *The biopsychology of development.* New York: Academic Press, 1971.

Hooker, D. The prenatal origin of behavior. *Porter Lectures* (Series 18). Lawrence: Univ. of Kansas Press, 1952.

Hunt, J. V., & Rhodes, L. Mental development of preterm infants during the first year. *Child Development,* 1977, *48,* 204–210.

Hutt, S. J., & Hutt, C. *Direct observation and measurement of behavior.* Springfield, Ill.: Thomas, 1970.

Jeffrey, W. E., & Cohen, L. B. Habituation in the human infant. *Advances in Child Development and Behavior,* 1971, *6,* 63–97.

Jones, H. E. Reaction time and motor development. *American Journal of Psychology,* 1937, *50,* 181–194.

Katona, F., & Berenyi, M. Differential reactions and habituation to acoustical and visual stimuli in neonates. *Activitas Nervosa Superior,* 1974, *16,* 305.

Knobloch, H., Rider, R., Harper, P., & Pasamanick, B. Neuropsychiatric sequelae of prematurity: A longitudinal study. *Journal of the American Medical Association,* 1956, *161,* 581–585.

Lewis, M. Individual differences in the measurement of early cognitive growth. In J. Hellmuth (Ed.), *Exceptional infant: Studies in abnormalities* (Vol. 2). New York: Brunner/Mazel, 1971.

Lipsitt, L. P. The newborn as informant. In R. B. Kearsley & I. E. Sigel (Eds.), *Infants at risk: Assessment of cognitive functioning.* New York: Wiley, 1979.

Lipton, E. L., Steinschneider, A., & Richmond, J. B. Autonomic function in the neonate. II: Physiological effects of motor restraint. *Psychosomatic Medicine,* 1960, *22,* 57–65.

Lipton, E. L., Steinschneider, A., & Richmond, J. B. Swaddling, a child care practice: Historical, cultural and experimental observations. *Pediatrics,* 1965, *35* (Suppl.), 519–567.

Lubchenco, L. O., Delivoria-Papadopoulos, M., & Searls, D. Long-term follow-up studies of prematurely born infants. II. Influence of birth-weight and gestational age on sequelae. *Pediatrics,* 1972, *80,* 509–512.

Luria, A. R. [*The nature of human conflicts or emotions, conflict and will.*] (W. H. Gantt, Ed. and trans.), New York: Liveright, 1932.

Mann, I. *The development of the human eye.* New York: Grune & Stratton, 1969.

Miles, W. R. Measures of certain human abilities throughout the life span. *Proceedings of the National Academy of Sciences of the U.S.A.,* 1931, *17,* 627–633.

Neligan, G. A., Kolvin, I., Scott, D. Mcl., & Garside, R. F. *Born too soon or born too small.* Philadelphia: Lippincott, 1976.

Parmelee, A. H., & Haber, A. Who is the "risk infant"? *Clinical Obstetrics and Gynecology,* 1973, *16,* 376–386.

Parmelee, A. H., & Schulte, F. J. Developmental testing of preterm and small for date infants. *Pediatrics,* 1970, *45,* 21–28.

Parmelee, A. H., & Sigman, M. Development of visual behavior and neurological organization in pre-term and full-term infants. *Minnesota Symposia on Child Psychology,* 1976, *10,* 119–155.

Pettersen, L., Yonas, A., & Fisch, R. O. The development of blinking in response to impending collision in preterm, full term, and postterm infants. *Infant Behavior and Development,* 1980, *3,* 155–165.

Philip, B. R. Reaction-times of children. *American Journal of Psychology,* 1934, *46,* 379–396.

Rose, S. A., Gottfried, A. W., & Bridger, W. H. Cross-modal transfer in infants: Relationship to prematurity and socioeconomic background. *Developmental Psychology,* 1978, *14,* 643–652.

Rose, S. A., Gottfried, A. W., & Bridger, W. H. Effects of haptic cues on visual recognition memory in full term and preterm infants. *Infant Behavior and Development,* 1979, *2,* 55–67.

Rose, S. A., Schmidt, K., & Bridger, W. H. Cardiac and behavioral responsivity to tactile stimulation in premature and full-term infants. *Developmental Psychology,* 1976, *12,* 311–320.

Schaefer, M., Hatcher, R. P., & Barglow, P. D. Prematurity and infant stimulation: A review of research. *Child Psychiatry and Human Development,* 1980, *80,* 195–198.

Schulman, C. A. Effects of auditory stimulation on heart rate in premature infants as a function of level of arousal, probability of CNS damage and conceptional age. *Developmental Psychobiology,* 1969, *2,* 172–183.

Sigman, M., Kopp, C. B., Littman, B., & Parmelee, A. H. Infant visual attentiveness in relation to birth condition. *Developmental Psychology,* 1977, *13,* 431–437.

Sigman, M., & Parmelee, A. H. Visual preferences of 4-month-old premature and full-term infants. *Child Development,* 1974, *45,* 959–965.

Sostek, A. M., Quinn, P. O., & Davitt, M. K. Behavior, development and neurologic status of premature and full-term infants with varying medical complications. In T. Field, A. M. Sostek, S. Goldberg, & H. H. Shuman (Eds.), *Infants born at risk.* Washington, D.C.: Spectrum, 1979.

Teberg, A., Hodgman, J. E., Wu, P. Y. K., & Spears, R. L. Recent improvement in outcome for the small premature infant. *Clinical Pediatrics,* 1977, *16,* 307–313.

Thompson, R. F., & Spencer, W. A. Habituation: A model phenomenon for the study of neuronal substrates of behavior. *Psychological Review,* 1966, *173,* 16–43.

Tilford, J. A. The relation between gestational age and adaptive behavior. *Merrill–Palmer Quarterly,* 1976, *22,* 319–326.

Werner, J. S., & Siqueland, E. R. Visual recognition memory in the preterm infant. *Infant Behavior and Development,* 1978, *1,* 79–94.

Wiener, G. Scholastic achievement at age 12–13 of prematurely born infants. *Journal of Special Education,* 1968, *2,* 237–250.

Wiener, G., Rider, R. V., Oppel, W. C., & Harper, P. A. Correlates of low birth weight: Psychological status at eight to ten years of age. *Pediatrics Research,* 1968, *2,* 110–118.

Winer, B. J. *Statistical principles in experimental design* (2nd ed.). New York: McGraw-Hill, 1976.

10

Mother-Infant Interactions in the Premature Nursery: A Sequential Analysis[1]

PETER MARTON
KLAUS MINDE
JOHN OGILVIE

Premature infants are at risk for a number of physical and psychological problems (Drillien, 1973). Advances in the field of neonatology have resulted in an increasing survival rate for these infants, thereby creating a growing need for empirical evidence on which to base their clinical management. In order to meet this need, research has moved away from the earlier simple follow-up studies whose aim was merely to categorize the sequelae of preterm birth. These studies found that there were often varied outcomes for similar biological insults in the neonatal period (Kopp & Parmelee, 1979). As a result, current hypotheses recognize that the process of development for these infants not only is influenced by the original biological trauma but also is often modified by more complex experiential factors. Three major clusters of contributing factors have been outlined: (*a*) the parents—their histories, personalities, and social context; (*b*) the infant—his physical substrate and its effect on his developmental competence and temperament; and (*c*) medical interventions in the neonatal period, which influence the biological outcome of the infant and set the context for early parent–infant interaction. These factors are seen as operating as a system, and the aim of much research has been to delineate their interplay and relative contributions (Klaus & Kennell, 1976; Kopp & Parmelee, 1979; Sameroff & Chandler, 1975). Parent–infant interaction has been recognized as one such important contributor to the development of the premature infant. The shift in emphasis from biological to social variables has produced a change in research methodology as well, requiring new techniques of data analysis to measure interactional phenomena.

[1] This work was supported by Grant No. 542 from the Ontario Mental Health Foundation and Grant No. 606–1360–44A1 from Health and Welfare Canada and the Laidlaw Foundation.

PRETERM BIRTH AND
PSYCHOLOGICAL DEVELOPMENT

179

The present chapter will review briefly some of the issues and pertinent findings about parent–infant interaction with premature infants. We will also review some of the principal strategies used to analyze parent–infant interaction. Additionally, we will present a procedure for sequential analysis of large blocks of concurrent, time-based observational data. Finally, we will illustrate this statistical procedure with some data obtained from observation of the interaction of mothers with their premature infants (birthweight < 1501 gm) in a neonatal intensive care unit.

Review of Research on Parent-Infant Interaction

Prematurity and Abuse

Premature infants have been found to be overrepresented in samples of abused children or those diagnosed with psychosocial failure to thrive (Elmer & Gregg, 1967; Fomufod, Sinkford, & Lovy, 1975; Klein & Stern, 1971; Schmitt & Kempe, 1975). Klaus and Kennell (1976, p. 3) attribute this to a disruption of the bonding process by medical procedures that require separation of mother and infant during a sensitive period. A cogent discussion of bonding and attachment in the full-term infant is available elsewhere (Campbell & Taylor, 1979). Bonding will be discussed here in relation to the premature infant only.

Barnett, Leiderman, Grobstein, and Klaus (1970) proposed that early contact of the mother with her premature infant was a necessary component of good clinical practice, since separation during the first few days postpartum was thought to attenuate the strength of the emotional bond between mother and infant. These authors also paved the way for the entry of parents into the premature nursery by demonstrating that this was not associated with increased infection on the ward. Two parallel series of studies were conducted—one at Stanford (e.g. Leifer, Leiderman, Barnett, & Williams, 1972) and one at Case Western Reserve (e.g., Kennell, Trause, & Klaus, 1975)—investigating the effects of early contact with the infant on the quality of mother–infant interaction.

At Stanford, Leifer *et al.* (1972) found no differences in maternal behavior during feedings (both in hospital and later at home) between mothers having early contact with their premature infants (after 2–3 days) and a group having later contact (3–12 weeks). A comparison group of mothers of full-term infants differed from both premature groups in the length of time spent in ventral contact and smiling during the first month at home. However, after the first month, no differences in behavior were found until 9 months. At this point, slight differences reemerged. Mothers of full-terms smiled at their infants more. Also, mothers having had early contact with their premature infants touched them more than did mothers initially separated from their premature infants. These differences were no longer observed at 11 months. It must be noted that this was predominently a white, middle-class sample of mothers and that early contact may be more crucial for families at greater psychosocial risk. In another report, these investigators also found that at least primiparous mothers of premature infants, while separated from their infants, expressed lower confidence in their caretaking competence than mothers of full-terms (Leiderman, Leifer, Seashore, Barnett, & Grobstein, 1973). Again, these differences disappeared after the first month at home.

The results of the studies at Case Western Reserve (Kennell *et al.,* 1975) were somewhat different. In one study, these authors examined mothers of premature infants who were allowed contact as soon as they were able and mothers who had contact with their infants only after a 3-week delay; they found that mothers in the early-contact group looked more at their infants during feedings in the hospital. Early-contact mothers also were found to hold their infants closer to their bodies during hospital feedings. These differences were attributed to greater maternal bonding. The fact that the specific differences found between early- and late-contact mothers were not consistent over time or across studies makes interpretation extremely difficult.

Some data are available regarding maternal visiting patterns to the premature nursery following mother's discharge from hospital. If the frequency of maternal visiting can be considered a measure of maternal bonding, some confirmation for the hypothesis that poor bonding increases the likelihood of abuse is provided by Fanaroff, Kennell, and Klaus (1972), who found that mothers who visited their infants infrequently in hospital showed a higher incidence of later abuse. Similarly, Minde, Trehub, Corter, Boukydis, Celhoffer, and Marton (1978) and Minde, Marton, Manning, and Hines (1980) found that mothers who were infrequent visitors were both less active and less responsive when they did visit their infants. However, neither of these studies examined the relative visiting patterns of early- and late-contact mothers. Therefore, although it may be possible to associate poor bonding with abuse, to date there is little to confirm a link between poor bonding and early separation of mother and infant. The studies presented above suggest that the effects of separation are of shorter duration, less consistent, and less pervasive than expected. Also, Campbell and Taylor (1979) have noted that the finding of a relation between abuse and prematurity has been based on retrospective studies with small samples of abused and control children. Douglas and Gear (1976) report results of a large-scale follow-up study in which they failed to find evidence of long-term disturbance in low-birthweight infants separated from their parents for several weeks. This study examined all children born in England during the first week of March 1946, thereby casting further doubt on the effects of early separation.

Although separation is one salient factor of prematurity, there are a number of other correlates that may play a causal role in the parenting relationship. Such factors as poverty, social and psychological deprivation, and an atypical child are also associated with abuse (Kempe & Helfer, 1972).

Parents of abused premature infants have been found to differ from those of nonabused prematures in the following ways: greater incidence of gestational illness (ten Bensel & Paxson, 1977); abnormal pregnancy, labor, and delivery (Lynch, 1975); increased maternal illness during the first year postpartum (Lynch, 1975; not replicated, Lynch & Roberts, 1977); social isolation, parental history of abuse and neglect, inadequate child spacing, and parental personality problems (Hunter, Kilstrom, Kraybill, & Loda, 1978). The relation of such parental factors to child abuse in general has been discussed at length in the literature on abuse (e.g., Kempe & Helfer, 1972). Although clearly documented, the clinical utility of these factors is limited, because in identifying families at risk, there is a prohibitively high rate of false positives. For example, Hunter *et al.* (1978), in applying these risk factors to families with infants in a neonatal intensive care unit, found that only 25% of the families that they had designated as being at risk actually abused their infants. Such a pattern of results would suggest that these parental factors, although clearly correlates of abuse, are not sufficient to trigger it when considered in isolation. Nonetheless, our own research points clearly to the importance of parental factors in the development of a disordered parenting relationship (Minde, Marton, Manning, & Hines, 1980). Mothers who visited their infants less frequently and who were less responsive in their interactions with their infants during hospital visits were also found to have poorer relations with their own parents and to receive less support from their spouses than the more responsive mothers. Mothers appear to enter the parenting relationship with a set, created by their life history and current social support systems, which is then modified by the infant's behavior and medical status.

Recent studies indicate that the child who is the target for abuse is often atypical or has aversive properties when compared to nonabused siblings. For example, several studies have found that many of the abused children are retarded (e.g., Schmitt & Kempe, 1975). Frodi, Lamb, Leavitt, Donovan, Neff, and Sherry (1978), in an interesting study found that, in general, adults' physiological reactions to the crying of preterm infants indicated that this cry was more aversive than the cry of a full-term infant. This suggests that such an infant may be more likely to trigger abuse.

Field and her colleagues (Field, 1977; Field, Hallock, Ting, Dempsey, Dabiri, & Shuman, 1978) looked at early indicators of developmental risk in preterm and postterm infants. Their research design permits a comparison of the relative contribution of early separation and atypical behavior of the infant to the quality of the early mother–infant relationship. The preterm group was separated for several days, whereas the postterm and a comparison group of full-terms were separated for only a few hours. When observed at 3½ months after their expected date of confinement, mothers in the two groups at risk behaved similarly to one another, but differed from the full-term group. During feeding and structured play, mothers of infants at risk were found to spend more time as the active initiators of exchanges with their infants. Since only the preterm group was separated, this argues that separation per se was not the critical factor in determining the pattern of the interaction. It was also found that both pre- and postterm infants were rated by their mothers as being more irritable and also were found to be less responsive on the Brazelton interactive process score. These differences between the groups at risk and the full-term group suggest alternately that it is the difficult temperament and lack of responsiveness of the infants that seemed to result in the different pattern of mother–infant interaction.

Further confirmation for this interpretation is found in a study by Brown and Bakeman (1980), who report similar differences between the interaction patterns of preterm infants and full-term infants with their respective mothers. They observed mothers and infants during a feeding in hospital a few days prior to discharge. In general, the preterm infants were found to be more difficult to feed and care for, and additionally to be less responsive and rewarding than full-term infants. Of particular interest is the finding that, although from 1 month to 3 months of age the behavior of the preterm infants approached that of the full-terms, the interaction patterns of mother and infant remained the same. Thus, throughout the predischarge observations and observations at 1 and 3 months, mothers of preterm infants carried the responsibility for initiating and maintaining the interaction more than the mothers of full-term infants.

Therefore, in this brief review we have considered the role of separation, parental factors, and infant factors in the development of an abusive relationship. It appears that in most cases none of these factors taken individually is a sufficient cause of abuse. Rather, they can be conceptualized as operating in a cumulative fashion, with each factor influencing the other. An important contribution of interaction research should be to clarify the process through which a disordered parenting relationship develops. It has been hypothesized that abuse is an extreme point along a continuum of disorders of parent–infant interaction (Sameroff & Chandler, 1975). Although this review has focused so far on the relation between prematurity and abuse, milder forms of parenting disorders also have implications for the emotional and cognitive development of the preterm infant.

Maternal Behavior and Developmental Competence

It is an accepted principal of development that the mother is an important early source of stimulation for the infant and in this way promotes his cognitive development. Since the preterm infant is at risk for later cognitive deficits, investigators have focused on mother–infant interaction, searching for maternal behaviors that can be associated with good outcome for the premature infant. The potential importance of the mother as a source of stimulation for her preterm infant has been noted by Minde and his colleagues, who found that mothers' visits represent a meaningful portion of their infants' interaction with caretakers in an intensive and post-intensive care unit (Marton, Dawson, & Minde, 1980; Minde, Trehub, Corter, Boukydis, Celhoffer, & Marton, 1978). Ward personnel were found to interact with these infants at a rate of 8 min per hour, whereas mothers touched their infants at an average rate of 24 min per hour. Hence, in a single 1-hour visit, the mother adds at least 20% to an infant's daily contact.

One area of investigation examined whether early contact in the nursery would facilitate mother–infant interaction and thus lead to improved cognitive development for preterm infants.

The two studies described in the preceding section (Kennell et al., 1975; Leiderman et al., 1973) that manipulated early contact in the premature nursery have presented, as preliminary findings, data showing better cognitive performance for early-contact infants, which they attributed to more optimal mother–infant interaction. Leiderman et al. (1973) found the early-contact infants to have higher Bayley scores at discharge. Kennell et al. (1975) found that at 42 months early-contact infants had higher scores on the Standford-Binet. Also, these latter scores were correlated with the amount of maternal looking at the infant observed during feedings at 1 month. However, these results have not been replicated by later studies. For example, Leiderman and his colleagues found no differences between the early- and later-contact groups of infants either at 3 months or at 15 months (Leiderman et al., 1973; Leiderman & Seashore, 1975).

Other investigators have attempted to use the quality of early mother-infant interaction as a predictor of later developmental outcome. Field et al. (1978) found that premature infants had lower Bayley scores than full-term infants at 8 and 12 months. Although the interactions of pre- and postterm infants with their mothers were rated as more difficult than the interactions with full-terms, these ratings were made at a different time (4 months of age), and the authors failed to specify the relationship between the degree of interactional difficulties within groups and their individual performance on the Bayley scales. Therefore, it is not possible to conclude whether the poor interaction was merely a correlate of cognitive deficits or was a contributing factor. This relationship remains unclear, since Brown and Bakeman (1979) compared premature and full-term infants and found differences in mother–infant interactions in the neonatal period but none in Bayley scores at 12 months.

Parmelee and his colleagues (Beckwith, Cohen, Kopp, Parmelee, & Marcy, 1976; Cohen & Beckwith, 1976, 1977) have investigated the relationship between specific patterns of mother–infant interaction and developmental competence of premature infants. Higher Gesell Developmental Quotient (D.Q.) scores at 9 months were found to be associated with maternal responses that may be characterized as providing less physical restraint and encouraging infants' independent postural balance and locomotor skills. Mothers who were more contingently responsive to their infants' social signals promoted greater infant sensorimotor skills. It was also noted that the particular infant behaviors to which mothers responded changed throughout the first year.

In conclusion, it appears that optimal mother–infant interaction may enable the premature infant to compensate for some of the hazards of a stormy perinatal course. However, the specific parameters of such optimal patterns of interaction are just beginning to be examined.

Most of the research in this area has been descriptive, linking interactional phenomena with later outcome on measures of cognitive and social development. More detailed molecular analyses can provide clarification of the process of interaction and permit specification of the developing relationship between parents and their premature infants.

In our own work (e.g., Minde *et al.*, 1978; Minde, Marton, Manning, & Hines, 1980; Minde, Shosenberg, Marton, Thompson, & Ripley, 1979), we have used behavioral observations that provide a detailed, continuous record of the developing relationship, in order to trace the course of the interaction process between the mother and her premature infant during the first year of life. We hope that this will allow us to determine the role of the various factors influencing this process.

The analysis of interaction, however, poses a number of methodological difficulties. To date, no universally acceptable statistical procedures exist for performing a sequential analysis on the type of detailed data produced by continuous observations of a relatively large number of concurrent events. The aim of this chapter is to outline a procedure that we have devised to analyze this type of data. In order to provide a perspective for this proposed method of analysis, we will present a brief review of the principal methods used to analyze interaction between parents and infants in the first year of life.

Review of Research on Methods of Analyzing Interaction

Although a great deal of research purports to investigate interactional phenomena, few studies actually present analyses of interactional data. The majority of "interactional" studies merely present data describing the behavior of one or both partners observed during an interaction (e.g., Lamb, 1977). To be truly interactional, data must at least reflect changes in behavior of one organism in response to changes in the behavior of another. More complete analyses, additionally, should give some indication of the chronological sequence of behaviors or the direction and magnitude of influence. Analysis procedures not meeting these criteria will not be covered in the following summary.

There are three principal approaches currently in use to analyze interaction in mother–infant dyads. The first is a descriptive approach, in which a single salient dimension thought to illustrate the interactional state of the dyad is derived from observations of discrete behavior categories. Changes in this state are subsequently scaled along a continuous dimension. For example, Brazelton and his colleagues (e.g., Brazelton, Tronick, Adamson, Als, & Wise, 1975; Tronick, Adamson, Wise, Als, & Brazelton, 1975) have coded the face-to-face interaction of mothers and their infants using 10 infant and 6 mother behavior categories. They have conceptualized five phases, made up of combinations of these discrete behaviors, to represent different states of the partners' mutual attentional and affective involvement, ranging from low to high involvement: (*a*) initiation; (*b*) mutual orientation; (*c*) greeting; (*d*) play–dialogue; and (*e*) disengagement. The interaction is described by tracing the cycling of the dyad through these phases over time.

A second approach is a statistical one, which uses a simple Markov-chain sequential analysis, in which behaviors of both members of the dyad are combined to define a few mutually exclusive and exhaustive discrete interactional states. The course of the interaction is traced in terms of the probability of transition from one discrete state to another (e.g., Bakeman & Brown, 1977; Lewis & Painter, 1974; Stern, 1974). Stern (1974), for example, uses this method to examine mother and infant face-to-face play. Mother and infant gazing is observed, producing four possible dyadic gazing states: (*a*) neither gazing at the other; (*b*) infant gazing at mother, mother gazing away; (*c*) infant gazing away, mother gazing at infant; and (*d*) both gazing at each other. A transition matrix is tabulated, showing the probability within a specified time interval of any dyadic state proceeding to any other dyadic state, including itself. The transition matrix can be converted into a state transition diagram for visual inspection.

A more comprehensive approach is a lag sequential analysis, as proposed by Sackett (1979) and Bakeman (1978). The behavior of each member of the dyad is first classified into any number of mutually exclusive and exhaustive categories. Then the occurrence of specific sequences of any single pair of behaviors of the mother and infant are examined over time. In this method, analysis requires first the determination of those behavior pairs that co-occur beyond chance expectation. The binomial z score is used to test this relationship. Sequential relations between significant behavior pairs are then determined by holding each behavior of the pair constant, in turn, as antecedent and examining the probabilities of occurrence for the consequent behavior conditional on the occurrence of the antecedent at increasingly distant time intervals. Examples applying this procedure to mother–infant interaction are not yet available.

Unfortunately, none of these procedures allowed us to adequately analyze the interactional components of our data, which consisted of a continuous record of a relatively large number of concurrent mother and infant behaviors. Complex observational data such as ours are becoming more common, primarily because of the ready availability of electronic recording devices that permit the acquisition and ready transfer to computers of vast quantities of data for storage and analysis (Celhoffer, Boukydis, Muir, & Minde, 1977). This has led to the creation of multicategory codes and the simultaneous recording of a relatively large number of ongoing behaviors. Such multicategory concurrent behavioral records are valuable for understanding the specific determinants of interaction because they provide a molecular description of the behaviors of mothers and their infants. However, all of the procedures presented in the preceding discussion impose limitations on the investigator that force the simplification of the data to permit analysis, thereby obscuring many interesting variables. A discussion of the problems associated with each of the procedures follows.

The descriptive approach (e.g., Brazelton *et al.,* 1975) provides clear descriptions of variations in interactional patterns at the global level. However, the method requires external validation of the dimension and scaling intervals selected, and statistical procedures for both describing and testing the results obtained are not readily determined. In addition to these difficulties, this method is clearly inadequate to handle the specificity of the type of data described earlier, since it must reduce the information to a single global dimension.

The Markov sequence analysis is the most commonly used method to describe patterns of mother–infant interaction, since it both permits examination of a greater number of dyadic events and is more amenable to quantitative analysis than the unidimensional descriptive approach. Nevertheless, this approach is unwieldy, in that every different combination of events is treated as a unique state, and thus the number of states that must be considered increases exponentially with the addition of each new behavior. For example, even four infant and four mother behaviors, if they are not mutually exclusive and can occur concurrently, can lead to 16 potential simple states and 48 potential combined states to be considered. This necessarily severely limits the number of behaviors that can be analyzed. Therefore, this approach, too, requires that for analysis the information contained in a complex record of behaviors be reduced to a few simple conditions. The product of the analysis is a matrix of transitional probabilities from one state to another. Interpretations of these probabilities into meaningful statements about interaction are not readily apparent. Furthermore, comparisons between subjects or groups is currently limited to visual inspection of patterns of transitional probabilities.

The lag sequential approach will be discussed in greater detail, because it comes closest to adequately analyzing multicategory behavioral data. The advantages of this procedure are that, first, unlike the other procedures described, it permits the examination of relationships between discrete behaviors. Second, the lag concept is a useful procedure that readily permits statistical analysis of the direction and magnitude of influence. However, the procedure has been developed to deal adequately only with mutually exclusive events, that is, coding systems in which only one category for an interaction is applicable at any one time. A serious problem with this approach is the choice of the underlying statistical model used to test the significance of relationships. The binomial test z score imposes the restriction that repeated observations over time be independent. In most applications, this assumption is violated. Although Bakeman (1978) suggests that this difficulty can be overcome by disregarding the probability levels ordinarily associated with binomial test z scores, and merely using the z score as an index for decision making, no data are presented on the validity of decisions made based on this index. A more critical problem associated with this test is that the binomial test z-scores, derived by:

$$z = \{[P(\text{observed})] - [P(\text{expected})]\}/ [SD (\text{expected})],$$

where $[SD (\text{expected})] = (\{[P(\text{expected})][1 - P (\text{expected})]\} /N)^{1/2}$ (derived, for example, by Gottman and Bakeman (1979) as:

$$z = \frac{N(\text{co-occurrences observed}) - [N(\text{behavior A})][P(\text{behavior B})]}{\{[N(\text{behavior A})][P(\text{behavior B})][1 - P(\text{behavior B})]\}^{1/2}}$$

yields biased results when the chance probability is derived from the same data set as the one being tested. In order to perform an unbiased test, this chance probability should be derived theoretically or estimated from a data set other than the one under consideration (Hays, 1963). An example will illustrate this problem.

Where $N(\text{observations}) = 30$, $N(\text{behavior A}) = 27$, $N(\text{behavior B}) = 10$,

$$z = \{[N(\text{co-occurrences})] - [(27)(10/30)]\} /[27)(10/30)(1 - 10/30)]^{1/2}$$

For a valid z test, the number of co-occurrences can theoretically range from 0 to 27, and thus, the probability of co-occurrences can range from 0 to 1. However, in the present example, the range of the number of co-occurrences is limited from 7 to 10, since the maximum number of non-co-occurrences possible is limited to 3 out of the 30 events. Hence the estimated probability here can range only from $\frac{7}{27}$ to $\frac{10}{27}$ or from .26 to .37.

Thus, z can only take on the following values:

$$N(\text{co-occurrences}) = (7 - 9)/2449 \ , \ (8 - 9)/2449 \ , \ (9 - 9)/2449 \ , \ (10 - 9)/2449$$

$$z = \quad - .817 \quad , \quad - .408 \quad , \quad 0 \quad , \quad + .408$$

[z must be ≥ 1.96 for $P \leq .05$]

Thus, in this example, the hypothesis of independence of the two behaviors could never be disproven.

Note that the problem does not disappear even if N is large. Suppose that $[N(\text{observations})] = 300$, $[N(\text{behavior A})] = 270$, $[N(\text{behavior B})] = 100$.

$$70 \leq \text{co-occurrences} \geq 100$$

$$- \frac{(70 - 90)}{9} \leq z \geq \frac{(100 - 90)}{9}$$

That is, $- 2.58 \leq z \geq 1.29$

Thus, even with a large number of observations, it cannot always be concluded that one behavior is dependent on the other, since it can be seen that the test is skewed, in this case toward detecting situations where the number of co-occurrences is less than expected by chance. This presents a considerable problem, since although the test is skewed the direction of bias cannot be predicted a priori.

Thus, although this procedure deals most comprehensively with the data, care must be exercised in the interpretation of results because of the likelihood that the assumptions of the statistical model will be violated to some extent in most applications.

In developing a sequential analysis procedure to fit our data, we have adopted the same overall strategy of first determining significant co-occurrences among behaviors and then lagging the significant behavior pairs over time. However, we have selected what we hope are more suitable statistical models and have adapted sampling procedures to satisfy the assumptions.

Time-Lag Sequential Analysis for Concurrent Behavior

We will first describe in general the procedure we have developed to perform a sequential analysis on data from continuous behavioral observations in which 10 mother and 12 infant behavior categories are recorded concurrently (see Table 10.1). Following this, the procedure will be illustrated with data obtained from our observations of mothers and infants in the neonatal intensive care unit during the first few visits. Such observations yield a rich data base in which we may examine 120 simple mother–infant behavior combinations and an astronomical number of possible combinations of multiple events. An example of one such record is presented in order to facilitate conceptualization of the nature of the data (see Figure 10.1). The data consist of information regarding the times of onset and offset and duration of specific behavioral categories such as infant eye opening and mother touching. Hence the categories represent the presence of behavioral conditions rather than frequency counts of specific events. In order to quantify these data, we divide the continuous record into convenient time slices (see Figure 10.2). In practice, we have found 5 sec to provide an optimal analogue to the continuous record. Thus, duration is translated into frequency counts by enumerating the number of intervals in which a behavior is present. In order to ensure that this pro-

TABLE 10.1
Behavior Categories for Mothers and Infants

Infant behavior categories

    Eyes scan
    Eyes open
    Arm movement
    Leg movement
    Head movement
    Mouthing
    Hand to mouth
    Vocalizing
    Crying
    Grimacing
    Yawning
    Smiling

Maternal behavior categories

    Looking
    Looking en face
    Vocalizing to baby
    Vocalizing to others
    Smiling
    Noninstrumental touch
    Instrumental touch
    Holding
    Feeding
    Standing more than 3 ft away

cedure does not distort the record, we compare the true relative durations (duration of behavior/total duration of observation) to the relative durations derived from the time-slice counts (N slices behavior is present/N slices total observation).

In order to determine the behaviors in the interaction that play a causal role, we identify those mother and infant behaviors that co-occur significantly more often than expected by chance. To overcome some of the difficulties associated with the binomial z score, we have selected chi-square because it is an appropriate statistic for determining dependence in qualitative data and provides a fairly robust unbiased test when the underlying assumptions are met. Similar to the binomial score, this test also assumes that observations on the same subject are independent. However, in this application, we know that this is not the case. Therefore, in order to satisfy this assumption of the test and thus make use of the probability levels associated with it, for this preliminary step only, we impose independence on the data by sampling from the continuous record. It was found that by selecting data from every tenth time interval of the continuous record, we could make a reasonable approximation to independence, with known error and without sacrificing an inordinate amount of data. Table 10.2 presents conditional probabilities at vary-

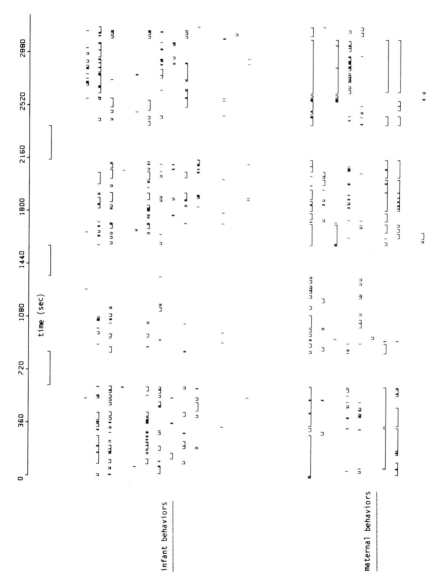

FIGURE 10.1. *The continuous behavior record representing mother-infant interaction during one nursery visit.*

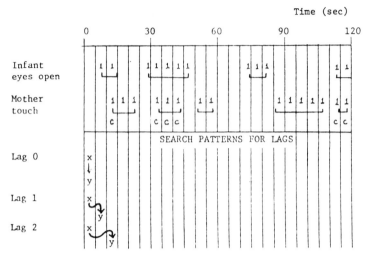

FIGURE 10.2. *Sampling from the continuous record: a hypothetical example. Eyes open, N = 12; mother touches, N = 14; co-occurrences, N = 6; slices, N = 24. Each slice = 5 sec.*

TABLE 10.2

Probability of Reocurrence of Maternal and Infant Behavior Categories at Selected Intervals

Behavior	Chance probability	Probability of reoccurrence at interval				
		1	5	10	15	20
Infant						
Eyes open	.220	.900	.740	.660	.610	.540
Arm	.350	.780	.520	.450	.400	.380
Leg	.370	.780	.490	.430	.390	.360
Head	.130	.650	.290	.210	.170	.140
Vocalize	.002	.290	.060	.000	—	—
Grimace	.006	.480	.020	.000	—	—
Smile	.006	.460	.080	—	—	—
Hand to mouth	.060	.820	.650	.560	.510	.450
Cry	.0005	.500	.000	—	—	—
Yawn	.008	.380	.020	.000	—	—
Mouth	.140	.650	.340	.310	.290	.240
Mother						
Look	.710	.930	.800	.730	.670	.620
Look en face	.130	.840	.500	.400	.380	.360
Hold	.020	.850	.710	.600	.530	.470
Vocalize to baby	.090	.680	.320	.240	.210	.190
Vocalize to other	.200	.690	.360	.330	.290	.260
> 3 ft	.005	.790	.310	.100	.070	.000
Touch	.360	.950	.820	.730	.660	.610
Smile	.160	.850	.610	.550	.510	.460
Instrumental touch	.003	.610	.070	.000	—	—

ing intervals for each behavior category, given a prior occurrence at time 0. It can be seen that most behaviors at lag 10 approach closely their chance level of occurrence and that little is gained by sampling more stringently (e.g., by halving the data, lag 20). An advantage of this method is that it allows us to determine the reliability of the results by repeating the analysis, up to 10 times, to examine the intervals ignored thus far. This can be accomplished by repeating the analysis, using as origin the second time interval, then the third, fourth, and so on.

Chi-square tests (corrected for continuity) are then calculated for all possible mother–infant behavior pairs. The chi square test has an additional requirement that all cells of the 2 × 2 table produced have a minimal expected cell frequency of 5 (Hays, 1963). Therefore, those behavior pairs that fail to meet this requirement are ignored. Those behaviors for which the chi-square test approaches conventional significance levels are considered to be mutually dependent. The observed and expected number of co-occurrences are examined to determine whether the dependence relationship can be considered to be mutually facilitative or inhibitory. Additionally, the phi coefficient (Hays, 1963) is used to indicate the strength of the association.

The following example is given to illustrate the application of the chi-square test to determine whether a maternal behavior (e.g., mother smiles) and an infant behavior (e.g., infant smiles) are mutually dependent.

Consider two hypothetical cases: (*a*) one in which, during 50 time intervals, the number of infant smiles is 30, the number of maternal smiles is 30, the number of co-occurrences is 25, and the number of nonoccurrences is 15; and (*b*) one in which, during 36 intervals, the number of infant smiles is 30, the number of maternal smiles is 30, the number of co-occurrences is 25, but the number of nonoccurrences is only 1. Figure 10.3 illustrates the 2 × 2 chi square tables for both sets of conditions. The tables contain both observed and expected frequencies for mother and infant behaviors. Expected frequencies are based on the number of events that would be expected to occur by chance if the behaviors were independent, given the number of mother and

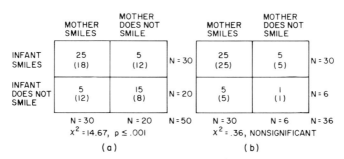

FIGURE 10.3. *A 2 × 2 chi-square table illustrating a hypothetical relation between mother smiles and infant smiles. (a) The behaviors are mutually dependent. (b) The behaviors are mutually independent.*

infant events. Differences between observed and expected frequencies are compared, and given the magnitude of these differences, the test gives an estimate of the probability that the two behaviors are mutually dependent.

Having identified those mother and infant behaviors that are mutually dependent, we then restore the record to its continuous state. The examination of the sequential relation between mother and infant behaviors is carried out on the complete record in which every time interval is considered. In order to determine the direction of influence of mother and infant during an interaction sequence, a time-lag procedure is carried out. That is, for each mother–infant behavior pair that co-occurs significantly, first the infant behavior is held constant and the conditional occurrence of the maternal behavior is determined at consecutive 5-sec intervals further away in time. Next, the conditional probabilities of these events are computed. Similarly, the counts and conditional probabilities for the infant behavior conditional on the antecedent maternal behavior are determined. To illustrate this procedure, a plot of a hypothetical relation between an infant behavior (smile) and a maternal behavior (smile) lagged over time is presented in Figure 10.4.

First, it should be noted that at the co-occurrence point (lag 0) the probability of a maternal smile conditional on an infant smile is greater than its chance level, and therefore, it can be concluded that maternal smiling is influenced by infant smiling. With increasing time after the occurrence of an infant smile, the probability of a maternal smile decreases, indicating that the degree of influence of the infant behavior diminishes with time. This function decays gradually over time, until it returns to chance level at lag 15, indicating that the mother is no longer being influenced by the smile which occurred at lag 0.

A comparison of this plot with the one in which the infant behavior is conditional upon the occurrence of the maternal behavior at lag 0 provides an indication of the direction of influence. By examining the points at which the

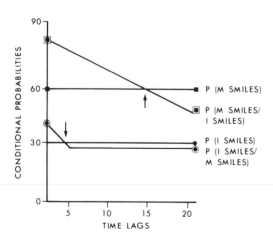

FIGURE 10.4. *Plot of conditional probabilities (P) obtained from time lags for a hypothetical case in which mother (M) smiles in response to infant (I) smiles.*

two functions return to chance level (lag 15 versus lag 5), as well as the magnitude of the increase of the conditional probability beyond the chance level, we can determine the sequence of events that occurred most often during the observation. In this example, the sequence that held most consistently was mother smiles in response to an infant smile.

A trend analysis is then performed on these data, comparing the two sets of conditional probabilities over time intervals, using a repeated measure analysis of variance (Winer, 1971, pp. 514–539). This analysis indicates the type of function that best describes the relation between the mother and infant variables. It also tests whether the two data sets display significantly different trends, thus enabling us to decide on the sequential relation. Visual inspection of the data, plotted over time intervals, allows us to estimate the relative difference in time when the consequent behaviors are no longer influenced (i.e., return to their simple chance level). Thus, our method determines first those behavior pairs that are mutually dependent (chi-square). Second, it allows us to determine the type of function that best describes the conditional relations over time (lagged conditional probabilities). Finally, the difference in temporal pattern is tested, allowing us to determine the direction of influence (trend analysis).

Our Study

To further illustrate the information that can be obtained with this type of analysis, we will apply it to some of our data obtained in a study of the interaction of mothers and their very low birthweight infants. A more complete presentation of these data can be found in a forthcoming publication (Marton, Minde, Trehub, & Corter, 1980).

Method

SUBJECTS

Our study sample consisted of 32 very low birthweight infants and their mothers. Selection criteria for the infants were the following: birthweight less than 1501 gm, singleton birth, weight appropriate for gestational age, absence of physical malformation, and absence at 72 hours of age of such serious medical complications as respiratory distress requiring respiratory assistance, sepsis, convulsions, or severe acid base imbalance. Criteria for the parents were that they intended to keep their infants and lived within 15 miles of the hospital in which the study was conducted. The sample thus constituted a group of very small premature infants who had a relatively good medical prognosis and were unlikely to have suffered gross cerebral damage. The background characteristics of this sample are described in Table 10.3.

TABLE 10.3[a]
Background Data for Study Sample

Mothers[b]	
Age (yr)	
Mean	28
Range	16–38
Marital status	
Married	26
Single	6
Parity	
Primipara	8
Multipara	24
Previous abortions	
or miscarriages	
1	11
More than 1	6
Lost infant of less than	5
3 months of age	
Socioeconomic class	
1 + 2	6
3	8
4 + 5	18

Infants[a]	
Sex	
F	17
M	15
Birthweight (gm)	
Mean	1160
Range	680–1490

[a] From K. Minde, P. Marton, D. Manning, & B. Hines. Some determinants of mother-infant interaction in the premature nursery. *Journal of the American Academy of Child Psychiatry,* 1980.
[b] $N = 32$.

SETTING

The study was conducted in the Neonatal Intensive Care Unit of the Hospital for Sick Children, Toronto, Canada. This unit has an annual admission rate of about 1200 infants, about 300 of whom weigh less than 1501 gm and 100 less than 1000 gm at birth. It has a nursing staff of approximately 150, placing it among the largest neonatal units in North America. In this unit parental visiting and stimulation of the infants are actively encouraged.

PROCEDURE

Mother–infant interaction was observed during maternal visits to the nursery and during the first 3 months at home. An attempt was made to observe up to two visits per week. The duration of visits was determined by the parents, up to a maximum of 40 min. Two observers, one recording infant behaviors and the other recording maternal behaviors, continuously categorized behavior interaction, with the observational code already described above, using an event recorder. The behaviors are recorded on a casette tape and then are directly entered into a minicomputer for storage and analysis. This system, which has been described in detail elsewhere (Celhoffer *et al.,* 1977), is able to simultaneously record up to 64 events. A detailed descriptive record is thus available with a machine accuracy of ¼ sec and an average observer reliability of at least 85%.

Results

Since we were concerned with whether mother–infant interaction was possible at this initial stage of acquaintance, we chose to analyze first the interaction of mothers and their very low birthweight infants during the first five visits to the neonatal intensive care unit. Throughout these visits, the infant remained in an isolette; however, mothers were permitted to touch and speak to their infants through the portholes.

To clarify our results, we divided our sample of mothers into three subgroups on the basis of maternal activity level during the first five nursery visits, a dimension that we have found to have meaningful correlates. These groupings have been found to be associated with differences in psychosocial history, in frequency of contact with the infant, and in responsivity to the infant during visits (Minde *et al.,* 1978; Minde, Marton, Manning, & Hines, 1980). The subgrouping was done by calculating the median of each maternal behavior for the initial five nursery visits. Subsequently, each mother's behavior was scored as falling either above or below the particular median of that observation. If the mother scored above the median on more than 75% of all behaviors during all observations, she was placed in the "high-activity" category. If she fell below the median on 75% of all behaviors during these observations, she was placed in a "low-activity" group. If she fit neither of these extreme groupings, she was designated as a "medium-activity" mother. Six mothers were assigned to the high, 11 to the low, and 15 to the medium group.

For this sequential analysis, the longest observed visit made within the mother's first five visits to the nursery was selected. The data consist of a total of 583 min of observation. Each observation record was divided into consecutive 5-sec time slices. Behaviors were noted as being present or absent within a time slice. By summing the number of these time slices in which a behavior was present, the continuous time information was transformed into frequency counts of behaviors. Data for statistical analysis of dependencies between behaviors were obtained by sampling from every tenth time slice.

To determine which mother–infant behaviors were mutually dependent, chi square analyses were performed on the co-occurrence of each simple mother–infant behavior combination and several multiple behavior clusters. Because

TABLE 10.4
Dependencies between Selected Maternal and Infant Behaviors

Infant	Mother	χ^2	Phi	Relation[a]
Eyes open	Touches	36.50**	.21	+
Moves arm, leg and head	Smiles	5.16*	.08	+

* $p \leq .05$
** $p \leq .001$
[a] (+) = mutual facilitation, (−) = mutual inhibition.

the sampling procedure eliminates a great proportion of data, the counts were summed over observations to ensure an adequate N for this analysis. The two behavior pairs that we have selected to illustrate this analysis are (*a*) infant moves arm, leg, and head (a stretch) and mother smiles; and (*b*) infant has eyes open and mother touches. The first pair serves as a check on our method, since the direction of influence should logically be infant stretch facilitates mother's smile. The relation of mother touch–infant eyes open is then analyzed, since this relation is theoretically of interest. As shown in Table 10.4, both behavior pairs are dependent and are mutually facilitative. This indicates that for the sample as a whole when the infant's eyes are open the mother is likely to be touching and also that when the infant is engaged in a gross motor stretch the mother is likely to be smiling at the infant. To clarify the sequential relation, we then lagged these behavior pairs over 20 5-sec time lags. The conditional probabilities were derived and were analyzed for trend over time with a three-way analysis of variance with repeated measures (antecedent condition × activity groups × time lags). The results of the trend analysis are presented in the following discussion. These results can be conceptualized more clearly while referring to Figures 10.5 and 10.6.

For the infant stretch–mother smile behavior combination, the following results were found:

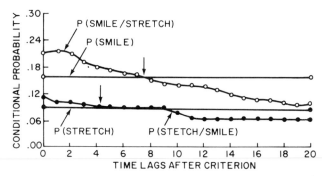

FIGURE 10.5. *Conditional probabilities (P) of infant stretch and mother smile for the entire sample lagged over 5-sec intervals.*

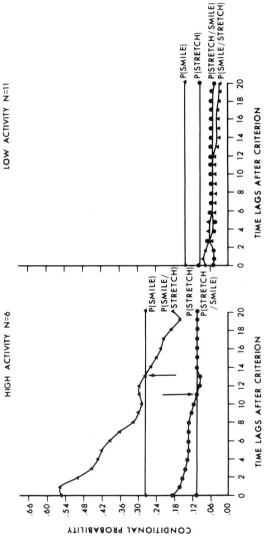

FIGURE 10.6. Conditional probabilities (P) of infant stretch and mother smile lagged over 5-sec intervals. (Reprinted from K. Minde, P. Marton, D. Manning, & B. Hines. Some determinants of mother-infant interaction in the premature nursery. Journal of the American Academy of Child Psychiatry, 1980, 19, 17.)

1. A main effect for time lags ($F = 5.81, p < .001, df = 20, 920$) indicates that the conditional probabilities change over time. A significant linear slope ($F = 11.76; p < .001, df = 1,46$) shows that this change can be described by a line sloping toward chance. We can interpret this to mean that infant stretch and mother smile influence each other so that they co-occur more frequently than we would expect and that, as time increases away from the point of co-occurrence, this influence decreases linearly toward chance.

2. A main effect for antecedent condition ($F = 6.07, p < .02, df = 1, 46$) was found and means that the conditional relations are different for the two antecedent conditions, if mother smiles and if infant stretches. The interaction of antecedent conditions with time lags ($F = 1.59, p < .05, df = 20, 920$) indicates that, overall, the difference for the two antecedents varies over time. This interaction also has a linear component that approaches significance ($F = 2.65, p < .11, df = 1, 46$). Thus, overall the sequence of events is that mothers smile more often after a stretch than vice versa. The influence of the infant's stretch on the mother decays linearly over time.

3. A main effect for maternal activity groups ($F = 3.37, p < .04, df = 2, 46$) was found and implies that the degree of responsivity of mothers and infants in the two groups varies. Visual inspection of Figure 10.6 shows that the high-activity mothers are responsive, whereas the low-activity mothers are not. To simplify presentation, the medium group is omitted from this figure. The responsivity of the three groups was found to differ generally over time ($F = 1.63, p < .01, df = 40,920$) and also to differ over time for each of the two antecedent conditions ($F = 1.30, p < .1, df = 40,920$). This implies that the high-activity mothers responded to the infant's stretch with a smile and that this tendency decreased over time. However, the low-activity mothers did not show such a response.

The results obtained are the ones we would logically expect, that is, that an infant's stretch is responded to with a smile and not that mothers' smiles are responded to by preterm infants with a gross motor stretch. This corroborates our methodology. Furthermore, the utility of the method is demonstrated by the additional potential for identifying different patterns among subgroups of parents. Thus through this analysis, we have been able to (a) identify that a relation exists between maternal and infant behavior; (b) compare the magnitude as well as trace the pattern of change of this influence; (c) detect differences in responsivity among groups of mothers; and finally (d) identify the sequence of events.

A similar presentation of results is provided for the relation between infant has eyes open and mother touches. Interpretation is facilitated by examining Figures 10.7 and 10.8. Fewer data were available for this analysis (only 18 dyads), since a number of infants were undergoing phototherapy and for protection had patches taped over their eyes or because observations of the eyes were restricted by other equipment (for example, oxygen hoods). Unfortunately, this reduced the power of the trend analysis (antecedent conditions × activity groups × time lags). Again, the influence of the antecedent

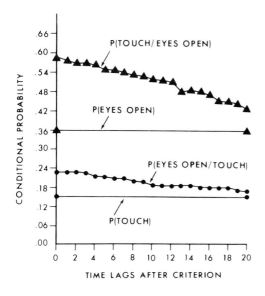

FIGURE 10.7. *Conditional probabilities (P) of infant eyes open and mother touch for the entire sample lagged over 5-sec intervals.*

behaviors (infant eyes open and mother touches) varied over time ($F = 2.01$, $p < .005$, $df = 20,840$) and diminishes with a considerable linear component ($F = 2.64, p < .11, df = 1, 42$). An examination of the dependencies of these two behavior pairs showed that these relations held more strongly for the high-activity group than for the low-activity group ($F = 4.34, p < .025$, df $= 2, 30$) (see Figure 10.8). Furthermore, an interaction of activity groups with antecedent conditions over time lags was found to approach significance ($F = 1.26$, p $< .138$, $df = 40, 600$). This result indicated that high-activity mothers

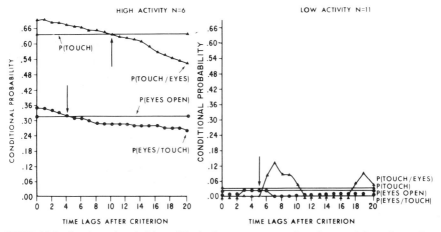

FIGURE 10.8. *Conditional probabilities (P) of infant eyes-open and mother touch lagged over 5-sec intervals. (Reprinted from K. Minde, P. Marton, D. Manning, & B. Hines. Some determinants of mother-infant interaction in the premature nursery.* Journal of the American Academy of Child Psychiatry, *1980, 19, 16.)*

tended to touch their infants when the eyes were open, whereas low-activity mothers failed to respond to this signal.

Discussion and Summary

Previously, we have used a detailed coding system to describe the behavior of mothers toward their premature infants. This has allowed us to identify characteristic maternal activity patterns and to evaluate both their role as predictors of the later caretaking relationship and the influence of determining factors. However, this type of data presents a number of difficulties for the analysis of sequential relationships. Sequential analysis procedures currently in use were not found to be appropriate, and thus, we were led to develop a procedure whose assumptions would suit this type of data.

The method of analysis that we have presented allowed us to determine the direction of influence of a series of mother–infant behaviors. For example, a gross motor stretch (arm, leg, and head movement) and eye opening by the infant serve as social signals for the mother and elicit such responses from her as smiling or touching. We have noted differences in maternal responsivity to these early social signals, and these differences can be related to specific maternal characteristics, such as the general activity level of the mother. Our data seem to document that even at such an early stage, when the infant is still in an isolette, patterns of interaction are developing. To date, we have identified some variables that influence the mother to modify her behavior in response to cues received from her infant.

Our confidence in the validity of these conclusions is increased by the corroboration provided by other, more global measures. For example, these differences in maternal responsivity have been found to be associated with differences in visiting patterns to the nursery and to psychosocial background variables, such as the mother's feeling of support from her family of origin and her spouse.

It appears that a mother enters the nursery with a predetermined set that influences her interactional style. The nature of her background and personal history influences the intensity with which a mother will interact with her infant and the degree to which she will be responsive. The specific events surrounding the birth seem to play a less direct role. Our data show that the high-activity mothers, who as a group had more positive interpersonal histories, are more responsive to the signs of their infant and that the interaction is more easily steered by the infant; whereas the low-activity mothers are less responsive to the infant's cues. This may mean that mothers who in the past had fewer positive interpersonal experiences may need greater stimulation from their infants to engage in activity with them. We have been unable to identify during these early visits any consistent responses to maternal stimulation and consider this to be a reflection of the relative immaturity of the infant's central nervous system.

The analyses of interaction presented here were derived from the first five nursery visits. We are currently examining interaction patterns during later hospital visits and the early months at home in order to determine whether levels of responsivity are consistent. A question of particular concern is whether low-activity mothers become more responsive over time. Furthermore, as the infant matures, we can expect a broader range of infant behaviors and the beginning of responding to maternal behavior. We hope to determine whether the early differences in maternal responsivity will be reflected in differences in the pattern of the infant's emerging behaviors.

At this point, the analysis of interaction in behavioral observation data seems to require as much art as it does technical skill. Nevertheless, the method proposed and illustrated in this chapter seems to yield meaningful information based on valid statistical principles that provide guidelines for decision making. In addition, our method has the advantage of permitting the analysis of concurrent events and thus enables us to retain the intricate nature of the interaction.

Acknowledgments

This work could not have been done without the continuing generous assistance of P. Swyer, director of perinatology, and all the staff and the mothers of the Neonatal Intensive Care Unit, The Hospital for Sick Children, Toronto, Canada.

The final revisions of this chapter were made after the untimely passing of John Ogilvie. His contributions to the initial conception of the sequential analysis procedures and their presentation in this chapter are gratefully acknowledged. Any errors that have crept into subsequent revisions must be attributed to the other authors.

Gratitude is also expressed to Bruce Schneider for statistical consultation and to Daniel Geurin for the development of computer programs.

References

Bakeman, R. Untangling streams of behavior. In Sackett, G. (Ed.), *Observing behavior Vol. 2. Data collection and analysis methods.* Baltimore: University Park Press, 1978.

Bakeman, R., & Brown, J. Behavioral dialogues: An approach to the assessment of mother–infant interaction. *Child Development,* 1977, *48,* 195–201.

Barnett, C., Leiderman, P. Grobstein, R., & Klaus, M. Neonatal separation: The maternal side of interactional deprivation. *Pediatrics* 1970, *45,* 197–205.

Beckwith, L., Cohen, S., Kopp, C., Parmelee, A., & Marcy, T. Caregiver–infant interaction and early cognitive development in preterm infants. *Child Development,* 1976, *47,* 579–587.

Brazelton, T., Tronick, E., Adamson, L., Als, H., & Wise, S. Early mother-infant reciprocity. In *Parent–infant interaction* (Ciba Foundation Symposium, 33). Amsterdam. Elsevier, 1975.

Brown, J., & Bakeman, R. Relationships of human mothers with their infants during the first year of life: Effects of prematurity. In R. Bell & W. Smotherman (Eds.). *Maternal influences and early behavior.* Holliswood, N.Y.: Spectrum, 1980.

Campbell, S., & Taylor, P. Bonding and attachment: Theoretical Issues. *Seminars in Perinatology,* 1979, *3,* 3–13.

Celhoffer, L., Boukydis, C., Muir, E., & Minde, K. A portable computer-compatible event recorder for observing behaviour. *Behaviour Research Methods and Instrumentation,* 1977, *9,* 442–446.

Cohen, S., & Beckwith, L. Maternal language in infancy. *Developmental Psychology,* 1976, *12,* 311–372.

Cohen, S., & Beckwith, L. Caregiving behaviors and early cognitive development as related to ordinal position in preterm infants. *Child Development,* 1977, *48,* 152-157.

Douglas, J., & Gear, R. Children of low birthweight in the 1946 cohort. *Archives of Diseases of Children,* 1976, *51,* 820-827.

Drillien, C. Fresh approaches to prospective studies of low birth weight infants. *Research Publications Association for Research on Nervous and Mental Diseases,* 1973, *51,* 198-209.

Elmer, E., & Gregg, G. Developmental characteristics of abused children. *Pediatrics,* 1967, *40,* 596-602.

Fanaroff, A., Kennell, J., & Klaus, M. Follow-up of low birthweight infants: The predictive value of maternal visiting patterns. *Pediatrics,* 1972, *49,* 287-290.

Field, T. Effects of early separation, interactive deficits, and experimental manipulations on infant-mother face-to-face interaction. *Child Development,* 1977, *48,* 763-771.

Field, T., Hallock, N., Ting, G., Dempsey, J., Dabiri, C., & Shuman, H. A first-year follow-up of high-risk infants: Formulating a cumulative risk index. *Child Development,* 1978, *49,* 119-131.

Fomufod, A., Sinkford, S., & Lovy, V. Mother-child separation at birth: A contributing factor in child abuse. *The Lancet,* 1975, *2,* 549-550.

Frodi, A., Lamb, M., Leavitt, L., Donovan, W., Neff, C., & Sherry, D. Fathers' and mothers' responses to the faces and cries of normal and premature infants. *Developmental Psychology,* 1978, *14,* 490-498.

Gottman, J., & Bakeman, R. The sequential analysis of observational data. In M. lamb, S. Suomi, & G. Stephenson (Eds.), *Social interaction analysis: Methodological issues.* Madison: Univ. of Wisconsin Press, 1979.

Hays, W. *Statistics.* New York: Holt, 1963.

Hunter, R. S., Kilstrom, N., Kraybill, E. N., & Loda, F. Antecedents of child abuse and neglect in premature infants: A prospective study in a newborn intensive care unit. *Pediatrics,* 1978, *61,* 629-635.

Kempe, C., & Helfer, R. *Helping the battered child and his family.* Toronto: Lippincott, 1972.

Kennell, J., Trause, M., & Klaus, M. Evidence for a sensitive period in the human mother. In *Parent-infant interaction.* (Ciba Foundation Symposium 33). Amsterdam: Elsevier, 1975.

Klaus, M., & Kennell, J. Mothers separated from their newborn infants. *Pediatric Clinics of North America,* 1970, *17,* 1015-1037.

Klaus, M., & Kennell, J. *Maternal infant bonding.* Saint Louis: Mosby, 1976.

Klein, M., & Stern, L. Low birthweight and the battered child syndrome. *American Journal of the Diseases of Children,* 1971, *122,* 15-18.

Kopp, C., & Parmelee, A. Prenatal and Perinatal Influences on Infant Behavior. In J. Osofsky (Ed.), *Handbook of infant development.* New York: Wiley, 1979.

Lamb, M. Father-infant and mother-infant interaction in the first year of life. *Child Development,* 1977, *48,* 167-181.

Leiderman, P., Leifer, A., Seashore, M., Barnett, C., & Grobstein, R. Mother-infant interaction: Effects of early deprivation, prior experience and sex of infant. In J. N. Nurnberger (Ed.). *Biological and environmental determinants of early behavior.* Baltimore: Williams and Wilkins, 1973.

Leiderman, P., & Seashore, M. Mother-infant neonatal separation: Some delayed consequences. In *Parent-infant interaction* (Ciba Foundation Symposium 33). Amsterdam: Elsevier, 1975.

Leifer, A., Leiderman, P., Barnett, C., & Williams, J. Effects of mother-infant separation on maternal attachment behavior. *Child Development,* 1972, *43,* 1203-1218.

Lewis, M., & Painter, S. An interactional approach to the mother-infant dyad. In M. Lewis & L. Rosenblum (eds.). *The effect of the infant on its caregiver.* New York: Wiley, 1974.

Lynch, M. Ill-health and child abuse. *The Lancet,* 1975, *2,* 317-319.

Lynch, M., & Roberts, J. Predicting child abuse: Signs of bonding failure in the maternity hospital. *British Medical Journal,* 1977, *1,* 624-626.

Marton, P., Dawson, H., & Minde, K. The interaction of ward personnel with infants in the premature nursery. *Journal of Infant Behavior and Development,* 1980 (in press)

Marton, P., Minde, K., Trehub, S., & Corter, C. The interaction of mothers and premature infants during the first six months of life. Ms in preparation, 1980.

Minde, K., Trehub, S., Corter, C., Boukydis, C., Celhoffer, L., & Marton, P. Mother–child relationships in the premature nursery: An observational study. *Pediatrics,* 1978, *61,* 373–379.

Minde, K., Marton, P., Manning, D., & Hines, B. Some determinants of mother–infant interaction in the premature nursery. *Journal of the American Academy of Child Psychiatry,* 1980, *19,* 1–21.

Minde, K., Shosenberg, N., Marton, P., Thompson, J., & Ripley, J. Self-help groups in a premature nursery—a controlled evaluation. *Journal of Pediatrics,* 1980, *96,* 933.

Sameroff, A. J., & Chandler, M. J. Reproductive risk and the continuum of caretaking casualty. In F. D. Horowitz (Ed.), *Review of child development research* (Vol. 4). Chicago: Univ. of Chicago Press, 1975.

Sackett, G. The lag sequential analysis of contingency and cyclicity in behavioral interaction research. In J. Osofsky (Ed.), *Handbook of infant development.* New York: Wiley, 1979.

Schmitt, B., & Kempe, H. Neglect and abuse of children. In V. Vaughan & R. McKay (Eds.), *Nelson textbook of pediatrics.* Philadelphia: Saunders, 1975.

Stern, D. N. Mother and infant at play: The dyadic interaction involving facial, vocal and gaze behaviors. In M. Lewis & L. Rosenblum (Eds.). *The effect of the infant on its caregiver.* New York: Wiley, 1974.

ten Bensel, R., & Paxson, C. Child abuse following early post-partum separation. *Journal of Pediatrics,* 1977, *90,* 490–491.

Tronick, E., Adamson, L., Wise, S., Als, H., & Brazelton, T. Mother–infant face to face interaction. In S. Gosh (Ed.), *Biology and Language.* London: Academic Press, 1975.

Winer, B. *Statistical principles in experimental design.* New York: McGraw-Hill, 1971.

11

Sensory Responsiveness and Social Behavior in the Neonatal Period: A Review of Chapters 9 and 10[1]

ANNELIESE F. KORNER

Over the last 25 years, a great deal of research has been done with newborn infants. This interest in the neonate has been based on many different fundamental research questions. For one, it was discovered that newborns are a great deal more competent than had been thought earlier. They are highly capable of responding to visual, auditory, tactile, vestibular-proprioceptive, gustatory, and olfactory stimuli, and they have a fairly large repertoire of motor responses. A good deal of recent research has also focused on individual differences among neonates and how these affect the infant's caregiver. This, in turn, led to the development of a variety of assessment procedures of newborns and methods of studying the earliest parent–infant interaction. Representative contributions to these areas of research can be found in volumes by Lewis and Rosenblum (1974) and by Osofsky (1979).

Until recently, most of the research with newborns was done with full-term infants. It is only since the early 1970s that investigators have begun to evaluate the behavioral repertoire of preterm infants. Relatively little is known, for example, of how the behavior of preterm and full-term infants differs at comparable ages. Yet the answer to this question not only has important practical implications for the differential handling requirements of these infants but is also of great theoretical importance. In a sense, the premature birth of an infant represents an experiment in nature that permits the study of the relative contribution of brain maturation and of extrauterine experience to developmental progress. Also, relatively little is known about the sensory receptivity of preterm infants or about the effect of preterm in-

[1] Preparation of this chapter was supported by the William T. Grant Foundation.

fants' behavior on parental response. The chapters in this volume by Friedman, Jacobs, and Werthmann and by Marton, Minde, and Ogilvie contribute a great deal toward answering some of these questions.

Chapter 9 by Friedman *et al.* reports part of a large study that compares the development of preterm infants at term with that of full-term infants. The comparison focuses on differences and similarities of these infants' responses to stimulation in three sensory modalities, namely, tactile, auditory, and visual. To my knowledge, this is the first study that makes this comparison across all three sensory channels. It was the aim of the authors to generate data that would provide scientific guidelines for planners of intervention programs that would help them decide whether to provide preterm infants with tactile, auditory, or visual stimulation.

The chapter begins with an excellent and succinct review of previous work that compared the sensory responsiveness of preterm and full-term infants to tactile, auditory, and visual stimuli. The authors then present their own study. In their sample of preterm infants, they included only very low-risk babies whose medical course was not marred by major complications. This in itself makes this study extremely valuable, since much of what we know about preterm infants is confounded by the effects of the many medical complications that these infants usually experience. Preterm infants whose medical course is relatively free of complications are very difficult to find. Thus, the authors' collection of information on 45 such infants provides a very valuable data base that permits us to examine the effects of prematurity itself rather than of its complications. What adds further to the value of this study is that the authors have succeeded in making an excellent match in conceptional age between the infants born prematurely and their full-term controls at the time both groups of infants were studied (40.1 and 40.2 weeks conceptional age, respectively, with a standard deviation of 1.2 for each). This allows a comparison of the functioning of the two groups that is uncontaminated by even subtle age differences.

The authors' methodology was impeccable in testing the tactile, auditory, and visual responsiveness of their subjects. They used a strictly controlled laboratory approach in conducting their experiments. In each condition, they snuggly swaddled the infants. They took comparable measures across the three sensory modalities so as to maximize the possibility of a meaningful comparison among the infants' responses. In each modality they measured (*a*) quickness of response, or response latency; (*b*) degree of responsiveness to the first three trials; (*c*) presence of response decrement between the initial and final trials; and (*d*) duration of time to reaching a response decrement criterion. To compute their results, the authors made 12 comparisons between pre- and full-term infants, using the above four response measures for each of the three sensory modalities.

The authors found no significant differences in responsiveness to tactile stimulation between the pre- and full-term infants. In the auditory modality, full-terms tended to respond more quickly to the first stimulus presentation and tended to respond more frequently or more vigorously during the first three trials. They also took significantly longer to reach the response decrement criterion. The most marked differences in functioning were seen in the visual modality. Full-terms were significantly quicker to respond to visual stimulation and took significantly less time to reach the response decrement criterion than did the preterm infants. The authors concluded from this evidence that relatively few differences in sensory functioning emerged between the preterm and full-term infants ("of 12 comparisons, only 3 were statistically significant") and that those differences that were found were not evenly distributed across the three sensory modalities. They hypothesized from the distribution of the statistically significant comparisons that there might be an inverse relationship between the maturity of a sensory system at preterm birth and the damage it suffers due to preterm exposure to the extrauterine environment. The authors concluded their chapter, suggesting that planners of intervention programs would do well to study ways of facilitating the optimal auditory and visual development of preterm infants, since their functioning in these areas is more affected.

In their discussion, the authors gave several reasons why they found what they consider only a small number of differences in the sensory functioning of the preterm and full-term infants. The authors' interpretation of their results seems somewhat overly conservative. They not only found 3 significant differences in 12 comparisons, but the results in 7 out of the 9 remaining nonsignificant comparisons were in the expected direction. It is likely that more significant differences might have been found under different circumstances. In addition to the reasons given by the authors, different stimulus conditions to which the infants were exposed might have highlighted more numerous significant differences in the functioning of the two groups. For one, relatively stong tactile and auditory stimuli were used, a fact that may have made the response of preterm and full-term infants more uniform. An 80 dB sound for 2 sec and the 5.46 filament of the Semmes-Weinstein Aesthesiometer should be strong enough stimuli to be highly perceptible to both prematurely born and full-term infants. One wonders if softer tones and filaments would not have highlighted a greater number of differences between the two groups. Also, as the authors mentioned, the differences in sensory functioning between the preterm and full-term infants might have been more pronounced had the subjects been unswaddled during the administration of the stimuli. Through swaddling, the preterm infants may have been enabled to function more nearly like full-term infants. The authors mentioned that they made observations of the spontaneous behavior of their subjects for a mean of 15–19 min while they were unswaddled and that in these observations the behavior of the preterm infants was characterized by significantly greater irritablility. My own observations of preterm infants and those of other investigators suggest that these infants are also considerably more restless than full-term babies. By swaddling their subjects, the authors may have provided an external aid to the organization of the infants' behavior by restricting their motility and calming the infants.

The pattern of the group differences found in response to the sensory stimuli was indeed very interesting and of great theoretical significance. To recapitulate, the authors found no significant differences between the preterm and full-term infants in response to tactile stimuli, one difference in the auditory responsiveness, and two in the infants' visual performance. The pattern fits well into Gottlieb's (1971) theoretical framework on the ontogeny of the maturation of the sensory functions. According to Gottlieb, in many species, including mammals, cutaneous or tactile responsivity is the earliest to develop *in utero,* followed closely by vestibular and then auditory responsiveness. Response to visual stimuli is a relatively late acquisition. It thus makes good theoretical sense for preterm infants to be able to respond to tactile and auditory stimuli more nearly like full-term babies than is the case in the visual sphere, where some of their immaturity becomes more apparent. Had the authors not accomplished the feat of testing the infants' responses in three different sensory modalities, they would never have found this interesting maturational pattern.

The authors interpreted their results as suggesting that there is a negative relationship between the maturity of a given sensory system at the time of the preterm birth and the amount of insult that that system may suffer by virtue of premature exposure to the extrauterine environment. In my view, the notion of an *insult* to the as yet immature auditory and visual sensory systems need not be invoked to explain the results. One could argue that the premature birth, the deprivation of the intrauterine stimulation that presumably is conducive to the normal growth and development of the fetus, and the exposure to a highly unnatural extrauterine environment may have disrupted or retarded the natural maturation of those sensory functions that were as yet not quite mature at the time of the premature birth. One may thus interpret the results as highlighting a *lag* in the preterm infants' overall central nervous system maturation, brought about by the circumstances of their birth. Supporting this view is the additional evidence that the preterm infants were significantly more immature in their spontaneous behavior as well as in their weight. Even though both preterm and full-term infants were tested at identical conceptional ages, the mean weight of the prematurely born infants was 2936.9 gm and that of the full-terms was 3272.1 gm.

If one accepts this alternate interpretation of the findings, planners of intervention studies may want to address the problem of how to facilitate the more normal maturation of the infants' general central nervous system functioning rather than attempt to ameliorate specific sensory functions. It is this general aim that we had in mind when we began to provide waterbed flotation to small preterm infants in order to compensate for the vestibular-proprioceptive stimulation so prevalent *in utero* (Korner, Kraemer, Haffner,

& Cosper, 1975; Korner, 1979). At term, a flotation environment is of course no longer age relevent. At that time or even slightly before, swaddling may be a highly appropriate and useful intervention to help organize the preterm infant's immature behavior. Evidence is accumulating that any means that restrain the infant's erratic motility will also increase, at least temporarily, the maturity of their functioning. The prone position, for example, which inhibits movements significantly (Brackbill, Douthitt, & West, 1973), enables infants to sleep more and cry less (Michel & Goodwin, 1979), and it improves the infant's oxygenation (Martin, Herrell, Rubin, & Fanaroff, 1979). Sucking on a pacifier, which reduces the infant's motility, enhances visual performance (e.g., Gregg, Haffner, & Korner, 1976; Wolff & White, 1965). Swaddling of full-term infants has been shown to reduce motor activity and heart rates and to increase sleep (Lipton, Steinschneider, & Richmond, 1965). The fact that the authors found such marked differences between their term and preterm subjects when they observed their spontaneous behavior, while noting only much subtler differences in response while the infants were swaddled, suggests that preterm infants too may benefit from swaddling. Perhaps, before embarking on an intervention study using swaddling, it would be prudent to assess the sensory responsiveness of preterm infants with and without swaddling, using each infant as his own control. If, as I would predict, the infants performed more maturely while swaddled, a systematic study of the behavioral and developmental effects of intermittent swaddling would be very much worthwhile.

Chapter 10, by Marton *et al.*, makes multiple contributions, some of which are highly innovative, all of which are most interesting. The chapter begins by stressing the fact that, for predicting the developmental outcome of preterm infants, it is not sufficient to consider only the biological insults and the physical and medical complications so frequently experienced by these infants. Environmental factors and particularly the parent–infant interaction contribute very heavily to the developmental outcome of these infants. The authors then succinctly and cogently review the literature on the relation between prematurity and child abuse and between the developmental competence of the infants and maternal handling. Next, a review is presented of current methods of capturing dyadic interactions that deal with the chronological sequence of behaviors and/or the direction and magnitude of their influence. A summary is then given of three of the most recent analytic approaches that meet these criteria of analysis: a descriptive approach (e.g. Brazelton, Tronick, Adamson, Als, & Wise, 1975), a Markov-chain sequential analysis (e.g., Lewis & Painter, 1974; Stern, 1974), and a lag sequential approach (e.g., Bakeman, 1978; Sacket, 1979). The advantages and problems of each of these approaches are analyzed. The authors then outline a method of their own that includes some of the features of the lag sequential analysis but, unlike any of the other methods of analysis, permits continuous recording of *concurrent* mother and infant behaviors. The chapter concludes with an illustration of this method of analysis of the interaction between small preterm infants and their mothers. The data presented, aside from illustrating a new method of data analysis, represent in themselves a substantive contribution to our understanding of the earliest mother–infant interaction.

Regarding the content of their findings, the authors have shown very convincingly that small preterm infants already emit signals to which mothers respond predictably. When these small infants open their eyes, mothers are apt to touch them, and when they move or stretch, mothers are apt to smile. The direction of influence clearly is from infant to mother, with the infant committing a definite act. In previous studies (Brown & Bakeman, in press; Field, 1977) with much older preterm infants, the findings were quite different, in that mothers mostly responded to what infants *did not do*. These older infants born prematurely were so unresponsive to their mothers' ministrations that the mothers were forced to be much more active and aggressive in their interaction with their infants than mothers of full-term babies.

One might well ask what it is about a small preterm infant's stretch or open eyes that evokes such a positive response in mothers. I suspect, both types of behaviors on the infant's part make mothers feel that their babies are more real and more human. Parallels of this phenomenon exist with both much younger and much older infants. To many pregnant women, the baby inside them becomes a reality only after quickening or when the fetus starts to move. With 4-week-old infants, many mothers express the feeling that their babies are becoming human or persons, because, at that time, the babies begin to look around much more, particularly at the mothers (Robson, 1967).

The authors not only demonstrated that a young preterm infant already emits signals to which the mother responds predictably, they also found that the mother's basic personality contributes heavily in how actively she responds. Clinically, one would of course expect this to be the case, but unfortunately in most research studies, the mother's basic personality is not considered in assessing the mother–infant interaction. Most commonly, the mother–infant interaction is studied purely by recording what the mother does on the one hand and what the child does on the other, without concern with the degree to which the underlying temperament or personality of each partner contributes to this equation. As a consequence, the behaviors observed may capture interactions that are in large part situationally determined behaviors. To capture some of the mother's personality characteristics, the authors took extensive psychiatric histories of the mothers. They found that the nature of her background and personal history influences the intensity with which she actively responds. It seems that the mother's life history and her social support systems influence her interactional style with her baby far more than do the specific events surrounding the birth of the baby. The authors' data show that mothers whose interactional style was characterized by high activity had, as a group, more postitive interpersonal histories than did the mothers who did not respond actively to their infants' cues. This approach to studying the underlying reasons for certain interactional patterns is distinctly novel and, in my view, immensely worthwhile.

In proposing their scheme of interactional data analysis, the authors introduce a new order of complexity in an already complex field. By adding the capability to record and analyze *concurrent* behaviors to the already existing methods of interactional analysis, they have made it possible to capture more minutely than has been done before what exactly is going on between mother and child. In the authors' words, their observations yield a rich data base in which they can "examine 120 simple mother–infant behavior combinations and an astronomical number of possible combinations of multiple events [p. 189." In my view, this capability may be of great importance for some applications but may be unessential for others. Obviously, it is the research questions that should dictate what level of precision of observation and analysis is optimal to answer the questions raised. Unfortunately, we live in an era where this truism is frequently forgotten. With the advent of computers and other electronic equipment, we are constantly tempted to capture as much as we possibly can, whether or not our questions really warrant the collection of voluminous microscopic and sequential data. We then find ourselves in the paradoxical position of having to cope with the enormity of the data collected and with the task of meaningfully reducing the data to manageable proportions. The authors' description of the steps they took to deal with their large data base highlights this problem very well. The data collected consisted of observations of the mother–infant interaction during maternal visits to the nursery and during the first 3 months at home. To capture the mother–infant interaction during its most initial phase, the authors chose to analyze the data from the mother's first five visits to the intensive care nursery. They then selected the longest of the first five maternal visits for analysis. Each observation record was then divided into consecutive 5-sec time slices. Data for statistical analysis of dependencies between behaviors were then obtained by sampling from every tenth time slice. In these types of analytic approaches, decisions have to be made each step of the way as to how to reduce the masses of data, and much depends on whether or not, among the enumerable options, the intuitively right decisions are made to extract the most meaning from the data. The task is a very difficult one, requiring not only a great deal of statistical sophistication but also a keen sense of what types of research questions are best answered through such an elaborate approach to data collection and data analysis.

What types of questions then might best be studied through these new approaches to data collection and data analysis? In my view, studies dealing with the mutual stimulus regulation between two partners or with the synchrony or asynchrony of their interactions are ideally suited for these new methods of approach. In these studies, it is often the split-second events that elucidate the essence of the interaction. For instance, the studies by Brazelton *et al.* (1975), by Tronick, Adamson, Wise, Als, and Brazelton (1975), and by Stern (1974)

that address the issue of face-to-face interaction and visual gaze behavior between mother and child are prime examples of how split-second events can
capture the essence of synchronous or asynchronous interactions. Other applications for these new methodological approaches come to mind, some of
which have never been attempted. For example, little is known about the
origins of the defense mechanisms and the acquisition of individual differences in cognitive and/or coping styles. With regard to the origins of the
defense mechanisms, I would postulate that congenital differences in sensory
threshold levels will, to a large extent, determine the extent to which an individual will need to protect against becoming overwhelmed by both internal
and external stimuli. Experientially, sensitive and responsive maternal
ministrations will have a powerful effect on the extent to which the infant's
original tendencies can be modulated. The mother–infant synchrony will
largely be a function of how well the mother is able to adjust the dosage and
the tempo of her ministrations to the needs of her particular infant. Only
split-second observations are apt to capture this interplay. Observations such
as Stern's (1974) on mutual gaze behavior and gaze aversions therefore not
only are a source of the most microscopic details of the mother–infant interaction but also may yield data on the earliest manifestations of the infant's
defense mechanisms and coping styles.

In their chapter, Marton *et al.* did not tell us about the many types of questions they will ask in addressing the large data base they have collected. Their
new methods of analysis hold great promise for capturing some of the
minutest details of sequential dyadic interaction. It will be of great interest to
read their future publications to see what types of questions they will address
with their new approach of data collection and data analysis.

References

Bakeman, R. Untangling streams of behavior. In g. Sackett (Ed.), *Observing behavior* (Vol.
2). *Data collection and analysis methods.* Baltimore: University Park, 1978.

Brackbill, Y., Douthitt, T. C., & West, H. Psychophysiologic effects in the neonate of prone
versus supine placement. *The Journal of Pediatrics,* 1978, *82* (1), 82–84.

Brazelton, T., Tronick, E. Adamson, L., Als, H., & Wise, S. Early mother–infant reciprocity. In
Parent-infant interaction (Ciba Foundation Symposium 33) Amsterdam: Elsevier Publishing
Company, 1975.

Brown, J., & Bakeman, R. Relationships of human mothers with their infants during the first
year of life: Effects of prematurity. In R. Bell & W. Smotherman (Eds.). *Maternal influences
and early behavior.* Holliswood, N. Y.: Spectrum, 1979, (in press).

Field, T. Effects of early separation, interactive deficits, and experimental manipulations on infant–mother face-to-face interaction. *Child Development,* 1977, *48*, 763–771.

Gottlieb, G. Ontogenesis of sensory function in birds and mammals. In E. Tobach, L. R.
Aronson, & E. Shaw (Eds.), *The biopsychology of development.* New York: Academic Press,
1971.

Gregg, C. L., Haffner, M. E., & Korner, A. F. The relative efficacy of vestibular–proprioceptive stimulation and the upright position in enhancing visual pursuit in neonates. *Child Development,* 1976, *47,* 309–314.

Korner, A. F. Maternal rhythms and waterbeds: A form of intervention with premature infants. In E. B. Thoman (Ed.), *Origins of the infant's social responsiveness.* Hillsdale, N. J.: Erlbaum 1979.

Korner, A. F., Kraemer, H. C. Haffner, M. E., & Cosper, L. Effects of waterbed flotation on premature infants: A pilot study. *Pediatrics,* 1975, 56 (3), 361–367.

Lewis, M., & Painter, S. An interactional approach to the mother–infant dyad. In M. Lewis & L. Rosenblum, (Eds.), *The effect of the infant on its caregiver.* New York: Wiley, 1974.

Lewis, M., & Rosenblum, L. A. (Eds.), *The origins of behavior: The effect of the infant on its giver.* New York: Wiley, 1974.

Lipton, E.L., Steinschneider, A., & Richmond, J. B. Swaddling, a childcare practice: Historical, cultural and experimental observations. *Pediatrics* 1965, *35* (Supplement), 521–567.

Martin, R. J., Herrell, N., Rubin, D., & Fanaroff, A. Effect of supine and prone positions on arterial oxygen tension in the preterm infant. *Pediatrics,* 1979, *63,* 528–531.

Michel, G. F., & Goodwin, R. Intrauterine birth position predicts newborn supine head position preferences. *Infant Behavior and Development,* 1979, *2,* 29–38.

Osofsky, J. D. (Ed.). *Handbook of infant development.* New York: Wiley, 1979.

Robson, K. S. The role of eye-to-eye contact in maternal–infant attachment. *Journal of Child Psychology and Psychiatry,* 1967, *8,* 13–25.

Sackett, G. The lag sequential analysis of contingency and cyclicity in behavioral interaction research. In J.D. Osofsky (Ed.), *Handbook of infant development.* New York: Wiley, 1979.

Stern, D. N. Mother and infant at play: The dyadic interaction involving facial, vocal and gaze behaviors. In M. Lewis & A. L. Rosenblum (Eds.), *The Effect of the Infant on its Caregiver.* New York: Wiley, 1974.

Tronick, E., Adamson, L., Wise, S., Als, H., & Brazelton, T. Mother–infant face-to-face interaction. In S. Gosh (Ed.), *Biology and language.* London: Academic Press, 1975.

Wolff, P. H., & White, B. L. Visual pursuit and attention in young infants. *Journal of the American Academy of Child Psychiatry,* 1965, *4,* 473–484.

IV

Cognitive and Visual Development in the Early Months

12

Processing of Relational Information as an Index of Infant Risk[1]

ALBERT J. CARON
ROSE F. CARON

Early Cognitive Assessment: Pro and Con

There is a by now familiar litany used to rationalize studies of infants at risk. It begins by citing evidence that neonatal complications jeopardize the infant's later intellectual functioning, goes on to assert that early assessment and intervention are needed to avert the cumulative effects of deficiency, and ends by proposing that the performance of high-risk babies on such and such a cognitive task is likely to provide a reliable index of current and future handicap.

We have no particular quarrel with this rationale—indeed we have used it ourselves—but we are uncomfortably aware of the dilemma posed by any attempt to realize its objectives. The problem, thoroughly aired in recent volumes on assessment (Kearsley & Sigel, 1979; Lewis, 1976a; Minifie & Lloyd, 1978), stems from the embarrassing finding that standard infant psychometric tests have poor predictive validity for all but the most seriously compromised babies. When grossly defective cases are excluded, test scores of infants up to 18 months of age account for only fractional portions of the variance in their childhood IQs. Thus, while early measurement may contribute to the detection of severe retardation, it appears to have little prognostic value for the more subtle and more frequently encountered handicaps of marginal mental deficiency and specific learning disability.

Recognition of this state of affairs has prompted students of early develop-

[1] The preparation of this chapter was supported in part by Social and Behavioral Sciences Research Grants 12-5 and 1-16 from the National Foundation—March of Dimes, in part by USAHS Grant MH-25360-06, and in part by an award from the W.T. Grant Foundation.

PRETERM BIRTH AND
PSYCHOLOGICAL DEVELOPMENT

ISBN 0-12-267880-X

ment to challenge long-held conceptions of mental measurement. Lewis (1976b), for example, calls for the abandonment of attempts to use infant tests to predict an essentially mythical IQ and cautions against their application in the evaluation of early intervention procedures. Elaborating on this theme, McCall (1976) argues that intelligence is not a unitary factor that remains fixed over time but rather that infant and childhood intellect are qualitatively distinct, the former reflecting momentary state and attentional variables, the latter, abstract verbal and symbolic reasoning abilities. And reinforcing these sentiments from an evolutionary perspective, Scarr-Salapatek (1976) contends that infant sensorimotor intelligence is mediated by systems that are much older phylogenetically than those underlying conceptual–verbal intelligence. As such, she concludes, sensorimotor intelligence is subject to less phenotypic variability (is more heavily "canalized") than verbal intelligence and hence not especially useful as a predictor of mature mental functioning.

Those of us who come to the problem of infant assessment by way of experimental research may well wonder, in the light of these pronouncements, what our own proper course should be. Should we perhaps finesse the early infant period and begin our studies in the third year of life, when mature intellective ability has presumably crystallized? Lewis (1976b) seems to suggest such an alternative. Or, if we insist on testing the young infant, should we disregard the predictive validity of our instruments and be content with their capacity to diagnose concurrent developmental status? As McCall (1976) points out, weight in infancy correlates poorly with adult weight, and yet pediatricians still make use of it to diagnose infant pathology.

Given the bare facts of the matter, these are not unreasonable suggestions. Nevertheless, as we contemplated our own assessment program, we found various grounds for resisting them. To begin with, the discovery that apples and oranges in infancy are unrelated to pears and grapefruits in childhood may say less about the nature of intellectual development than about our scientific preconceptions concerning infant mentality. We are alluding here to the fact that the bulk of past thinking regarding early cognition, whether psychometric or Piagetian, was cast in peripheral sensorimotor terms. While such a view is understandable from a historical perspective, it is becoming increasingly clear that circular reactions, eye–hand coordination, and the like do not exhaust the intellective capability of the young baby. This is not to gainsay the epigenetic view of development espoused by Piaget, for obviously the mentality of the inarticulate infant is of a different order from that of the verbal child. But to say that is not to say what these earlier abilities are or how they relate to later functions.

Another reason for our reluctance to downgrade the clinical utility of infant assessment derives from the distinctive developmental orientation of the experimental tradition. Whereas psychometric testing often presupposes a concept of intelligence as unitary and unchanging, experimental research is more closely aligned with a process-centered model of cognitive development wherein discrete functions are seen to build upon prior, rudimentary capacities. The emphasis on functional continuity between early and later abilities shifts the problem of validity from establishing correlations between gross outcome measures at different ages (predictive validity) to demonstrating that deficiency in a particular process at one period leads to disability in related capacities at a subsequent period (construct validity). We are just now in a position, analytically and empirically, to forge such connections between infant and childhood cognition (see, for example, Bornstein & Kessen, 1979), and, while this effort may be fraught with difficulties of its own, it would seem premature to abandon it.

This brings us to our final reason for resisting the counsel of our colleagues. If we take our cue from contemporary cognitive theory, particularly in the area of language development, as well as from research in infant perception and cognition, we gain a different perspective on the intellective potential of the young infant. These sources give us reason to believe that information processing of a relatively high order occurs in early infancy, that it is possible to measure it, and that it may indeed be intimately linked to later childhood mental functioning. In our view, two capacities seem to be importantly implicated: (*a*) the ability to process invariant information (i.e., to isolate the constant from the changing), and (*b*) the ability to process invariant relational information in particular. It is the study of relational information processing that constitutes the core of our own research program, and in the sections that follow, we shall review in turn the evidence that directed us to this particular cognitive function, the tasks and procedures currently being developed to measure it, and finally, some preliminary but nonetheless provocative experimental findings.

Relational Concepts: Pathway from Preverbal to Verbal Intellect

Theoretical Perspectives

What then are the specific theoretical and empirical considerations that led us to examine the infant's ability to process relational information? As to theory, converging trends from a number of disciplines—perception, memory, psycholinguistics, comprehension—point to the centrality of relational information in the formation and organization of cognitive representational systems. In perception, James Gibson (1950) has long held that the visual apparatus is attuned not to static images projected on the retina, but to the high fidelity, invariant relational information contained in temporal sequences of retinal images (e.g., parallax and texture density gradients). Eleanor Gibson (1969) has since extended this theme to all of perceptual development, which she conceives as a hierarchical progression from the detection of isolated features (itself based on relational comparison) to invariant configurations of features defining individual objects and ultimately to invariant relationships between different objects in event contexts.

These speculations are further reinforced by inferences from early language development. We know, for example, that the child utters his first words at about 12 months of age and begins to combine words to form sentences about 6 months later. If we ask, as students of semantic development are now asking, what cognitive prerequisites he or she must possess in order to perform these acts meaningfully, the first thing to be noted is that most words do not refer to particular objects in the world but to categories or classes of objects— *dog* refers to all four-legged animals of a certain type, *car* to all vehicles sharing certain characteristics. Thus, it is generally agreed that to comprehend categorical terms the child must already have the capacity to perceive equivalences between their instances on a nonlinguistic basis (Brown, 1973; Macnamara, 1972; Nelson, 1977; Slobin, 1974). There is considerable evidence, as we shall soon see, that young infants can conceptualize in this manner and do so long before the appearance of language.

In turning from words to sentences, we encounter an even more sophisticated aspect of early categorization. Semantic analysis reveals that to comprehend (and produce) sentences the child must not only be able to segment the environment into distinctive object and event classes, but also be able to integrate them in terms of such abstract relational concepts as agency of an action, recipient, possession, location, temporal sequence, and causation, that is, in terms of the multiple relationships encoded by the syntactic conventions of language. Again, this implies that an infant who understands utterances of even a rudimentary nature ought already to have acquired the relevant relational concepts preverbally.

When we shift from the semantics to the pragmatics of early language development, we find an even closer link with the infant's emerging ability to cognize relationships. Bates (1979) has noted that the onset of communicative intention (the use of vocalizations as signals) occurs about the same time objects begin to be employed as tools (9 months). Bates conjectures that such social and nonsocial tool use may both involve the same underlying analytic capacity—the comprehension of causal interdependence—and in this regard she cites evidence that language-delayed children are also delayed in understanding means–ends relationships (Snyder, 1975). It may well be, then, that the concept of causal agency, though not reflected in productive speech until the third year, originates in the first year and is a fundamental precursor of communicative behavior.

Beyond language, the relational idiom now permeates almost every aspect of cognitive psychology. Thus, semantic memory is currently regarded as a repository of thematic as well as taxonomic knowledge (Mandler, 1979). Under such rubrics as "frames" (Minsky, 1975), "scripts" (Schank & Abelson, 1977), and "schematic memory" (Mandler, 1979), the organization of thematic material is viewed primarily in relational terms, that is, as networks of object concepts bound by spatial, temporal, causal, and actional relationships. This development, in turn, has given renewed impetus to "constructivist" approaches to cognition, in the sense that "what the head knows" powerfully influences via inferential (relational) links "what the head sees, understands, and remembers" (Bransford & Franks, 1971; Flavell, 1977; Franks, 1974; Hochberg, 1979; Paris & Lindauer, 1977). Bransford and McCarrell (1974) have elevated these ideas to a general relational theory of meaning that stresses that nothing is ever comprehensible in isolation but only in relation to other things and ultimately to one's total storehouse of acquired knowledge. And finally, even the classical view of learning as acquired stimulus–response associations is beginning to give way to learning conceived as "knowledge" of contingent relationships (Bolles, 1975). Clearly, the dominant cognitive metaphor has shifted from association to meaning, from mind-as-transmitter to mind-as-organizer of events.

Empirical Perspectives: Normal Infants

A summary of the pertinent developmental research lends substance to the view that young infants are able to detect invariant properties, both absolute and relational, of otherwise dissimilar events. Using a modification of the standard habituation paradigm, McGurk (1972) provided the first clear demonstration to this effect. After habituating his subjects to a form that changed in orientation from trial to trial (e.g., ?, ↖, ↗, ⟶), he found that they generalized habituation (showed little recovery) to the same form in an entirely new orientation (↳) but dishabituated to an altered form in the new orientation (↓). By contrast, infants who saw a single orientation of the figure during habituation, dishabituated equally to both test stimuli. McGurk's "conceptual" habituation procedure has since been used to show that infants of 6 months or younger can respond to a wide range of invariant properties across a number of changing parameters, for example, constant object shape across changing colors, sizes, and orientations (Caron, Caron, & Carlson, 1979; Ruff, 1977; Schwartz, 1975); constant color across changes in wavelength (Bornstein, 1976); chromaticity across varying hues (Bornstein, 1979); and invariant object rigidity across movement transformations (Gibson, Johnson, & Owsley, 1977). These studies provide clear evidence that the preverbal infant is prone to perceive the world categorically.

Research on the processing of relational information per se has been confined largely to discrimination of arrangements of visual elements as in geometric forms and human faces, although there has also been some work on the perception of auditory patterning. As to form, there is a general consensus that, prior to 2–3 months of age, the infant is responsive to high-contrast edges and angles but is insensitive to their overall organization (Haith & Campos, 1977; Salapatek, 1975). After 3 months, infants become able to discriminate one configuration from another when both patterns consist of different arrangements of the same simple components (Cornell, 1975; Fagan, 1977; Milewski, 1979; Ruff, 1976; Schwartz & Day, 1979; Vurpillot, Ruel, & Castrec, 1977). In the experiment by Vurpillot *et al.*, for example, 4-month-old infants were first habituated to a large cross made up of nine smaller crosses. They were then tested with a square pattern made from the same nine crosses versus a cross pattern made from nine small squares. When the size of the elements was small, the infants dishabituated to a change in the shape of the pattern but not to a change in the elements. It has since been demonstrated (Milewski, 1979) that such configurations can be abstracted not only across shifts in element shape but also across shifts in element position and inter-element distance (contour density).

Detection of patterns composed of disparate items appears to occur somewhat later. Thus, infants shown a cross inside a circle tend to perceive it as an assemblage of individual components—cross *and* circle—until about 5 months of age, at which point it becomes encoded as a compound—cross *within* circle (Bower, 1966; Cornell & Strauss, 1973; Miller, 1972; Miller, Ryan, Sinnott, & Wilson, 1976). A similar timetable seems to hold for naturally occuring stimuli such as the human face. Identical elements such as the eyes appear to get organized between 2 and 4 months (Ahrens, 1954; Maurer & Barrera, 1978), but integration of all the features into a total face configuration does not occur until about 5 months (Caron, Caron, Caldwell, & Weiss, 1973). Beyond 5 months, infants become increasingly capable of abstracting more subtle features of faces, for example, sex (Cornell, 1974) and facial identity (Cohen, 1977; Fagan, 1978).

The ability of infants to process relationships between events distributed over time is reflected in (*a*) habituation studies of responsiveness to configurations in the auditory modality; and (*b*) conditioning studies that index sensitivity to contingent relationships between successively presented events. With regard to the latter, it has become quite clear that infants from birth are able to modify their own behavior as a function of contingent feedback, and that several months later, they can learn the predictive relationship between distinctive cues and consequences (Caron & Caron, 1978; Hulsebus, 1973). With respect to the habituation of auditory stimuli, it has been shown that infants can respond to the temporal order of tones of different pitch (Chang & Trehub, 1977; Horowitz, 1972; McCall & Melson, 1970). Most pertinent is the study by Chang and Trehub (1977). Five-month-old subjects were first habituated to a six-tone melody and were then shifted either to a transposition of the pattern five semitones above or below the original or to a control pattern comprised of the novel tones in scrambled order. Dishabituation did not occur for the transposed stimulus but was clearly evident for the scrambled stimulus, indicating that the infants had processed the tonal configuration rather than the absolute pitch of the individual tones. To date, no attempt has been made to extend these findings to younger age groups.

A final group of experiments merits consideration in the present context, namely, those concerned with infant perception of dynamic relationships between independent entities. They indicate that marginally verbal children (14–18 months) are able to discriminate the action roles underlying complex event sequences (Gilmore, Suci, & Chan, 1974, Golinkoff, 1975; Golinkoff & Kerr, 1978). Golinkoff and Kerr (1978), for example, habituated infants to filmed sequences of a man, *A*, pushing another man, *B*, while at the same time alternating the direction of action from trial to trial ($A\longrightarrow B$, $B\longleftarrow A$, $A\longrightarrow B$, etc.). Following habituation, *B* was now shown pushing *A*. The demonstrated recovery of response indicated that infants had abstracted the basic role information regardless of the position of the actors and the direction of the action. The fact that the reversals were perceived by infants who were unable to produce two-word utterances also suggests that these cognitive categories are developed prior to their linguistic encoding.

Overall, these studies indicate that the recognition of constancy across change is probably the rule rather than the exception in normal infant perception and that it occurs quite early in life. The research suggests, too, that interrelationships between elements may be among the first features to be so abstracted. Since much of the critical information in the world is patterned, and since organized material imposes less of a burden on memory, the functional importance of this mechanism can hardly be overestimated.

Relational Information Processing in Risk Infants

Although research on the cognitive capacities of preterm and risk infants has begun to accumulate, there have been no investigations directly concerned with relational information processing per se. Indirect evidence, however, may be gleaned from a series of studies by Fantz and his colleagues who attempted to determine whether visual recognition memory is related to infant risk category (Fagan, Fantz, Miranda, 1971; Fantz, Fagan, & Miranda, 1975; Fantz & Miranda, 1977; Miranda, 1976; Miranda & Fantz, 1973, 1974). The results clearly establish that Down's syndrome infants, a group for whom retardation is virtually certain, are delayed relative to normal infants in the development of recognitive capacity. Particularly relevant to our purposes is the finding that Down's babies are inferior to normals in distinguishing and recognizing such configural patterns as faces and arrangements of elements (Fantz *et al.,* 1975; Miranda, 1976; Miranda & Fantz, 1974).

As regards the preterm infant, however, the research is less conclusive. Fagan *et al.* (1971) reported that preterm infants showed a reliable preference for multidimensionally novel stimuli at the same conceptional age as full-term infants (51 weeks). On the other hand, Sigman and Parmelee (1974) found that at 59 weeks conceptional age, preterms, unlike full-terms, exhibited no preference for multidimensionally novel stimuli. They suggested that the deficient performance of their preterm subjects may have been due to a higher incidence of fetal complications in their sample, but given the methodological differences between the two studies, attribution of performance differences to the risk status of the samples is questionable. Another possibility is that stable differences between normal and preterm infants in early infancy will not be manifested in efficiency of information processing or memory capacity per se but rather in the *content* of information processing, specifically, in the ability to encode relational information. In this regard, it is noteworthy that 1-year-old preterms were found to be deficient relative to full-term infants in the ability to detect invariant shape information across tactual and visual modalities (Rose, Gottfried, & Bridger, 1978). Sensitivity to spatial relationships between temporally distributed inputs would seem to be a particular requirement for success on this task.

The Present Research Program

Goals and Methods

The foregoing ideas and facts provide the working assumption of our own research, namely, that vulnerability to future cognitive deficit will manifest itself early in life as difficulty in abstracting relational information. This proposition has been translated into a number of interrelated goals. A preliminary aim is to increase our knowledge about the ability of normal, full-term babies to abstract various kinds of relational patterns, in particular to determine when these capacities emerge and how they can best be facilitated. A further objective is to compare the performance of normal and high-risk samples on age-graded tasks and to identify which subcategories of risk infants are deficient on which types of problems. Finally, we expect to relate specific aberrations in infancy to particular linguistic and cognitive disabilities in early childhood.

In pursuit of the first objective, we have to date been trying to locate tasks in the visual modality that can be solved by a majority of healthy, full-term infants at specified ages between 12 and 24 weeks. Figure 12.1 presents in schematized form a variety of problems that are currently in various stages of investigation. The problems are similar in that they each contain stimuli that may be encoded in either absolute or relational terms, that is, in terms of the absolute properties of their elements (color, size, shape, etc.) or in terms of the relationship holding between elements (e.g., "little above big" in first row of Figure 12.1). The distinction drawn here between absolute and relational properties has much in common with Garner's (1978) differentiation of "componential" and "configural" aspects of stimuli. As Garner has noted, the latter depend on the former and yet are more than simply their summation.

The choice of specific relationships has been guided not only by the em-

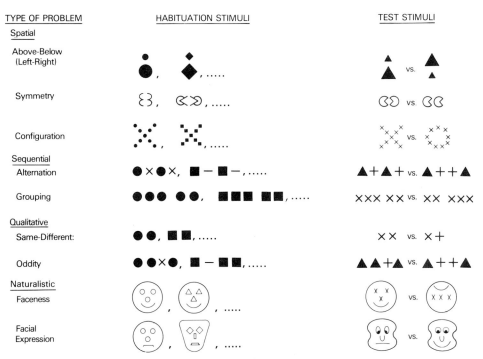

FIGURE 12.1. *Examples of relational problems.*

pirical considerations reviewed earlier but also by recent evidence that hemispheric specialization—parallel-spatial processing in the right hemisphere, sequential-analytic processing in the left—may begin quite early in life and thus provide a clue to the specific character of future disabilities (Witelson, 1977). Consequently, we have sampled relationships that appear to require analysis (those labelled "sequential" and "qualitative" in Figure 12.1)[2] as well as those of a spatiogestalt type. At a more technical level, it should be noted that the construction of the actual stimuli for each problem is an exacting task. The figures must be sufficiently attractive to recruit attention but not so attractive that the infant becomes bogged down in detail to the exclusion of the relational features. A further complication is that the same stimulus may be differentially attention-getting at different ages. These obstacles may be turned to our advantage, however, since, by manipulating the relative salience of relational and component features, the difficulty level of tasks may be scaled for purposes of test construction or training.

Our general procedure, which has been modeled after McGurk's technique, can best be explained with reference to Figure 12.1. On the initial habituation

[2] Ultimately, we expect to employ time-distributed input (both visual and auditory) to provide more extensive assessments of left-hemisphere functioning.

trial, a stimulus is presented (e.g., ⊙), which, as mentioned, may be encoded either absolutely (circular shapes) or relationally (little above big). On succeeding trials, either the same stimulus may be repeated or its component features may be varied from trial to trial while the relational feature is held constant (e.g., ⊙, ◌, ◌, . . .), that is, infants may be shown either one or more exemplars of the relational concept. Following habituation, a new set of components is presented, once in the habituated configuration (△) and once in a novel configuration (△). If an infant has abstracted the relational feature during habituation, he should generalize the habituated response (i.e., show little response recovery) to the familiar configuration at test and dishabituate (recover responding) to the novel configuration. This response pattern constitutes the operational definition of relational abstraction. By contrast, recovery to both test stimuli would imply either that the component features alone had been processed (in the case of equal recovery) or that the relational feature had been processed but responding to components had not fully abated (in the case of still stronger recovery to the novel configuration). Nonrecovery to both test stimuli, on the other hand, would mean that neither property had been encoded during habituation (assuming that the baby had not become generally fatigued or otherwise disinterested in the situation).

Preliminary Investigation

At this point, we would like to describe a preliminary experiment in which the performance of term and preterm infants was compared on four of the problems represented in Figure 12.1. Given that the specific stimuli and procedures are still being refined, and that the preterm cases, because of limited numbers, could not be divided according to category of illness, the results are perhaps more illustrative than definitive.

SUBJECTS

The term infants were healthy, thriving babies from a middle-class, suburban milieu (median maternal educational level, 15+ years). Perinatal complications were minimal, and 5-min Apgar scores were typically 9 or above. The median birthweight was 3430 gm (7 lb. 9 oz.). Four percent of the sample was black and 1% of Hispanic origin. The preterm infants came primarily from two hospitals in the Washington, D.C., area. All had been in intensive care for complications of varying severity. Gestational ages (as measured by the Dubowitz scale) ranged from 27 to 36 weeks (median, 33 weeks) and birthweight varied from 910 to 2580 gm (median, 1620 gm—3 lb. 8 oz.). These families, too, were predominantly middle class, although the maternal educational level was somewhat lower than that for the full-term sample (median, 13 years). Ten percent of the babies were black and 3% Hispanic. Both sexes were about equally represented in the term and preterm samples and were evenly distributed within experimental conditions.

HABITUATION **TEST**

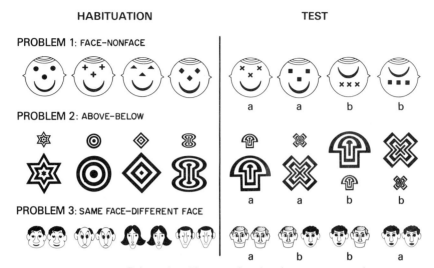

FIGURE 12.2. *Relational problems employed in the present research.*

TASKS

The four problems (face–nonface, above–below, same face–different face, neutral–smiling face) were administered at 52, 58, 61, and 64 weeks conceptional age, respectively. Groups of term and preterm infants were shown four exemplars of each of the first three concepts (Figure 12.2) and six exemplars of the last concept (Figure 12.3) during habituation. Following habituation, two new figures were presented at test, each appearing once in the familiar configuration (e.g., above) and once in the novel configuration (below). In

HABITUATION STIMULI

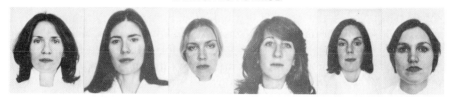

TEST STIMULI

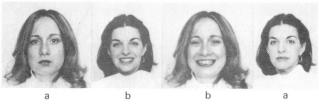

a b b a

FIGURE 12.3. *Neutral versus smiling-face problem.*

Problems 1 and 2, the order of testing was a, a, b, b; in Problems 3 and 4, a, b, b, a. To determine the extent to which test performance was a function of exposure to the multiple exemplars during habituation, control term infants were habituated to a single exemplar of each concept (each habituation stimulus being used equally often).

PROCEDURES

Visual fixation was measured from a television monitor by the corneal reflection technique (Fantz, 1961), each trial terminating when the infant looked away from the stimulus for at least .5 sec. Habituation, which was calculated on line, was defined *relatively* as a 50% decrement from initial looking levels (based on blocks of three trials) or *absolutely* as a decline to 8 sec or less of total fixation on three trials (to prevent those few subjects whose initial looking was brief from having to undergo prolonged habituation). In order to provide a check on the infant's terminal level of alertness, each session began and ended with the presentation of the same attractive art slide. Infants were excluded from the study who were either insufficiently exposed to the habituation stimuli (less than 10 sec of overall fixation) or gave evidence of being "turned off" at test (looked less than 8 sec at all four test stimuli).

DEPENDENT MEASURES

A number of response measures were examined, the most important of which were two scores based on test performance: (*a*) a *configural discrimination* score, that is, total fixation to the two novel configurations (N) relative to the two familiar configurations (F); and (*b*) a *component discrimination* score, that is, total fixation to the two familiar configurations relative to the last two habituation trials (H). The configural discrimination score was computed as the ratio $N/(N + F)$, a value of 50% meaning that the infant had responded equally to the novel and familiar patterns at test, and a value in excess of 50%, that he had attended longer to the novel than to the familiar patterns (thus implying that he had processed the relational feature during habituation). The component discrimination score measured the extent to which habituation had generalized to the new instances of the familiar concept at test. Calculated as $F/(F + H)$, a score of 50% or less meant that the infant had generalized (not dishabituated) to the new instances relative to his terminal habituation level. A score greater than 50% indicated that responding had recovered to the new exemplars and therefore that the infant had perceived these figures more in terms of their novel components than their familiar configuration.

To compare rate of information processing between groups, two additional scores were analyzed: (*a*) total fixation during habituation; and (*b*) number of trials to habituation. Finally, to assess general attentiveness at test, total test fixation was examined.

RESULTS

Single-versus multiple-exemplar comparisons. In accord with McGurk's (1972) findings, it was anticipated that exposure to multiple instances of a relational concept during habituation would enhance the ability of infants to detect the invariant relational property and, correspondingly, diminish their attention to elemental details. It was expected, therefore, that term infants who were so exposed would have higher configural discrimination scores and lower component discrimination scores than term infants shown a single conceptual exemplar. The results (see last two columns of Tables 12.1 and 12.2) bear out this expectation. On all four problems, the configural discrimination scores of the multiple-exemplar groups (see Table 12.1) were significantly above chance (50%), whereas the configural scores of the single-exemplar groups exceeded chance on only one problem (face–nonface).The single and multiple groups differed reliably from one another on all but the face problem, and on two problems (above–below and neutral–smile), a greater proportion of cases exceeded chance[3] in the multiple- than in the single-exemplar condition.

When we turn to the component discrimination scores (see Table 12.2), the effects are just the reverse. Here the single-exemplar groups responded beyond chance on three of the four problems (face–nonface again being the exception), and the multiple-exemplar groups, only on the same–different problem (although even on this task significantly more single- than multiple-exemplar cases discriminated the new components). While only one other between-group difference (the parametric comparison on the above–below problem) reached significance on the component measure, the overall findings clearly demonstrate that exposure of infants to multiple instances of an invariant configuration increases the perceptual salience of the configuration and reduces that of its components.[4]

The previous results do not appear to have been influenced by differences in rate of habituation or in general attentiveness at test (see Table 12.3). The single-exemplar groups, as might have been expected, tended to habituate more rapidly than the multiple-exemplar groups (significantly so on the face and same–different problems), but on the above–below problem (where their

---

[3] Defined as a score beyond a .05 critical ratio (C.R.) based on all cases combined—approximately 56% for all problems.

[4] The fact that exposure to one exemplar was sufficient to produce conceptual transfer on the face problem suggests that the face was a much more salient configuration for the 12-week-olds than the above–below, same–different, and neutral–smile patterns were for the 18-, 21-, and 24-week-olds, respectively. Examination of the figures themselves would seem to bear out this conclusion, and this of course raises the further question of whether the face details were at all discriminable by the 12-week-olds. While we have no direct evidence on this point, the significant recovery of the preterm infants to the test faces suggests that these transformations were in fact perceived. We also have unpublished data that indicate that minute element changes following habituation to assemblages of random shapes can be detected by 3-month-olds.

TABLE 12.1

Comparisons of the Configural Discrimination Scores of Term and Preterm Infants and of Single- and Multiexemplar Term Groups on Four Relational Problems

Problem	Preterm (multiexemplar)		Term (multiexemplar)		Term (single-exemplar)
Face–nonface					
(12 weeks)					
Mean configural score $\left[\frac{N}{N+F} \right]$	47.2	††	63.4***		59.2*
Number exceeding chance (50%)	7	‡	15		11
Total number	22		22		20
Above–below					
(18 weeks)					
Mean configural score	53.6	†	62.2***	††	39.8
Number exceeding chance	8	‡	16	‡‡	2
Total number	22		22		14
Same–different					
(21 weeks)					
Mean configural score	49.4	†	57.5**	†	49.2
Number exceeding chance	5	‡‡	12		9
Total number	22		22		22
Neutral–smile					
(24 weeks)					
Mean configural score	56.0		62.5***	†	53.6
Number exceeding chance	10	‡	19	‡‡	11
Total number	20		22		24

* $P < .05$ (one tail, relative to chance)
** $p < .01$
*** $p < .001$
† $p < .05$ (one tail, between means)
†† $p < .01$
‡ $p < .05$ (one tail, between proportions)
‡‡ $p < .01$

TABLE 12.2

Comparisons of the Component Discrimination Scores of Term and Preterm Infants and of Single- and Multiexemplar Term Groups on Four Relational Problems

Problem	Preterm (multiexemplar)	Term (multiexemplar)		Term (single-exemplar)
Face–nonface (12 weeks)				
Mean component score $\left[\frac{F}{F+H}\right]$	57.6*	53.9		53.8
Number failing to generalize (exceeding 50%)	12	11		8
Total number	22	22		20
Above–below (18 weeks)				
Mean component score	56.8*	53.3	†	66.2**
Number failing to generalize	14	11		11
Total number	22	22		14
Same–different (21 weeks)				
Mean component score	56.4*	60.1*	‡	66.6***
Number failing to generalize	11	11		18
Total number	22	22		22
Neutral–smile (24 weeks)				
Mean component score	55.5*	54.2		61.3**
Number failing to generalize	10	11		15
Total number	20	22		24

* $p < .05$ (one tail, relative to chance)
** $p < .01$
*** $p < .001$
† $p < .05$ (one tail, betwwen means)
‡ $p < .05$ (one tail, between proportions)

TABLE 12.3

Comparisons of Rate of Habituation and Overall Attentiveness at Test of Term and Preterm Infants and of Single- and Multiexemplar Term Groups, on Four Relational Problems

Problem	Preterm (multiexemplar)		Term (multiexemplar)		Term (single-exemplar)
Face–nonface (12 weeks)					
Total fixation: Habituation (sec)	193.2	**	221.0	**	109.6
Number habituation trials	13.0	*	7.3		7.3
Total fixation: Test (sec)	37.7		73.0		46.0
Above–below (18 weeks)					
Total fixation: Habituation (sec)	62.0		72.6		111.9
Number habituation trials	9.7		9.0		9.1
Total fixation: Test (sec)	17.6		21.1		28.4
Same–different (21 weeks)					
Total fixation: Habituation (sec)	49.3	*	73.4	**	37.4
Number habituation trials	7.3		11.0	**	6.6
Total fixation: Test (sec)	23.7		26.6		22.0
Neutral–smile (24 weeks)					
Total fixation: Habituation (sec)	55.7		65.8		55.9
Number habituation trials	8.4		9.1		7.5
Total fixation: Test (sec)	22.9		20.9		24.3

* $p<.05$ (two tail, between groups)
** $p<.01$

discrimination scores differed most dramatically from those of the multiple-exemplar infants), they tended, if anything, to habituate more slowly. Overall fixation during test was comparable for both groups on all four problems.

Term–Preterm Comparisons. If preterm infants, though exposed to multiple exemplars, nonetheless have greater difficulty abstracting invariant relational properties than full-term infants, then they too would be expected to yield lower configural discrimination scores and higher component discrimination scores than full-term infants shown multiple exemplars. The data provide striking support for this prediction as well (see left-hand columns of Tables 12.1 and 12.2). In contrast with term infants, the configural discrimination scores of the preterm infants failed to exceed chance on any of the four problems (see Table 12.1). On three of these, their scores were significantly below those of the term infants, and on all four, the proportion of cases exceeding chance discrimination was lower than that in the full-term groups. The preterm infants, on the other hand, recovered uniformly to change in components (see Table 12.2). Although they did not dishabituate reliably more than the term infants, their overall pattern of responding at test was clearly less conceptual.[5] Whereas 71% of all term infants responded significantly more to configural than to component change, only 36% of preterms so responded. Conversely, 37% of preterms dishabituated to change in components alone, as against 19% of full-terms.

Again, the overall pattern of attending during habituation and test (see Table 12.3) provides no consistent clue to the differences between term and preterm infants in test performance. Although previous research suggested that preterm infants might be generally less efficient than term infants in processing information, our data are not in agreement with this expectation. On no problem were preterm infants slower to habituate than term infants; indeed, if anything, they tended to be somewhat faster. On the face problem, the preterm group did require a significantly greater number of trials to habituate, but on the same–different problem, they required significantly fewer. With regard to overall attentiveness during test, only on the face problem was there a significant difference (preterm infants fixating less). The bulk of this difference, however, was confined to the two scrambled face patterns, the intact test faces recruiting equivalent attention from term and preterm groups (23.9 versus 22.1 sec, respectively).

Concluding Comment

The differences in performance of term and preterm infants are impressive, particularly if one considers that the preterm groups were quite variable with respect to neonatal complications and undoubtedly included some infants who

---

[5] In this respect their performance parallels that of term infants 6 weeks younger than each of the present term groups, as recently obtained in our laboratory.

were only of marginal risk. More importantly, the findings suggest that preterm dysfunction may be viewed not as a deficiency in information processing per se but as a deficiency in the *content* of information processing. Our preterm subjects were able to discriminate change in stimulus components at test but failed to detect change in stimulus configurations. In short, they had encoded part of the stimulus information during habituation—the elemental part—but were insensitive to the invariant relationships linking these elements.

However promising the results, many questions remain to be answered before the clinical utility of our procedures can be established. As noted previously, it would be important to determine whether performance varies with severity of neonatal complications, particularly with the incidence of symptoms (seizures, intracranial bleeding, etc.) that index central nervous system disorders. It would also be of interest to know whether our techniques are sensitive to less direct risk factors such as medication, nutrition, and socioeconomic status. Most importantly, we would like to examine the relationship between performance in infancy and cognitive dysfunction in childhood. Given the emphasis on content in our procedures, we are especially curious about the differential predictability of different types of relational tasks. For example, will infants who have difficulty processing spatial relationships be more deficient in visual problem solving as children, and will infants who are delayed in processing sequential relationships show future dysfunctions in linguistic tasks?

In addition to issues of diagnosis, we have a residing interest in the remedial potential of our procedures. Our findings bear out McGurk's (1972) observation that attributes of stimuli are better perceived as invariants in the context of variation, and they also extend this principle to relational features. We intend, therefore, to examine whether the relational processing of impaired infants can be improved by exposure to multiple instances of a variety of relationships, and whether the resulting gains are maintained in childhood. If infancy is a crucial period in mental development, such that delays have cumulative debilitating effects, then the consequences of early intervention could be far reaching. Needless to say, these considerations apply not only to remedial efforts with handicapped infants but also to pedagogic work with healthy infants.

It is apparent that much has yet to be learned about the development of relational encoding per se. Existing research has focused almost exclusively on discrimination of visually presented spatial configurations, both abstract and naturalistic. There have been virtually no visual studies involving qualitative relationships between features (alternation, oddity, part–whole, etc.). Likewise, there has been hardly any auditory research using the morphemic, prosodic, or syntactic configurations found in natural speech. Finally, there has been far too little experimentation with young infants in the crucial area of event relationships. Infants live in a dynamic world in which things act and can be acted upon, and in this ferment, fundamental physical and social relationships begin to be discerned. It has been argued (Nelson, 1979; Rosch, 1978) that even the first object concepts of infancy are based on such dynamic relationships, and that the earliest holophrastic utterances of children are efforts to communicate broader relational knowledge. In the last analysis, only the systematic investigation of such issues can lead to the emergence of a viable diagnostic and remedial armamentarium applicable to the mentality of infants.

Acknowledgments

The research described herein was conducted with the collaboration of Gordon B. Avery and Juarlyn L. Gaiter of the Division of Neonatology, Children's Hospital National Medical Center; Anita M. Sostek and Mary Kate Davit, Division of Newborn Medicine, Georgetown University Hospital; Lawrence J. Grylack, Division of Neonatology, Columbia Hospital for Women, and the staff of the Child Development Center, Georgetown University Hospital, in Washington, D.C. The able assistance of Johanna Glass and Sandra Weiss is also gratefully acknowledged.

References

Ahrens, R. Beitrage zur entwicklung des physiognomie und mimikerkennes. *Zeitschrift für Experimentell und Angewandte Psychochologie,* 1954, *2,* 412-454.

Bates, E. The emergence of symbols: Ontogeny and phylogeny. In W. A. Collins (Ed.), *Children's language and communication.* Hillsdale, N.J.: Erlbaum, 1979.

Bolles, R. C. *Learning theory.* New York: Holt, 1975.

Bornstein, M. H. Infants' recognition memory for hue. *Developmental Psychology,* 1976, *12,* 225-245.

Bornstein, M. H. Effects of habituation experience on posthabituation behavior in young infants: Discrimination and generalization among colors. *Developmental Psychology,* 1979, *15,* 348-349.

Bornstein, M. H., & Kessen, W. (Eds.). *Psychological development from infancy: Image to intention.* Hillsdale, N.J.: Erlbaum, 1979.

Bower, T. G. R. Heterogeneous summation in human infants. *Animal Behavior,* 1966, *14,* 395-398.

Bransford, J. D., & Franks, J. J. The abstraction of linguistic ideas. *Cognitive Psychology,* 1971, *2,* 331-350.

Bransford, J. D., & McCarrell, N. S. A sketch of a cognitive approach to comprehension: Some thoughts about understanding what it means to comprehend. In W. B. Weimer and D. S. Palermo (Eds.), *Cognition and the symbolic processes.* New York: Wiley, 1974.

Brown, R. A first language. Cambridge, Mass.: Harvard Univ. Press, 1973.

Caron, A. J., Caron, R. F., Caldwell, R. C., & Weiss, S. Infant perception of the structural properties of the face. *Developmental Psychology,* 1973, *9,* 385-399.

Caron, A. J., Caron, R. F., & Carlson, V. R. Infant perception of the invariant shape of an object varying in slant. *Child Development,* 1979, *50,* 716-721.

Caron, R. F., & Caron, A. J. Effects of ecologically relevant manipulations on infant discrimination learning. *Infant Behavior and Development,* 1978, *1,* 291-307.

Chang, H., & Trehub, S. Auditory processing of relational information by young infants. *Journal of Experimental Child Psychology,* 1977, *24,* 324–331.

Cohen, L. B. Concept acquisition in the human infant. Paper presented at the meetings of the Society for Research in Child Development, New Orleans, March 1977.

Cornell, E. H. Infants' discrimination of faces following redundant presentations. *Journal of Experimental Child Psychology,* 1974, *18,* 98–106.

Cornell, E. H. Infants' visual attention to pattern arrangement and orientation. *Child Development,* 1975, *46,* 229–232.

Cornell, E. H., & Strauss, M. S. Infants' responsiveness to compounds of habituated visual stimuli. *Developmental Psychology,* 1973, *9,* 73–78.

Fagan, J. F. An attention model of infant recognition. *Child Development,* 1977, *48,* 345–359.

Fagan, J. F. Facilitation of infants' recognition memory. *Child Development,* 1978, *49,* 1066–1075.

Fagan, J. F., Fantz, R. L., & Miranda, S. B. Infants' attention to normal stimuli as a function of postnatal and conceptional age. Paper presented at the meetings of the Society for Research in Child Development, Minneapolis, 1971.

Fantz, R. L. The origin of form perception. *Scientific American,* 1961, *204,* 66–72.

Fantz, R. L., Fagan, J. F., & Miranda, S. B. Early visual selectivity as a function of pattern variables, previous exposure, age from birth and conception, and expected cognitive deficit. In L. B. Cohen & P. Salapatek (Eds.), *Infant perception: From sensation to cognition* (Vol. 1). New York: Academic Press, 1975.

Fantz, R. L., & Miranda, S. B. Visual processing in the newborn, preterm, and mentally high-risk infant. In L. Gluck (Eds.), *Intrauterine asphyxia and developing fetal brain.* Chicago, Ill.: Year Book Medical Publishers, 1977.

Fillmore, C. J. The case for case. In E. Back & R. T. Harms (Eds.), *Universals in linguistic theory.* New York: Holt, 1968.

Flavell, J. H. *Cognitive development.* Englewood Cliffs, N.J.: Prentice-Hall, 1977.

Franks, J. J. Toward understanding understanding. In W. B. Weimer and P. S. Palermo (Eds.), *Cognition and the symbolic processes.* New York: Wiley, 1974.

Garner, W. R. Aspects of a stimulus: Features, dimensions, and configurations. In E. Rosch and B. B. Lloyd (Eds.), *Cognition and categorization.* Hillsdale, N.J.: Erlbaum 1978.

Gibson, E. J. *Principles of perceptual learning and development.* New York: Appleton-Century-Crofts, 1969.

Gibson, E., Johnson, J., & Owsley, C. Perception of invariance over perspective transformations in five-month-old infants. Paper presented at the meetings of the Society for Research in Child Development, New Orleans, March 1977.

Gibson, J. J. *The perception of the visual world.* Boston: Houghton Mifflin, 1950.

Gilmore, L. M., Suci, G. J., & Chan, S. Heart rate deceleration as a function of viewing complex visual events in eighteen-month-old infants. Paper presented at the American Psychological Association meeting, 1974.

Golinkoff, R. M. Semantic development in infants: The concepts of agent and recipient. *Merrill-Palmer Quarterly,* 1975, *21,* 181–193.

Golinkoff, R. M., & Kerr, J. I. Infants' perception of semantically defined action role changes in filmed events. *Merrill-Palmer Quarterly,* 1978, *24,* 53–61.

Haith, M., & Campos, J. *Human infancy.* In M. R. Rosenzweig & L. W. Poerter (Eds.), *Annual review of psychology* (Vol. 28). Palo Alto: Annual Reviews, 1977.

Hochberg, J. Sensation and perception. In E. Hearst (Ed.), *The first century of experimental psychology.* Hillsdale, N.J.: Erlbaum, 1979.

Horowitz, A. B. Habituation and memory: Infant cardiac responses to familiar and discrepant auditory stimuli. *Child Development,* 1972, *43,* 43–53.

Hulsebus, R. C. Operant conditioning of infant behavior. In A. W. Reese (Ed.), *Advances in child development and behavior* (Vol. 8). New York: Academic Press, 1973.

Kearsley, R. B., & Sigel, I. E. (Eds.). *Infants at risk: Assessment of cognitive functioning.* Hillsdale, N.J.: Erlbaum, 1979.

Lewis, M. (Ed.). *Origins of intelligence: Infancy and early childhood.* New York: Plenum, 1976. (a)

Lewis, M. What do we mean when we say "infant intelligence scores"? A sociopolitical question. In M. Lewis (Ed.), *Origins of intelligence.* New York: Plenum, 1976. (b)

Macnamara, J. Cognitive basis of language learning in infants. *Psychological Review,* 1972, *79,* 1–13.

Mandler, J. M. Categorical and schematic organization in memory. In C. R. Puff (Ed.), *Memory, organization and structure.* New York: Academic Press, 1979.

Maurer, D., & Barrera, M. Normal and distorted faces: When do infants see the difference? Paper presented to the International Conference on Infant Studies, Providence, 1978.

McCall, R. B. Toward an epigenetic conception of mental development in the first three years of life. In M. Lewis (Ed.), *Origins of intelligence.* New York: Plenum, 1976.

McCall, R. B., & Melson, W. H. Amount of short term familiarization and the response to auditory discrepancy. *Child Development,* 1970, *41,* 861–869.

McGurk, H. Infant discrimination of orientation. *Journal of Experimental Child Psychology,* 1972, *14,* 151–164.

Milewski, A. E. Visual discrimination and detection of configurational invariance in 3-month infants. *Developmental Psychology,* 1979, *15,* 357–363.

Miller, D. J. Visual habituation in the human infant. *Child Development,* 1972, *43,* 481–493.

Miller, D. J., Ryan, E. B., Sinnott, J. P. & Wilson, M. A. Serial habituation in two-, three- and four-month-old infants. *Child Development,* 1976, *47,* 341–349.

Minifie, F. D., & Lloyd, L. L. (Eds.). *Communicative and cognitive abilities—early behavioral assessment.* Baltimore: University Park Press, 1978.

Minsky, M. A framework for representing knowledge. In P. Winston (Ed.), *The psychology of computer vision.* New York: McGraw-Hill, 1975.

Miranda, S. B. Visual attention in defective and high-risk infants. *Merrill-Palmer Quarterly,* 1976, *22,* 201–227.

Miranda, S. B., & Fantz, R. L. Visual preferences of Down's Syndrome and normal infants. *Child Development,* 1973, *44,* 555–561.

Miranda, S. B., & Fantz, R. L. Recognition memory in Down's Syndrome and normal infants. *Child Development,* 1974, *45,* 651–660.

Nelson, K. The conceptual basis for meaning. In J. Macnamara (Ed.), *Language learning and thought.* New York: Academic Press, 1977.

Nelson, K. Explorations in the development of a functional semantic system. In W. A. Collins (Ed.), *Children's language and communication.* Hillsdale, N.J.: Erlbaum, 1979.

Paris, S. B., & Lindauer, B. K. Constructive aspects of children's comprehension and memory. In R. V. Kail & J. W. Hagen (Eds.), *Perspectives on the development of memory and cognition.* Hillsdale, N.J.: Erlbaum, 1977.

Rosch, E. Principles of categorization. In E. Rosch & B. B. Lloyd (Eds.), *Cognition and categorization.* Hillsdale, N.J.: Erlbaum, 1978.

Rose, S. A., Gottfried, A. W., & Bridger, W. H. Cross-modal transfer in infants: Relationship to prematurity and socioeconomic background. *Developmental Psychology,* 1978, *14,* 643–652.

Ruff, H. A. Developmental changes in the infant's attention to pattern detail. *Perceptual and Motor Skills,* 1976, *43,* 351–358.

Ruff, H. A. The role of stimulus variability in infant perceptual learning. Paper presented at the meetings of the Society for Research in Child Development, New Orleans, March 1977.

Salapatek, P. Pattern perception in early infancy. In L. B. Cohen & P. Salapatek *Infant perception: From sensation to cognition* (Vol. 1). New York: Academic Press, 1975.

Scarr-Salapatek, S. Evolutionary perspective on infant intelligence: Species patterns and individual variations. In M. Lewis (Ed.), *Origins of intelligence.* New York: Plenum, 1976.

Schank, R. C., & Abelson, R. P. *Scripts, plans, goals, and understanding.* Hillsdale, N.J.: Erlbaum, 1977.

Schwartz, M. Visual shape perception in early infancy. Unpublished doctoral dissertation, Monash University, 1975.

Schwartz, M. & Day, R. H. Visual shape perception in early infancy. *Monographs of the Society for Research in Child Development,* 1979, *44,* (7, Serial No. 182), 1–58.

Sigman, M., & Parmelee, A. H. Visual preferences of four-month-old premature and full-term infants. *Child Development,* 1974, *45,* 959–965.

Slobin, D. I. Cognitive prerequisites for the development of grammar. In C. A. Ferguson & D. I. Slobin, (Eds.), *Studies of child language development.* New York: Holt, 1974.

Snyder, L. Pragmatics in language-deficient children: Prelinguistic and early verbal performatives and presuppositions. Unpublished doctoral dissertation, University of Colorado, 1975.

Vurpillot, E., Ruel, J., & Castrec, A. L'organisation perceptive chez le nourrisson: Response au tout ou a ses elements. *Bulletin de Psychologie,* 1977, *327,* 396–405.

Witelson, S. F. Early hemisphere specialization and interhemispheric plasticity: An empirical and theoretical review. In S. J. Segalowitz & F. A. Gruber (Eds.), *Language development and neurological theory.* New York: Academic Press, 1977.

13

Examination of Habituation as a Measure of Aberrant Infant Development[1]

LESLIE B. COHEN

The need for early screening and detection of infants at risk for intellectual disabilities has become of increasing concern to professionals interested in child development and to society as a whole. Even though the belief has been widespread that cognitive abilities in the child or older infant can be predicted from the infant's prenatal and perinatal biological conditions (i.e., from so called high-risk factors), the research evidence has been equivocal at best (Sameroff & Chandler, 1975). In the present chapter, I will describe two experiments from our laboratory in Chicago that represent our first attack on this problem. For a number of years, we have been investigating the development of visual habituation in normal infants. The habituation paradigm has turned out to be an excellent device for examining early visual attention, recognition memory, and information-processing ability. The experiments to be described addressed two basic questions; first, is the habituation paradigm sensitive to differences between normal and retarded development, and second, if it is, do high-risk infants differ from normal ones in infant visual attention, memory or information processing?

However, before I describe any specific experiment, I would like to spend a few minutes discussing the habituation paradigm and our rationale for using it. If one repeatedly presents the same visual pattern to infants over 2 months of age, their fixation times typically will decrease or habituate. Furthermore, if a novel pattern is presented following habituation, fixation times will usually increase once again or dishabituate. Numerous investigators have used

[1] The research reported in this chapter was supported in part by National Institute of Health Grants HD–03858 and HD–05951 and by the Illinois Institute for Developmental Disabilities.

PRETERM BIRTH AND
PSYCHOLOGICAL DEVELOPMENT

this habituation–dishabituation procedure to study infant memory and visual information processing. The decrease in attention during habituation is assumed to result from the infant's growing recognition of the habituation stimulus. In other words, the infants are becoming bored with seeing the same stimulus over and over; but the only way they could have become bored is if they had recognized the stimulus as something they had seen before. Thus, the habituation phase of these experiments taps some aspect of the initial acquisition or encoding process.

The dishabituation phase of the experiments usually provides some indication of infants' information-processing or discriminative abilities. For example, we and others have reported experiments in which infants were habituated to one simple geometric pattern, such as red circle, and then were tested on patterns that had new colors or forms or both. The dishabituation that occured to any changed pattern indicated that the infants were processing and storing both color and form information and that they could discriminate between the colors and forms we had presented.

Up to the present time, the habituation–dishabituation paradigm has been used almost exclusively with normal infants. Since the paradigm provides a good measure of some basic perceptual and cognitive abilities, it seemed worthwhile to expand our research to include aberrant infants as well as normal ones. The future goal, of course, is to develop some infant assessment device sensitive to specific cognitive abilities that can be used with infants suspected of being deficient in those abilities.

Our first step was to compare the performance in a visual habituation task of a group of normal infants who can be assumed to be of normal intelligence with a group of infants diagnosed as retarded and who will almost certainly be subnormal in intellectual functioning. For a visual habituation task to be of any possible diagnostic significance, it must be able to discriminate reliably between two such divergent groups. Therefore, in the first experiment we compared the performance of Down's syndrome versus normal infants.

Eight Down's and 8 normal infants at each of three ages—19, 23, and 28 weeks—were given a simple habituation task. The Down's and normal infants were matched on the basis of age, sex, socioeconomic status (SES), and number of times tested. (Because of the limited availability of Down's infants, approximately 30% of them and their normal controls were tested more than once.)

All infants were examined in a mobile laboratory. The infant sat in his mother's lap, facing a 4 ft. × 4 ft. display screen. Fixation times were recorded in an adjacent control room by an observer who watched the infant's face and eyes via closed circuit television. We have demonstrated several times previously that this method has high interobserver reliability. Each trial began with a light blinking on and off in the center of the screen. As soon as the infant fixated the light, it went off and a pattern appeared on the left side of the screen. Infants were allowed one unlimited look at the pattern on each trial.

TABLE 13.1
Experimental Procedures for Study of Down's Syndrome and Normal Infants[a]

Pretest	Habituation	Posthabituation	Posttest
SH, SH	CH, CH, ...	CH	CH, CH, SH, SH
SH, SH	CH, CH, ...	CH	SH, SH, CH, CH

[a] SH-shapes; CH-checkerboard.

When they turned away, the pattern went off, and the blinking light reappeared to start the next trial.

The stimuli and experimental procedure are presented in Table 13.1. Subjects were first given a pretest consisting of two trials with multicolored shapes. They were then habituated to a 24 × 24 black-and-white checkerboard pattern. This habituation phase continued until each subject's fixation time dropped to one-half of what it had been on the first three trials. At that point, one more checkerboard was presented as a posthabituation test to determine if the infant's fixation time remained low following criterion. Finally, a post test was given with the checkerboard and shapes presented twice in a counterbalanced order. Since the study was exploratory in nature, several aspects of the data that might be sensitive to differences between Down's and normal infants were examined.

The main results of the study are shown in Table 13.2. One place to look for differences between Down's and normal infants is in the number of trials

TABLE 13.2
Number of Habituation Trials and Mean Fixation Time for Down's Syndrome and Normal Infants

		Number of habituation trials	Mean fixation time (sec)			
			Pretest	Habituation 1, 2	Posttest	
	N		SH, SH [a]	CH, CH [a]	CH, CH [a]	SH, SH [a]
19 weeks						
Down's	8	8.6	12.5	13.9	12.9	11.3
Normal	8	8.9	2.6	3.2	1.4	2.1
23 weeks						
Down's	8	9.4	9.1	13.3	4.5	5.7
Normal	8	10.1	1.7	2.1	1.0	2.0
28 weeks						
Down's	8	6.6	3.9	7.7	3.8	5.1
Normal	8	7.6	2.4	2.8	1.2	2.6

[a] SH = shapes; CH = checkerboard.

needed to reach our criterion of habituation. If Down's infants have greater difficulty remembering information they have seen before, they should take longer to habituate than normal infants. As you can see from the second column of Table 13.2, that difference did not occur. At all three ages, the number of habituation trials for Down's and normal subjects was approximately the same. If anything, the Down's infants took slightly fewer trials, although that difference was not significant. A second possible difference between the groups is that, although Down's infants may take as few trials to habituate as normal infants, the time it takes Down's infants to process a stimulus on each trial might be longer. Once again, examining Table 13.2 one can see that throughout the experiment, at every age, Down's infants had longer fixation times than their normal controls. Differences between Down's and normal fixation times were significant at 19 weeks, $F(1/14) = 21.45$, $p < .001$; at 23 weeks, $F(1/14) = 17.49$, $p < .001$; and at 28 weeks, $F(1/14) = 7.38$, $p < .02$. Although we did not test it directly, it is also clear from Table 13.2 that, whereas normal infants look about the same duration of time across all three ages, the Down's infants decrease their fixation times as they become older. We have found the same decrease to hold for normal infants between the ages of 8 and 18 weeks.

Probably the most critical test of the present experiment is a comparison of performance on the initial shapes and checkerboards versus performance on the final shapes and checkerboards. These data are given in the last four columns of Table 13.2. The column labeled "habituation" gives the mean fixation time for the first two habituation trials. We averaged across two trials to make the mean comparable to the two pretest trials with the shapes. Taking the normal infants first, at every age, the infants decreased their fixation time to the checkerboards from the early habituation trials to the posttest but maintained the same level of fixation to the shapes from pretest to posttest. This stimulus × pretest–posttest interaction was significant at 28 weeks, $F(1/6) = 6.00$, $p < .05$, and at 23 weeks, $F(1/6) = 24.54$, $p < .005$, and approached significance at 19 weeks, $F(1/6) = 3.99$, $p < .10$.[2] On the other hand, Down's infants showed an interesting developmental change. At 19 weeks, their fixation time did not drop off significantly to either stimulus from pretest to posttest. They did reach criterion during the habituation phase of the experiment, which meant that their fixation time to the checkerboard decreased temporarily to one-half of what it had been on the first three habituation trials. However, that decrease to criterion was apparently accidental since their fixation time to the checkerboard increased again when they were given the posttest. This pattern of results with the 19-week-old Down's infants highlights the importance of including the familiar habituation

---

[2] Several reported studies from our laboratory and from other laboratories substantiate the fact that by 19 weeks of age normal, middle-class infants are fully capable of habituating to a familiar pattern and of dishabituating to a novel one. See Jeffrey and Cohen (1971) and Cohen and Gelber (1975) for reviews of this literature.

stimulus in the posttest. Without such a stimulus, one might have concluded spuriously that the infants had habituated when in fact they had not.

At 23 weeks, the Down's infants did decrease their fixation time to the checkerboard from habituation to posttest. However, their fixation time to the shapes also decreased. There was a significant main effect of early versus late trials, $F(1/6) = 12.03, p < .02$, but no interaction with stimuli. At least two explanations may be posited for this general decrease in looking from beginning to end of the experiment. One is that the Down's infants were becoming tired and irritable and just would not look at anything. This explanation seems unlikely for three reasons. First, Down's infants are generally more attentive, better subjects, than their normal counterparts. Second, the 23-week-old Down's subjects were still looking approximately 5 sec per trial. If they had been cranky or sleepy, their fixation times would have been much lower. Finally, it is unlikely that the Down's infants would have become irritable at 23 weeks but would have maintained their interest at both 19 and 28 weeks. An alternative explanation for the performance of the 23-week-old Down's subjects is that they did in fact habituate, but what they remembered was something rather diffuse. They may have remembered that they had seen a picture but did not differentiate between the familiar (i.e., the checkerboard) and the novel picture (i.e., the shapes). We lean toward this latter interpretation.

At 28 weeks, for the first time, the behavior of the Down's infants began to approximate that of the normal ones. They decreased their looking to the checkerboard but maintained their looking to the shapes. For the first time with Down's infants, the interaction between stimuli and early versus late testing was statistically significant, $F(1/6) = 10.33, p < .02$. It is interesting to note, that the Down's infants appeared to habituate to the familiar stimulus and to dishabituate to the novel stimulus at the same time that their overall fixation time dropped to the same level as that of the normal infants. The exact relationship between fixation time and habituation is unknown, but these results would suggest that there is some relationship between the two.

Thus, the results of this first experiment indicate that the habituation paradigm is sensitive to differences between normal and retarded infants. The most obvious difference was in the duration of time infants would look. Somewhat less obvious, but more informative, was the pattern of habituation and dishabituation. Although the normal infants habituated to the familiar stimulus and dishabituated to the novel one at all three ages, the Down's infants appeared to go through a series of steps. At 19 weeks, they did not clearly habituate. At 23 weeks, they habituated but probably did not differentiate between two very different visual patterns, and finally, at 28 weeks, they showed both habituation and dishabituation.

Given the encouraging outcome of the first experiment, we decided to conduct a second study—this time with infants suspected of having some type of developmental delay, namely, high-risk preterm infants. We did not know what we were getting into. First, there were the technical problems: finding a hospital that would be cooperative; months waiting for the project to pass human subjects and other committees; a low return rate to the outpatient clinic by mothers of high-risk infants; and finally, a political dispute between the hospital and the state that closed down the clinic completely. I am sure these difficulties are common knowledge to those working with this type of population, but for us, it was a new experience.

Then, there is the definitional problem. Different studies have used different criteria for high-risk infants. We excluded from our experiment those infants whom Tjossem (1976) has labeled "established risk," those with such obvious mental or motor handicaps as Down's syndrome, cerebral palsy, and microcephaly. We concentrated on subjects who had an environmental and/or biological risk. We wanted to see if lower-class infants who had had some perinatal trauma but who had survived relatively intact would be delayed in their development of visual habituation and dishabituation.

The infants we tested had all been born in a local Chicago hospital. They were seen when they came back to the hospital for their regular clinic appointments. Based upon a total of 18 perinatal factors, the high-risk infants were assigned by a neonatal nurse into either "severe" or "mild" categories. A third group of healthy, lower-class infants born in the same hospital but with normal deliveries was also tested as a control. A subsequent multiple discriminant analysis of the nurses ratings indicated that the severe infants could best be distinguished from the combined normal and mild samples on the basis of severe respiratory distress. On the other hand, the normal infants could best be distinguished from the combined mild and severe ones on the basis of gestational age. Because the mild group was more heterogeneous in its perinatal sequelae, and because it did not differ from the normal controls in any measure of attention or habituation, I shall limit my discussion to the data from severe and normal infants.

We were able to test a total of 23 severe infants. Several were tested repeatedly during the first year of life. All these infants were born with some type of complication that required placing them in the hospital's intensive care nursery. All but three were preterm, which we defined as less than 37 weeks gestation at the time of birth. All but four had hyaline membrane disease and required respiratory assistance. Five had seizures, one had severe hypocalcemia, and one had congenital heart disease.

Table 13.3 highlights some of the differences between our normal and severe subjects. For comparison purposes, infants were grouped into three age categories: 20, 33, and 49 weeks. These categories were based upon corrected age rather than age since birth. Since the normal infants were full-term, age since birth and corrected age were the same. Corrected age for the severe infants was computed by subtracting 40 weeks from the hospital's estimate of each infant's conceptional age. As you can see from Table 13.3, the mean birthweight averaged about 3300 gm for the normal infants and was under 2000 gm for the severe infants. Mean gestational age at birth was 40 weeks for

TABLE 13.3
Characteristics of Three Age Groups of Normal and Severe Infants

Correct age [a]	Mean birthweight (gm)	Mean gestational age (weeks)	Number of females	Number of males
20 weeks				
Normal	3395	40	7	5
Severe	1956	33	2	9
33 weeks				
Normal	3277	39	10	4
Severe	1963	29	2	7
49 weeks				
Normal	3384	40	11	4
Severe	1662	31	3	36

[a] Corrected age refers to mean conceptional age of group at time of testing minus 40 weeks.

the normals and approximately 30 weeks for the severes. One potentially confounding factor in the experiment was the proportion of males and females in the two groups. As is typical, we had quite a few more males in our severe group and for some unknown reason, more females in our normal control group.

For reasons that will become apparent shortly, upon completion of this experiment, we also decided to run some 20-week-old middle-class infants on the same task. Table 13.4 indicates some of the demographic differences between our lower-class and middle-class populations. Approximately two-thirds of the lower-class infants came from single-parent families, whereas all of the middle-class infants had two parents living at home. The average number of years of education was fewer than 12 years for the lower-class parents and greater than 14 years for the middle-class ones. Our lower-class sample was almost entirely black, whereas our middle-class one was entirely white. Finally, the place of residence was predominately urban for both samples; although obviously the location in the city where the two groups lived was quite different.

Table 13.5 describes the experimental procedure used in the high-risk study. On the first trial, all the infants were shown a 24 × 24 black-and-white checkerboard pattern. They were then repeatedly shown a color photograph of a female face until they reached our criterion of habituation (three trials whose mean is one-half the looking time of the first three trials). Two posthabituation trials followed with the same face. A test was then given consisting of the same face, a novel face, a lion's face, and another checkerboard pattern.

TABLE 13.4

Demographic Characteristics of Subject Sample for High-Risk Study

	Percentage low SES	Percentage middle SES
Two-parent families (percentage)		
Father and mother	33	100
Mother only	67	0
Mean number years of education		
Mother	11.43[b]	14.3
Father	12.0[c]	14.5
Obtained college degrees (percentage)		
Mother	n.a.[d]	45
Father	n.a.[d]	33
Racial background (percentage)		
Black	98	0
White	2	100
Place of residence		
City	100	90
Suburban	0	10

[a] Lower-class values estimated from listing of father's name on medical records.

[b] Based on 77% of subjects who filled in mother's education level for medical records.

[c] Based on 30% of subjects who filled in father's education level for medical records.

[d] n.a. = not available.

TABLE 13.5

Experimental Procedures for High-Risk Study [a]

Pretest	Habituation	Posthabituation	Posttest
CH	F_1, F_1, . . .	F_1, F_1,	F_1, F_2, L, CH
CH	F_2, F_2, . . .	F_2, F_2,	F_1, F_2, L, CH

[a] F_1 = black face; F_2 = oriental face; L = line cartoon face; CH = checkerboard.

We decided to habituate the infants to photographs of female faces rather than to checkerboards as we had done in the Down's study for two reasons. First, we thought faces would be more interesting to the infants than checkerboards would be. Given our difficulty in obtaining infants in the first place, we did not want to take the risk of losing a sizable number because of inattention or boredom. The second reason was that instead of the rather gross test of discrimination we had used in the Down's study, in the present experiment we wanted to test for degree of generalizability of habituation. Therefore, our test stimuli included two quite different faces, one black and one oriental, and a colored drawing of a lion's face that retained the facelike quality but was very different from the other two faces. Since the checkerboard was presented at the end of the experiment as well as at the beginning, we could use performance on these trials as a test for fatigue or nonspecific generalization.

The results of the experiment are presented in Table 13.6. For the moment, concentrate only on the comparison between the high-risk and the full-term lower-class groups. At all ages, both of these groups habituated in approximately the same number of trials. Also, at all ages, the infants looked for significantly less time on the mean of the two posthabituation trials than they did on the mean of the first three habituation trials (20 weeks, $F(1/21) = 48.16$, $p < .001$; 33 weeks, $F(1/21) = 40.12$, $p < .001$; 49 weeks, $F(1/21) = 24.12$, $p < .001$). Analysis of the posttest data revealed that at 33 and 49 weeks of age both high-risk and full-term infants looked significantly longer at the novel face and at the lion than at the familiar face (33 weeks, $F(2/42) = 20.35$, $p < .001$; 49 weeks, $F(2/42) = 16.73$, $p < .001$). Either stimulus was sufficiently novel to produce recovery of the previously habituated response. The story was different at 20 weeks. Contrary to our expectations, neither group looked significantly longer at the novel test faces than at the familiar one. In fact, from inspecting the means, it appeared as though the severe infants were displaying more recovery than the full-term infants. However, the two group × test trials interaction did not approach significance.

In some respects, both groups of 20-week-old lower-class infants resembled the 23-week-old Down's subjects from the previously reported experiment. Both the lower-class and Down's infants appeared to habituate but then generalized or remained low to all test stimuli. This generalization, particularly by the lower-class normal subjects, surprised us, since previous research from our laboratory in Champaign had consistently shown that by 20 weeks of age middle-class infants could discriminate between photographs of faces and would fixate novel faces longer than familiar ones. Perhaps the particular faces used in the high-risk study or something about the experimental procedure was responsible for the failure to obtain recovery and discrimination at 20 weeks. In order to test this possibility, we ran an additional group of middle-class infants on the same task we had given the lower-class infants. All

TABLE 13.6
Number of Habituation Trials and Mean Fixation Time for High-Risk and Full-Term Infants

	N	Number of habituation trials	Mean fixation time (sec)				
			Habituation 1, 2, 3 Face₁	Posthabituation Face₁	Posttest Face₁	Posttest Face₂	Posttest Lion
20 weeks							
Severe							
Lower class	11	7.4	5.8	1.9	3.2	4.1	4.1
Full-term							
Lower class	12	6.1	17.8	3.7	4.1	4.6	3.0
Middle class	12	7.9	5.5	2.2	3.3	6.2	6.0
33 weeks							
Severe							
Lower class	9	7.3	3.1	1.1	1.3	2.9	2.6
Full-term							
Lower class	14	7.7	3.5	1.9	2.9	4.0	5.8
49 weeks							
Severe							
Lower class	8	7.0	3.3	1.9	2.8	4.6	4.4
Full-term							
Lower class	15	9.1	2.8	1.4	2.3	3.8	5.1

middle-class subjects were full-term and were equated with the full-term lower-class subjects on age and sex.

In Table 13.6, the third row under "20 weeks" provides the results for these middle-class controls. They too habituated in about the same number of trials as the lower-class infants and also showed a significant decrease in looking from the first three habituation trials to the posthabituation trials, $F(1/10) = 105.94$, $p < .001$. That is where the resemblance ends, however. In the posttest, unlike the lower-class subjects, the middle-class subjects clearly recovered to both novel faces. Their behavior closely resembled that of the 33- and 49-week-old lower-class infants. A 3 group × 3 test stimulus analysis of the data for 20-week-old infants yielded a significant groups × test stimuli interaction, $F(4/64) = 3.80$, $p < .01$. The interaction was produced by the fact that the full-term middle-class group looked longer at the novel face and lion face than at the familiar face, whereas the severe and full-term lower-class groups did not.

What conclusions can be drawn from these first attempts to investigate habituation in Down's syndrome and high-risk infants? Perhaps the first point is that one should be hesitant about drawing any definite conclusions. As is so often the case with research of this type, in both experiments the numbers were relatively small, some infants could be tested repeatedly whereas others could only be tested once, and counterbalancing of potentially confounding factors (such as sex of the infant in the high-risk study) was not always possible. Nevertheless, both experiments have provided some valuable new information. Both studies demonstrated the sensitivity of our habituation procedure for investigating early cognitive ability in aberrant populations. In the Down's study, we found that overall fixation time consistently differentiated Down's from normal infants. Even more important, with respect to habituation and recovery, we found Down's infants progressed through a three-stage sequence. At the youngest age, the Down's infants did not habituate; at the intermediate age, they did habituate but did not recover to a novel test stimulus; and at the oldest age, they showed both habituation and recovery. The last two stages were also found in the high-risk study. Like the 23-week-old Down's infants, the 20-week-old lower-class infants habituated but did not recover to a novel stimulus. Again, as in the Down's study, the lower-class infants did recover at older ages.

Considering both experiments together, normal middle-class infants showed both habituation and recovery at all ages. One obvious experiment to verify the three-stage developmental sequence of habituation would be to replicate either the Down's or high-risk study with younger normal middle-class infants. Some evidence already available indicates the difficulty of obtaining habituation in middle-class infants under 2 months of age (Jeffrey & Cohen, 1971) and the lack of discrimination between novel and familiar faces at 3–4 months (Fagan, 1976). Given this evidence, it seems likely that the same developmental sequence we found with Down's infants would occur in middle-class infants, but at an eariler age.

We are not claiming that at an early age Down's, lower-class, or even middle-class infants are incapable of habituation and discrimination under any circumstances. There are studies that report that under certain conditions even neonates can habituate (Friedman, 1972). We were trying to test the relative ease of habituation and discrimination at various ages rather than to show that, if one manipulates the stimuli and procedure enough, one can find some task on which any infant can habituate. If we had selected a procedure that showed all infants performing equally well at all ages, the procedure would have been useless as a diagnostic tool. Perhaps, the most encouraging aspect of the present experiments is that our task did produce differences across both age and population.

Finally, some specific comments are in order regarding the differences we did find and did not find in our high-risk study. We had expected to find that lower-class full-term infants performed better than lower-class severe infants. That result did not occur. The two groups were quite similar. Perhaps that similarity resulted from the fact that even our most severe infants were reasonably healthy by the time they participated in our experiment. Others (Parmelee & Haber, 1973; Sameroff & Chandler, 1975) have discussed the difficulty in making long-term predictions from perinatal condition. Perhaps the influence of the lower-social-class environment is so crucial that it may mask the effects of high-risk factors in the newborn. Our results do not prove this latter alternative, but they certainly do suggest the importance of social-class factors in later perceptual or cognitive development. Our findings were also consistent with a large collaborative project (Broman, Nichols, & Kennedy, 1975) that reported that social-class-related variables were more predictive of later IQ than were prenatal or perinatal variables.

Although a comparison of our middle-class and lower-class full-term infants did implicate social-class factors in the development of infant memory and discrimination, our study lacked one important group, a middle-class severe group, which is necessary for determining whether or not perinatal factors are also important. In fact, we are attempting to test infants in that group at the present time. If the middle-class severe infants perform like the middle-class full-term infants did, we will have demonstrated the general pervasive influence of social class. On the other hand, if the middle-class severe subjects perform like our lower-class subjects, we will have demonstrated that both social class and perinatal condition contribute to the development of infant memory and discrimination.

Whatever the outcome of this final study, our initial studies of aberrant infant populations have already demonstrated the feasibility of employing visual habituation techniques to investigate differences in early cognitive ability. Until now, our research has emphasized rather simple abilities, such as memory for repeated visual stimuli or discrimination of one stimulus from another. Some of our more recent research with normal infants also has shown habituation to be an effective means of investigating more complex processes, such as the ability to form a conceptual category from a variety of different exemplars (Cohen & Strauss, 1977). We are just beginning to examine the acquisition of conceptual categories in aberrant populations as well. Ultimately, what is needed is a series of tasks that tap different levels of perceptual and cognitive functioning in the infant and that can be given at a variety of ages. We and others working in the area of infant habituation may not have achieved that goal yet, but we are certainly making consistent progress toward it.

Acknowledgments

I wish to thank Nadine Caputo, Janice Aiello, and Judy DeLoache for their assistance in conducting this research.

References

Broman, S. H., Nichols, P. L., & Kennedy, W. A. *Preschool IQ: Prenatal and early developmental correlates.* New York: Wiley, 1975.

Cohen, L. B., & Gelber, E. R. Infant visual memory. In L. Cohen & P. Salapatek (Eds.). *Infant perception from sensation to cognition: Basic visual processes* (Vol. l). New York: Academic Press, 1975.

Cohen, L. B., & Strauss, M. S. Concept acquisition in the human infant. *Child Development,* 1977, *50,* 419–424.

Fagan, J. F. Infants recognition of invariant features of faces. *Child Development,* 1976, *47,* 627–638.

Friedman, S. Habituation and recovery of visual response in the alert human newborn. *Journal of Experimental Child Psychology,* 1972, *13,* 339–349.

Jeffrey, W. E., & Cohen, L. B. Habituation in the human infant. In H. Reese (Ed.), *Advances in child development and behavior* (Vol. 6). New York: Academic Press, 1971.

Parmelee, A. H., & Haber, A. Who is the risk infant? *Clinical Obstetrics and Gynecology,* 1973, *16,* 376–387.

Sameroff, A. J., & Chandler, M. J. Reproductive risk and the continuum of caretaking casualty. In F. D. Horowitz (Ed.), *Review of child development research.* Chicago: Univ. Of Chicago Press, 1975.

Tjossem, T. D. Early intervention: Issues and approaches. In T. D. Tjossem (Ed.), *Intervention strategies for high risk infants and young children.* Baltimore: University Park, 1976.

14

Lags in the Cognitive Competence
of Prematurely Born Infants[1]

SUSAN A. ROSE

Potential of New Measures for Assessing
Cognitive Development in Infancy

Until the 1970s, there had been relatively little effort to develop measures
for assessing the range of cognitive skills that might be available to the young
infant. The few measures widely used provide either a global index of
developmental status (e.g., Bayley scales) or a measure of specific competen-
cies that are acquired in their entirety during infancy (e.g., object permanence). They do not dovetail in any conspicuous way with learning or
memory paradigms that are commonly used to assess development at older
ages. In fact, there appears to be a discontinuity in the nature of the tasks comprising early and later tests of development. Whereas tests of later cognitive
development, such as the Stanford-Binet, are heavily saturated with
assessments of information processing, the infant scales, both the sensorimotor and the Piagetian, are heavily dependent on the development of
motor skills (Bower & Wishart, 1972; Gottfried & Brody, 1975; Kopp, 1975).
There appeared to us to be a need for measures of cognitive development in
infancy, particularly for clinical groups, to include other indexes of development. The need seemed particularly pressing for prematurely born infants in
view of the general failure of psychometric and Piagetian tests of sensorimotor development to discriminate these infants from nonrisk infants.
For example, once corrections are made for differences in length of gestation,
the performance of prematures on standard tests of infant development is ac-

[1] The research reported in this chapter was supported in part by National Institute of Health
Grant HD 13810, New York State Health Research Council (C-106138) Grant 238, and a Social
and Behavioral Sciences Research Grant from the National Foundation–March of Dimes.

PRETERM BIRTH AND
PSYCHOLOGICAL DEVELOPMENT

tually on a par with that of full-term infants (Fitzhardinge, 1975; Goldstein, Caputo, & Taub, 1976; Parmelee & Schulte, 1970; Tilford, 1976). Nevertheless, even despite recent advances in the medical management of these infants, lags and deficits continue to be reported by the school years (e.g., Fitzhardinge & Ramsay, 1973; Francis-Williams & Davies, 1974; Rubin, Rosenblatt, & Balow, 1973; Taub, Goldstein, & Caputo, 1977).

In our laboratory at Albert Einstein College of Medicine, we have been working on the development of measures we think may more closely reflect differences in cognitive development in infancy. Much of this work builds upon an area in which there have been major advances relevant to cognitive competence, namely, the study of infant visual perception (e.g., Cohen & Gelber, 1975; Fantz, Fagan, & Miranda, 1975). We now know that the young infant is capable of perceiving and remembering an astonishing amount about his visual world. One technique that has been used a great deal to study these abilities, and which we have used extensively, capitalizes on the infant's well-established tendency to selectively fixate new stimuli. In this technique, often called that of recognition memory, a stimulus is displayed for a period of visual inspection, then the now-familiar stimulus is presented simultaneously with a novel stimulus so the infant can inspect them both. Typically, the infant shows a differential preference for the novel stimulus, providing evidence for recognition memory (e.g., Fagan, 1970, 1972). Such differential responsiveness could not be the result of the particular stimulus, since each stimulus of every pair serves equally often as the familiar and novel one. The information taken in during familiarization is the only basis for the differential responsiveness. In effect, the process of recognition requires a match between the current input and the stored mental representation of previous input. The results of this technique have shown us that by 6 months of age the infant can remember complex abstract patterns, discriminate changes in the arrangements of elements that make up such patterns, and recognize photographs of faces (Fagan, 1974).

For our work with prematures, we of course wanted a measure that would be maximally sensitive to the infant's skill in processing information. A study we had done with full-term infants highlighted for us the exquisite sensitivity of the recognition memory paradigm (Rose, 1977). In that study, 6-month-old full-terms were tested with stimuli that were discrepant from the familiar stimulus in either pattern or dimension, or both pattern and dimension, that is, in either one or two respects. For example, an infant who had seen a photo of a sunburst on familiarization trials then saw, on test trials, the familiar photo paired with a photo of four diamonds (for a change in pattern), a wooden construction of the sunburst (for a change in dimension), or a wooden construction of the diamonds (for a change in both pattern and dimension). The results showed that in all cases, infants looked significantly longer at the novel stimulus, indicating they could detect each type of change. While they responded as much to a change in dimension as a change in pattern, they were even more attentive to stimuli that differed from the familiar stimulus in both respects (the percentages of visual fixation to the novel stimuli being 57%, 58%, and 64%, respectively). Thus, the magnitude of the novelty effect actually mirrored the degree of novelty present in the new stimulus, a finding that agrees with predictions from Fagan's theoretical model (1977). This close coupling of visual discrepancy and response magnitude was impressive and suggested that this paradigm might have the requisite sensitivity for detecting differences between risk and nonrisk infants.

A second experiment from the same study (Rose, 1977) had further implications for the direction our research effort with prematures was to take. There we found that full-term infants were able to extract information about invariances from both pictures and objects and to transfer this information across dimensions. For example, when they had been familiarized with an object, they were less attentive in the test phase to a picture of that object than to a picture of a different object. Since neither test stimulus had been seen previously, we could infer that the infant recognized the original pattern and treated it as familiar, despite a change in its dimension. Other results from this study clearly showed that the infants were not confusing the object with its photographic representation. Quite the contrary: They readily discriminated between the two. Thus, not only could they differentiate objects from the pictorial counterparts, but they could recognize the similarities that exist between the two. This ability of infants to recognize a photo and an object at first sight suggests that they can perceive the representational character of at least some stimuli very early in life and without any special training.

Cross-Modal Transfer

The first study that we did with prematures (Rose, Gottfried, & Bridger, 1978) was concerned with infants' ability to extract invariances in the face of even more radical differences in the stimuli. Here we investigated their ability to recognize an object when the information about it was obtained through different sense systems, that is, to extract information about an object in one modality and transfer it to another. Adults can accurately identify by touch alone objects they have only seen and recognize by sight objects they have experienced only by touch. The ability to make information in one sense modality available to another is termed *cross-modal transfer* (or intersensory equivalence). We decided to try to adapt the visual recognition memory design for the study of such cross-modal abilities in infancy. In doing so, the stimuli were presented either tactually or orally during familiarization and visually during testing. When the stimuli are presented in different modalities during familiarization and test, occurrence of recognition memory demonstrates cross-modal transfer (Gottfried, Rose, & Bridger, 1977).

Based on evidence in older groups, there were reasons to think that this measure might turn out to be sensitive to cognitive lags or deficits in infancy. First, this skill has been found deficient in a variety of populations with either known or presumptive disabilities (see review by Deutsch & Schumer, 1970; Friedes, 1974). Furthermore, this skill has been shown to correlate with intellectual performance in school-aged children (Das, Kirby, & Jarman, 1975). Some investigators have even suggested that cross-modal abilities are a critical underpinning of cognitive functioning in humans (Birch & Lefford, 1963, 1967; Ettlinger, 1967; Geschwind, 1965).

We have now tested three groups of 1-year-old infants: middle-class, full-terms, lower-class full-terms, and prematures (Rose *et al.*, 1978). The social class was varied in this study for two reasons. First, while we had evidence that full-term infants from middle-class backgrounds demonstrate cross-modal transfer (Gottfried *et al.*, 1977), the premature sample we had available was predominantly from lower-class backgrounds. There is evidence showing that older children from lower-class backgrounds (even those of presumably term birth) lag in the development of cross-modal skills (Connors, Schuette, & Goldman, 1967). Second, there is ample evidence that children from lower-social-class backgrounds are at risk for lags in cognitive development, although these lags generally are not detected until the preschool and school years (e.g., Birns & Bridger, 1977; Blank, Rose, & Berlin, 1978). Thus, in order to assess the effects of prematurity separate from those of social class, we tested full-term infants from different social-class backgrounds.

In the present study, socioeconomic status (SES) was determined by the level of parental education. If the infants' parents had completed an average of more than 12 years of education, the infants were considered middle SES; if the infants' parents averaged 12 years or less of schooling, the infants were considered lower SES. Prematures had a mean gestational age at birth of 33 weeks and a mean birthweight of 1650 gm. They were tested at corrected age, that is, age estimated from expected date of birth. The average educational level of parents of the prematures fell midway between that of the other two groups ($M = 12.5$).

Each infant was administered six tasks: three cross-modal (one oral–visual and two tactual–visual) and three intramodal (all visual–visual). The intramodal tasks served as controls to determine if failure on the cross-modal tasks was due to failure in discriminating stimuli within the visual modality. A different pair of objects was used in each task; members of a pair differed from one another primarily in terms of shape (see Figure 14.1). In the oral–visual task, the stimulus was placed in the infants's mouth for familiarization, whereas in the tactual–visual tasks, it was placed in the infant's hand. If the infant did not spontaneously palpate the object, the experimenter moved it about in the infant's hand. In each case, the experimenter shielded the object from the infant's view. During the familiarization period, one member of the stimulus pair was presented for 30 sec; during the test period, the infant was shown both members of the pair—the familiar and the

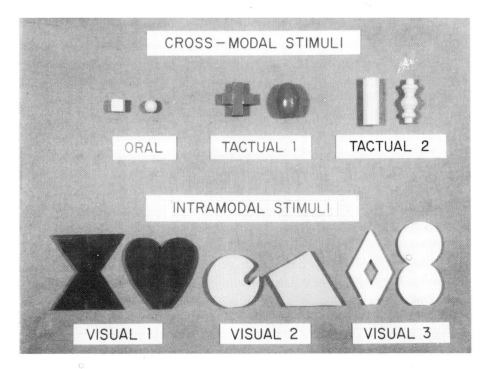

FIGURE 14.1. *Pairs of stimulus objects used in the cross-modal study. (From Gottfried, Rose, & Bridger, 1977).*

novel—for 20 sec (with left–right positions reversed after the first 10 sec). At the end of the visual test period, the infant was permitted to reach for one of the paired test stimuli.

Since differential responses by infants of this age customarily reflect a preference for the novel stimulus, a novelty percentage was derived for each infant by dividing the amount of fixation to the novel stimulus by the total fixation time (novel plus familiar). To determine whether these novelty percentages are significant in each condition, they were tested against a chance value of 50%, using one-tailed t tests.

The results are clear cut. The mean novelty percentages shown in Figure 14.2 illustrate the main findings, namely, each group showed visual recognition memory following visual familiarization, but only middle-class full-term infants showed visual memory after familiarization in a different modality. In all problems, the middle-class infants looked significantly longer at the novel as compared with the familiar stimulus and reached significantly more for the novel stimulus as well. Their percentages of looking at the novel stimulus ranged from 56% to 67% (all $p < .05$), and scores in the cross-modal and intramodal tasks were comparable. The results indicate that middle-class full-term infants can exhibit cross-modal transfer. They gain knowledge about the

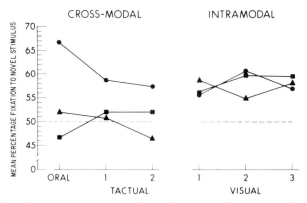

FIGURE 14.2. *Visual fixation to novel stimuli after oral and tactual familiarization (cross-modal tasks) and after visual familiarization (intramodal tasks). Circles show middle-class full-term infants; squares show lower-class full-terms, triangles show preterm infants. (Adapted from Rose, Gottfried, & Bridger, 1978.)*

shape of an object by feeling it and mouthing it, and they can make this information available to the visual system. They were able to do this after only 30 sec (or less) of handling or mouthing the object.

The results from the lower-class full-terms and the premature sample, however, are quite different. If we look at their scores, which are quite similar to one another, we see that, although these infants are capable of recognition memory within the visual modality, they consistently failed to show cross-modal functioning. As you can see in Figure 14.2, both groups looked significantly longer at the novel stimulus on all three visual–visual intramodal tasks (55–60%, all $p < .05$), but they consistently failed to look longer at the novel stimulus in the cross-modal tasks (scores ranged from 47% to 52%, $p > .05$). Analyses of variance for the intramodal and cross-modal tasks simply corroborate what you see in Figure 14.2: On the cross-modal tasks the middle-class full-term infants had significantly higher novelty scores than did infants in the other two groups, whereas on the intramodal tasks, there were no significant differences among the three groups. Overall, the reaching responses for the two risk groups were inconsistent in both the cross-modal and intramodal tasks.

I should point out that these results cannot be explained by differences in attentiveness during the familiarization period, since the groups did not differ in how much they handled the objects on the tactual tasks, and, of course, the fact that we tested at corrected ages indicates that we are not dealing with a simple maturational difference. Since the prognosis for lower-class prematures is sometimes reported to be poorer than for middle-class prematures (Sameroff & Chandler, 1975), we divided our sample of prematures by the same criterion used for full-terms and examined performance of the two subgroups separately ($N = 19$ middle class; $N = 8$ lower class). None of the comparisons we made showed any difference. Thus, while social class seems to be a potent factor for the full-terms, as far as we could tell, this factor did not interact in any way with prematurity in the present sample.

The explanation for these findings remains unclear. Although we think that we might be on the road to pinpointing a precise cognitive deficit in high-risk infants, we are not yet clear as to why these infants failed to show cross-modal transfer. We do think that their difficulty probably lies in one of three areas.

1. First, there may be *modality-specific deficits* in information processing, such as inferior registration, storage, or retrieval of tactual and oral information (Goodnow, 1971; Milner & Bryant, 1970; Rose, Blank, & Bridger, 1972; Rudel & Teuber, 1964). That is, inferior cross-modal performance may simply be a reflection of a poor ability to perceive, encode, and/or retain tactual information. So, for example, the risk infants might also fail tactual–tactual conditions, in which the objects had to be recognized tactually.

2. There may be *overall, nonspecific deficits* information processing that are common to all modalities (e.g., slower speed in gathering information and/or less refinement of the strategies used). In the data discussed earlier, both risk groups actually performed as well as the middle-class full-terms on the intramodal visual–visual tasks. However, the familiarization periods may have been suffiently long for all infants to process visual stimuli, which are ordinarily processed faster than tactual (Garvill & Molander, 1975; Lobb, 1965), but insufficiently long for the risk infants to process tactual stimuli. We do have data that suggest that, at younger ages, premature infants require longer familiarization times than full-term infants before they evidence visual recognition memory. It is possible that with increasingly longer familiarization times in the cross-modal conditions, the risk infants might actually show successful transfer.

3. The third possibility is that there may, of course, be a *deficit in sensory integration per se,* that is, in transferring information across sense systems. If cross-modal transfer involves the development or operation of a mediator, the risk infants may simply not have developed it yet and hence not know that the object they felt is the same as the object they see.

Effects of Manipulation on Visual Processing

We have also been studying another aspect of intersensory functioning, namely, the effect of temporally coordinated haptic cues on the visual perception of objects. We initiated these studies with the idea that visual memory would be enhanced if the infant were permitted to touch and manipulate the object while looking at it. That is, we thought that the infant might actually obtain more information about the form of an object by both touching and seeing it than by just seeing it. The Russian literature (Zaporozhets, 1965, 1973) and the work of Piaget (Piaget & Inhelder, 1948/1956) both suggest that active manipulation of an object leads to better schema development: Manipulation is thought to lie at the heart of representation and memory. However, a large body of work in this country with preschool-aged children, school-aged children, and adults actually shows that active manipulation does not facilitate visual recognition memory of objects (e.g., Abravanel, 1968; Butter & Zung, 1970; Weiner & Goodnow, 1970; although see Wolff, Levin, & Longobardi, 1972, for an exception to this general trend). Since infancy is a period during which the infant engages in a tremendous amount of manipulatory and exploratory activity, we thought that manipulation might have its most pronounced effect at this time. We have now studied this issue with infants aged 6–12 months in two separate experiments (Gottfried, Rose, & Bridger, 1978; Rose, Gottfried, & Bridger, 1979). Each used a methodology similar to that of the cross-modal study, in that each task consisted of a familiarization stage followed by a visual fixation test stage.

The essential difference between the cross-modal procedure and this procedure is the type of familiarization or sensory experience the infant receives. In these studies, we used three different familiarization conditions. In the *visual condition,* the infant was shown an object, and only visual inspection was permitted. In the *visual–haptic condition,* the infant was given the object so that he or she could see as well as actively manipulate and touch it. The third condition, the *visual–haptic control condition,* differed from the second only that the object was encased in a transparent box before it was presented to the infant. Since the infant's manipulation was now not in contact with the test object itself, he or she was unable to gain tactual information about its shape. This last condition served as a control to determine whether the haptic experience would affect performance by the tactual knowledge it provided about the shape of the object or simply by the manipulatory activity it permitted the infant. In particular, we were concerned that manipulation might increase the quality of the infant's visual attentiveness to the object and thus facilitate visual recognition memory, quite apart from any tactual information that was gained. We also took an important methodological step to actually ensure that each infant looked at the object the same amount of time: In all conditions, the familiarization phase lasted until the infant had accumulated 20 sec of looking directed at the frontal perspective of the object. Thus, any differences in recognition memory among the three tasks cannot be attributed to differences in visual attention directed to the stimulus.

In the first study (Gottfried *et al.,* 1978), we tested 108 middle-class full-term infants, 6, 9, and 12 months old. Infants were randomly assigned to one of three conditions, and each child was given three tasks per condition. The stimuli for these conditions are pictured in the first three columns of Figure 14.3. The major findings were that (*a*) 12-month-olds showed evidence of memory in all three conditions (62%, 56%, 55%, respectively); (*b*) younger infants (both 6 and 9 months old) showed evidence of memory only in the visual condition (61%, 52%, 51%, respectively); and (*c*) at all ages, the

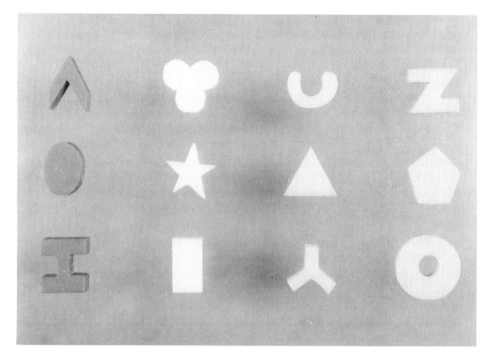

FIGURE 14.3. *Sets of stimulus objects used in examining the effect of visual and visual-plus-haptic familiarization on visual recognition memory. (From Rose, Gottfried, & Bridger, 1979.)*

infant's preference for novel relative to familiar stimuli was significantly greater in the visual condition than in the visual–haptic and visual–haptic control conditions, with the latter two not differing significantly from one another. Thus, contrary to our expectations, manipulatory activities did not facilitate the visual knowledge that infants gained about the object's shape. To our surprise, the results suggested instead that the addition of manipulation to visual familiarization interfered with subsequent visual recognition memory.

In the second study (Rose *et al.,*1979), we tested 6- and 12-month-old prematures and lower-class full-terms. In this study, each infant was tested in every condition, with but a single task being used in each condition. We also added a fourth condition in this study, a *visual control,* in which the object was visually inspected while inside the plastic box. This was to ensure that such encasement in no way hampered visual inspection. With these exceptions, the design was just like the first. The four sets of objects shown in Figure 14.3 served as stimuli.

As in the previous study, the full-term infants all weighed above 2500 gm at birth and had Apgar scores of 9 or 10. The 6-month-old group of prematures had a mean gestational age at birth of 33 weeks and a mean birthweight of

1610 gm; for the 12-month-old group, the comparable figures were 33 weeks and 1738 gm. Again, both groups of prematures were tested at corrected ages, so that they were, on the average, 6–7 weeks older chronologically than their full-term counterparts.

As can be seen Figure 14.4, the results for full-term infants at both 6 and 12 months replicated those of the initial study shown. (A comparison of these findings with those of the first study indicate that there were no social-class differences on these tasks.) At 6 months of age, the full term infants showed evidence of memory when familiarization involved only visual exposure. Although 12-month-old full-term infants showed memory in all conditions, the novelty percentages were somewhat attentuated in both conditions where manipulation of the object was permitted. Prematures, on the other hand, showed no evidence of memory in any of the conditions at 6 months, and at 12 months, they showed memory only in the visual conditions. At 12 months, the performance of the prematures is strikingly similar to that of the younger full-terms: Both groups show memory in the two visual conditions but not in conditions involving manipulation. Overall then, prematures showed lags both in the ability to process exclusively visual information and in the ability to deal with haptic and visual cues simultaneously.

These studies clearly show that haptic exploration of the objects did not facilitate visual recognition memory at either age or in either group. In fact, it actually interfered. Moreover, it made no difference whether the manipulation provided tactual information that was congruent with the visual impression of the object (visual–haptic) or discrepant from it (visual–haptic control). Yet, these interfering effects are puzzling, and their source remains unclear. They may be specific to the infant's manipulatory activities, or they may be due instead to factors that vary as the infant manipulates the object. In the course of manipulatory activity, the infant sees the object in many different visual perspectives. The possibility arises that the constant variation in perspective may have interfered with gaining or consolidating information about any single perspective. So, for example, if the object has been rotated

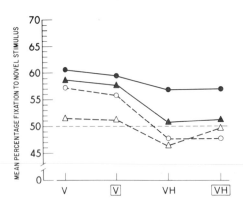

FIGURE 14.4 *Visual fixation to novel stimuli for full-term and preterm infants after four different types of familiarization. V, visual;* $\boxed{V}$, *visual control; VH, visual-plus-haptic;* $\boxed{VH}$, *visual-plus-haptic control. In control conditions, the stimulus object was encased in a clear transparent box during familiarization. Closed circles show 12-month-old and open circles show 6-month-old full-term infants; closed triangles show 12-month-old and open triangles show 6-month-old preterm infants. (Adapted from Rose, Gottfried, & Bridger, 1979.)*

during visual presentation, performance in the visual conditions might have been similarly depressed. Or, if tactual exploration were permitted, but the object was made to remain stationary and thus seen in only a single perspective, performance in the haptic condition might have improved. Another possibility is that any attempt to process information in more than one modality at a time is taxing for the young infant and that this effect shows up most clearly when the familiarization times are as short as they were in the present study.

Visual Recognition Memory

As can be seen in Figure 14.4, at 6 months of age, full-term infants showed evidence of visual recognition memory in the two visual conditions (visual and visual control), but preterms did not. We have completed a study that supports the idea that this result reflects, at least in large measure, differences in the speed of processing visual information. In this more recent study, comparable groups of 6-month-olds, full-term as well as preterm infants, were tested for visual recognition memory of patterns (Rose, 1980).

Each infant was given three problems in a fixed order, with stimuli similar to, but not identical with, those used by Fagan (1974). The stimuli for problem 1 consisted of abstract designs differing widely from one another (e.g., a glossy photograph of zig-zag black lines on a white background; a clover shape made up of nested black and white paper cutouts; and a random array of green, red, and blue geometric shapes cut from paper and pasted to a yellow background). Problem 2 used designs that displayed equal numbers of identical black elements arranged into different configurations, and problem 3 used achromatic photographs of human faces. Familiarization times were minimal, being 5, 10, and 20 sec, respectively. During familiarization the stimulus remained in view until each infant had looked at it for the specified amount of time, that is, all infants actually looked at the target for the same amount of time. Each phase was followed by a 10-sec test trial (with the position of novel and familiar stimuli reversed after 5 sec).

The results are clear cut. Full-terms showed recognition memory in problems 1 and 3, that is, infants looked significantly longer at the novel as compared with the familiar stimulus (60% and 65%, respectively). The premature group, on the other hand, failed to differentiate the novel from the familiar stimulus on either of these two problems (47% and 49%, respectively). The 10 sec of study time used in problem 2 appears to have been too brief for any of the infants, even the full-terms, to process those stimuli. It can be noted that the time taken to accumulate the specified study times did not differ between full-terms and preterms, suggesting that both groups were equally attentive during the familiarization.

A replication sample of prematures was tested, and the results were similar—chance responding on all problems. The replication included a fourth problem, in which a sunburst design and a pattern of diamonds was given with 5 sec of study time (a familiarization time we have found sufficient to elicit the novelty response in full-terms of this age). The prematures failed to show recognition memory on this problem as well. A second group of prematures was tested using longer study times (20, 20, 30, and 20 sec for problems 1, 2, 3, and 4, respectively). This group showed significant novelty responses on problems 1, 3, and 4 (62%, 63%, and 71%, respectively); 20 sec of study time proved still insufficient for differentiation of the novel from the familiar stimulus on problem 2. The improvement in performance obtained by lengthening study time in this study was notable. Such success suggests that the prematures were able to store and retrieve the visual information and to make the visual discriminations involved. They did, however, show a clear deficit in the speed of encoding the visual information about shape.

Conclusions

In sum, the studies that I have discussed here show that middle-class full-term infants can transfer information across modalities by 12 months of age. Neither prematures nor lower-class full-terms showed any evidence of cross-modal transfer. Even among those full-terms who can transfer tactual information across modalities, manipulation of objects that occurs concurrent with visual involvement did not appear to enhance infant's visual memory for shape. The infants appeared to have difficulty acquiring and/or encoding the visual information when they were permitted to manipulate the object. Being able to see and feel an object depressed performance even more so in prematures. While object manipulation may enhance knowledge of other characteristics, such as solidity, texture, and flexibility, it did not enhance visual recognition memory of shape. And finally, we now have evidence that prematures take longer than full-terms to encode visual information about objects and about two dimensional stimuli as well.

In conclusion, I would like to suggest that our own findings, as well as those from other investigators (e.g., Sigman & Parmelee, 1974; Sigman, 1977), point the way to conceiving of young infants as a cognitive organism. However limited their abilities, they clearly show at least a rudimentary capability for internally representing reality and for ordering and structuring the perceptual flux. Although the full story remains to be told, and the developmental course is largely uncharted, the outlines have been limned. Even for the newborn, the world is far from blooming, buzzing confusion that William James supposed it to be. The wealth of research that began in the 1950s, when the elegantly simple techniques of Fantz revealed that the newborn could see, is slowly giving us access to the infant's mind. This understanding is opening the way to detect basic disabilities earlier than ever before (see Kopp, Sigman, Parmelee, & Jeffrey, 1975; Miranda, 1976; Rose, Schmidt, & Bridger, 1976, 1980; Schmidt, Rose, & Bridger, 1980; Sigman, Kopp, Littman, & Parmelee, 1977; Werner & Siqueland, 1978, for work in the newborn period) and hopefully to understand their nature in greater depth than we have heretofore.

Acknowledgment

The author would like to express her appreciation to Holly Ruff for a critical reading of the manuscript.

References

Abravanel, E. The development of intersensory patterning with regard to selected spatial dimensions. *Monographs of the Society for Research in Child Development,* 1968, *33* (Serial No. 118).

Birch, H. G., & Lefford, A. Intersensory development in children. *Monographs of the Society for Research in Child Development,* 1963, *28* (5, Serial no. 89).

Birch, H. G., & Lefford, A. Visual differentiation, intersensory integration and voluntary motor control. *Monographs of the Society for Research in Child Development,* 1967, *32* (2, Serial No. 110).

Birns, B., & Bridger, W. H. Cognitive development and social class. In J. Wortis (Ed.), *Mental retardation and developmental disabilities* (Vol. 9) New York: Brunner/Mazel, 1977.

Blank, M., Rose, S. A., & Berlin, L. *The language of learning: The preschool years.* New York: Grune & Stratton, 1978.

Bower, T. G. R., & Wishart, J. G. The effects of motor skill on object permanence. *Cognition: International Journal of Cognitive Psychology,* 1972, *1,* 165–172.

Butter, E. J., & Zung, B. J. A developmental investigation of the effects of sensory modality on form recognition in children. *Developmental Psychology,* 1970, *3,* 276.

Cohen, L. B., & Gelber, E. R. Infant visual memory. In L. B. Cohen & P. Salapatek (Eds.), *Infant perception: From sensation to cognition* (vol. 1). New York: Academic Press, 1975.

Connors, C. K., Schuette, C., & Goldman, A. Informational analyses of intersensory communication in children of different social class. *Child Development,* 1967, *38,* 251–266.

Das, J. P., Kirby, J., & Jarman, R. F. Simultaneous and successive synthesis: An alternative modal for cognitive abilities. *Psychological Bulletin,* 1975, *82,* 87–103.

Deutsch, L. P., & Schumer, F. *Brain damaged children: A modality-oriented explanation of performance.* New York: Brunner/Mazel, 1970.

Ettlinger, G. Analysis of cross-modal effects and their relatioship to language. In F. L. Darley & C. H. Millikan (Eds.), *Brain mechanisms underlying speech and language.* New York: Grune & Stratton, 1967.

Fagan, J. F. Memory in the infant. *Journal of Experimental Child Psychology,* 1970, *9,* 217–226.

Fagan, J. F. Infants' recognition memory for faces. *Journal of Experimental Child Psychology,* 1972, *14,* 453–476.

Fagan, J. F. Infant recognition memory: The effects of length of familiarization and type of discrimination task. *Child Development,* 1974, *45,* 351–356.

Fagan, J. F. An attention model of infant recognition. *Child Development,* 1977, *48,* 345–359.

Fantz, R. L., Fagan, J. F., & Miranda, S. B. Early visual selection. In L. B. Cohen & P.

Salapatek (Eds.), *Infant perception: From sensation to cognition* (Vol. 1). New York: Academic Press, 1975.

Fitzhardinge, P. M. Early growth and development in low-birthweight infants following treatment in an intensive care nursery. *Pediatrics*, 1975, *56*, 162–172.

Fitzhardinge, P. M., & Ramsay, M. The improved outlook for the small prematurely born infant. *Developmental Medicine and Child Neurology*, 1973, *15*, 447–459.

Francis-William, J., & Davies, P. A. Very low birthweight and later intelligence. *Developmental Medicine and Child Neurology*, 1974, *16*, 709–728.

Friedes, D. Human information processing and sensory modality: Cross-modal functions, information complexity, memory and deficit. *Psychological Bulletin*, 1974, *81*, 284–310.

Garvill, J., & Molander, B. Verbal mediation in cross-modal transfer. *British Journal of Psychology*, 1971, *62*, 449–457.

Geshwind, N. Disconnection syndromes in animals and man (2 pts.) *Brain*, 1965, *88*, 237–294; 1965, *88*, 515–644.

Goldstein, K. M., Caputo, D. V., & Taub, H. B. The effects of prenatal and perinatal complications on development at one year of age. *Child Development*, 1967, *47*, 613–621.

Goodnow, J. Eye and hand: Differential memory and its effect on matching. *Neuropsychologia*, 1971, *9*, 89–95.

Gottfried, A. W., & Brody, N. Interrelationships between and correlates of psychometric and Piagetian scales of sensorimotor intelligence. *Developmental Psychology*, 1975, *11*, 379–387.

Gottfried, A. W., Rose, S. A., & Bridger, W. H. Cross-modal transfer in human infants. *Child Development*, 1977, *48*, 118–123.

Gottfried, A. W., Rose, S. A., & Bridger, W. H. Effects of visual, haptic, and manipulatory experiences on infants' visual recognition memory of objects. *Developmental Psychology*, 1978, *14*, 305–312.

Kopp, C. B. Development of fine motor behaviors: Issues and research. In N. R. Ellis (Ed.), *Aberrant development in infancy*. New Jersey: Erlbaum, 1975.

Kopp, C.B., Sigman, M., Parmelee, A. H., & Jeffrey, W. E. Neurological organization and visual fixation in infants at 40 weeks conceptional age. *Developmental Psychobiology*, 1975, *8*, 165–170.

Lobb, H. Vision versus touch in form discrimination. *Canadian Journal of Psychology*, 1965, *19*, 175–187.

Milner, A., & Bryant, P. Cross-modal matching by young children. *Journal of Comparative and Physiological Psychology*, 1970, *71*, 453–458.

Miranda, S. B. Visual attention in defective and high risk infants. *Merrill-Palmer Quarterly*, 1976, *22*, 201–228.

Parmelee, A., & Schulte, F. Developmental testing of preterm and small-for-date infants. *Pediatrics*, 1970, *45*, 21–28.

Piaget, J., & Inhelder, B. *The child's conception of space*. London: Routledge & Kegan Paul, 1956. (Originally published, 1948.)

Rose, S. A. Infant's transfer of response between two dimensional and three-dimensional stimuli. *Child Development*, 1977, *48*, 1086–1091.

Rose, S. A. Enhancing visual recognition memory in preterm infants. *Developmental Psychology*, 1980, *16*, 85–92.

Rose, S. A., Blank, M. S., & Bridger, W. H. Intermodal intramodal and retention of visual and tactual information in young children. *Developmental Psychology*, 1972, *6*, 482–486.

Rose, S. A., Gottfried, A. W., & Bridger, W. H. Cross-modal transfer in infants: Relationship to prematurity and socio-economic background. *Developmental Psychology*, 1978, *14*, 643–652.

Rose, S. A., Gottfried, A. W., & Bridger, W. H. Effects of haptic cues on visual recognition memory in fullterm and preterm infants. *Infant Behavior and Development*, 1979, *2*, 55–67.

Rose, S. A., Schmidt, K., & Bridger, W. H. Cardiac and behavioral responsivity to tactile stimulation in premature and fullterm infants. *Developmental Psychology*, 1976, *12*(4), 311–320.

Rose, S. A., Schmidt, K., Riese, M. L., & Bridger, W. H. Effects of prematurity and early intervention on responsivity to tactual stimuli: A comparison of preterm and fullterm infants. *Child Development,* 1980, *51,* 416–425.

Rubin, R. A., Rosenblatt, M. A., & Balow, B. Psychological and educational sequelae of prematurity. *Pediatrics,* 1973, *52,* 352–363.

Rudel, R., & Teuber, H. L. Crossmodal transfer of shape discrimination by children. *Neuropsychologia,* 1964, *2,* 108.

Sameroff, A.H., & Chandler, M.J. Reproductive risk and the continuum of caretaking casualty. In F.D. Horowitz, M. Hetherington, S. Scarr-Salapatek, & G. Siegel (Eds.), *Review of child development research* (Vol. 4). Chicago: Univ. of Chicago Press, 1975.

Schmidt, K., Rose, S.A., & Bridger, W.H. Effect of heartbeat sound on the cardiac and behavioral responsiveness to tactual stimulation in sleeping preterm infants. *Developmental Psychology,* 1980, *16,* 175–184.

Sigman, M. Early development of preterm and fullterm infants: Exploratory behavior in eight-month olds. *Child Development,* 1977, *47,* 606–612.

Sigman, M., Kopp, C. B., Littman, B., & Parmelee, A. H. Infant visual attentiveness in relation to birth condition. *Developmental Psychology,* 1977, *13,* 431–437.

Sigman, M., & Parmelee, A. H. Visual preferences of four-month old premature and fullterm infants. *Child Development,* 1974, *45,* 959–965.

Taub, H. B., Goldstein, K. M., & Caputo, D. V. Indices of neonatal prematurity as discriminators of development in middle childhood. *Child Development,* 1977, *48,* 797–805.

Tilford, J. A. The relationship between gestational age and adaptive behavior. *Merrill-Palmer Quarterly,* 1976, *22,* 319–326.

Weiner, B., & Goodnow, J. J. Motor activity: Effects on memory. *Developmental Psychology,* 1970, *2,* 448.

Werner, J. S., & Siqueland, E. R. Visual recognition memory in the preterm infant. *Infant Behavior and Development,* 1978, *1,* 79–94.

Wolff, P., Levin, J. R., & Longobardi, E. T. Motoric mediation in children's paired-associate learning: Effects of visual and tactual contact. *Journal of Experimental Child Psychology,* 1972, *14,* 176–183.

Zaporozhets, A. V. The development of perception in the preschool child. *Monographs of the Society for Research in Child Development,* 1965, *30* (2, Serial No. 100).

Zaporozhets, A. V. The development of perception and activity. *Early Child Development and Care,* 1973, *2,* 49–56.

Studies of Visual Recognition Memory in Preterm Infants: Differences in Development as a Function of Perinatal Morbidity Factors[1]

EINAR R. SIQUELAND

For several years at Brown University, we have been conducting laboratory studies in which we have employed visual reinforcement procedures to investigate the early development of visual exploration and recognition memory in infants. We found that, within a visual novelty paradigm, high-amplitude nonnutritive sucking (HAS) can be employed as a dependent variable to study developmental changes in the visual discrimination and recognition memory abilities of infants over the first weeks and months of postnatal development. Like researchers who have employed visual preference and habituation procedures, we assume that some type of visual recognition memory is involved when infants respond differentially to familiar and novel stimuli. A number of excellent reviews of the infant visual recognition literature are currently available (e.g., Cohen, 1976; Cohen & Gelber, 1975; Fagan, 1975; Olson, 1976), and a summary will not be attempted here. Our goal in this chapter is to focus primarily on the contributions of some of the more recent studies of infant visual recognition from our laboratory. These studies were undertaken with one eye on their implications for our understanding of early brain maturation and the other on their implications for our understanding of the early substrates of cognitive development. The assumption that emerging cognitive processes are involved in infant visual recognition follows from a commonly shared view that perceptual systems are basically hierarchical in nature. The

[1] The original research studies were supported by U.S. Public Health Service Center Grant HD–03386 to E. R. Siqueland. Some of the studies conducted with preterm infants, further data analyses, and preparation of the manuscript have been supported in part by U.S. Public Health Service Center Grant HD–11343, entitled "Diabetes Pregnancy: Effects on Mother and Her Offspring," to P. M. Galletti.

early processing stages used in stimulus encoding and simple pattern recognition provide the basis for later higher-order recognition processing that requires cognitive transformations of visual information. While maturational changes in the infant's visual system determine what attributes and features of visual stimuli can be discriminated, what visual information is extracted and retained depends on both developmental maturity and perceptual learning. The primary goals of our research have been to (a) determine more about the nature and order of changes in the abilities of full-term infants to visually encode, extract, and retain visual information as a function of age over the first weeks of postnatal development; (b) assess, with preterm infants, the influence of differences in maturational levels and postnatal visual experience on the development of these visual processing abilities; and (c) pinpoint developmental delays and deficits in these abilities that may be associated with premature birth status and perinatal medical risk factors in preterm infants.

The plan of this chapter, following a description of the experimental procedures employed in our HAS studies, is to (a) review briefly the major contributions of our previously published studies on the early beginnings of infant visual exploration and recognition memory; (b) present findings from more recent experiments on the early development of form recognition in full-term and preterm infants; and (c) discuss some initial findings that indicate that developmental delays and/deficits in the visual recognition performance of preterm infants are associated with differences in birth status and perinatal risk factors.

Only a brief description of the rationale and experimental procedures, common to all of our HAS studies of visual recognition, will be presented in this chapter. More detailed descriptions of the experimental procedures are provided in previous publications (Milewski, 1976; Milewski & Siqueland, 1975; Siqueland, 1969; Siqueland & DeLucia, 1969; Werner & Siqueland, 1978). In these studies, infants were presented with an experimental situation where their exposure to visual patterns was made contingent upon increases in their rates of HAS. In an operant reinforcement paradigm, the HAS behavior of infants controlled the onset and duration of their exposure to visual stimuli, rear-projected on a frontally positioned viewing screen. It is assumed that the typically observed initial increases and subsequent decreases in HAS rates of infants to an initially presented visual stimulus occurred with increased amounts of continued exposure to a familiar reinforcing stimulus. If a familiar visual stimulus was subsequently replaced with a novel stimulus without changes in the reinforcing contingencies, and the infant's HAS rate increased relative to that of a control condition in which continued exposure to the previous familiar stimulus occurred, discrimination of differences in some attribute(s) of the familiar and novel stimuli was inferred. Differential recovery in HAS rate to the presentations of familiar and novel stimuli during the posttest phase provided the measure of visual discrimination and recognition memory.

The familiarization procedures were identical in all of these studies and were designed to provide infants with optimal amounts of stimulus familiarization prior to assessing their visual recognition performance. Following 3 min of visual reinforcement training, subjects were required to meet a performance criterion of stimulus familiarization (i.e., 20% decrement in HAS rate for 2 consecutive min) prior to the presentation of either a novel or familiar stimulus during the posttest phase. Although the length of the familiarization period varied between subjects, depending upon individual differences in time to criterion, all infants were exposed to the initial familiar stimulus for a minimum of 5 min. With the exception of differences in the type of recognition task employed in the respective experiments, all other aspects of the experimental procedures were essentially identical. It is important to note that this feature of relatively long durations of stimulus familiarization, tailored to the performance of individual subjects, stands in marked contrast to the relatively brief and fixed amounts of stimulus familiarization typically employed in most preferential looking (PL) and habituation studies of infant visual recognition (Cohen & Gelber, 1975; Fagan, 1975).

Early Beginnings of Visual Exploration and Recognition Memory

In general, reviewers of the visual preference and habituation literature (e.g., Bond, 1972; Cohen & Gelber, 1975; Fagan, 1975; Olson, 1976) have concluded that it is difficult to demonstrate rudimentary forms of recognition memory with infants prior to approximately 2½ months of age. In reviewing preference paradigm studies, Fantz, Fagan, and Miranda (1975) and Fagan (1975) concluded that differences between familiar and novel stimuli must be large and multidimensional to be recognized as early as 2–3 months of age, but at later ages, differences between stimulus attributes may be increasingly smaller and unidimensional. In both habituation and preference studies, when experimenters have provided infants with relatively brief and fixed amounts of exposure to visual stimuli prior to testing for visual recognition, the typical finding has been that infants younger than 2½ months, in contrast to older infants, fail to demonstrate reliable stimulus novelty effects. However, in our studies, and in more recent habituation studies of visual recognition in which familiarization procedures have been tailored to the performance of individual subjects, evidence of visual recognition has been obtained at 1 month of age (Hunter & Ames, 1975; Milewski & Siqueland, 1975; Siqueland, 1969) and with newborns during the first days of postnatal life (Friedman, 1975; Werner & Siqueland, 1978). The previously obtained findings of marked changes in the visual recognition performance of full-term infants between 2 and 3 months of age would appear to be related to age differences in processing time or rate of habituation rather than to differences in visual memory capacity per se. When considerations are given to insure adequate amounts of stimulus familiarization, even preterm newborns demonstrate reliable stimulus novelty effects, at least when differences between novel and familiar visual stimuli at large and multidimensional (Werner & Siqueland, 1978). The results from this study with preterm newborns have some important implications for our understanding of the early beginnings of visual exploration and recognition memory in human infants.

The subjects in this study were 16 preterm newborns with an average birthweight of 2074 gm (SD 211), a mean gestational age of 35 weeks (SD 1.95) at birth, and a mean postnatal age of 6.5 days (SD 4.38). Using a HAS novelty paradigm similar to that employed in our previous studies with full-term infants (Milewski & Siqueland, 1975), a within-subjects experimental paradigm was used to assess the differential effects of familiar and novel visual stimuli on HAS performance of preterm infants during the posttest phase. The visual stimuli consisted of familiar and novel checkerboard patterns that differed simultaneously in the number, size, and color of the checkerboard form elements. The order of the novel and familiar test conditions (i.e., one session per day), as well as the four types of visual stimuli (i.e., red and white, or green and white, 2 × 2 or 4 × 4 checkerboards) were counterbalanced across the 16 subjects. The results obtained in this experiment are summarized in Figure 15.1 This figure shows the mean minute-by-minute HAS rates for the 16 subjects during baseline, the 5 min just prior to the posttest phase, and the novelty phase. Their performance during the novel and familiar stimulus testing sessions are plotted separately. The increases in HAS rate relative to baseline levels, as seen in both of the daily preshift-familiarization phases of this experiment, were statistically reliable. Furthermore, following the decrements seen in the HAS rates during the familiarization phases, these preterm newborns showed greater recovery in their HAS rates to

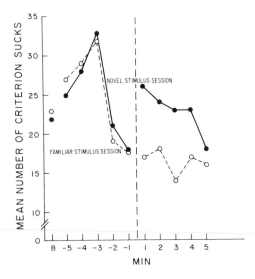

FIGURE 15.1. *The mean number of criterion sucks plotted for the novel and familiar conditions as a function of time. Time is measured with respect to the moment of the stimulus shift. Plotted are the 5 min prior to the shift and the first 5 min after the stimulus shift and no-shift conditions. B indicates the baseline minute prior to visual reinforcement. Closed circle shows novel stimulus session; open circle shows familiar stimulus session. (From Werner & Siqueland, 1978).*

novel relative to familiar visual stimuli during the first 2 min of the postshift phase. Statistical assessments of reliable stimulus novelty effects in these experiments were based on a measure of the amount of recovery in HAS rate during the posttest phase. Recovery scores were computed for each subject by subtracting the average response rate during the 2 min preceding the stimulus shift from the response rate during each of the 5 posttest min. Positive scores indicate recovery of HAS, while negative scores indicate further decrements in HAS during the posttest phase. When we examined the effects of stimulus novelty on the HAS recovery scores of individual subjects, we obtained findings consistent with the relatively robust novelty effects seen in the group performance measures in Figure 15.1. Twelve of the 16 subjects showed higher levels of HAS recovery to novel relative to familiar stimuli. When a replication experiment was conducted with 7 of the 16 subjects, we found that, whereas 6 of these subjects showed greater HAS recovery to novel stimuli over the first two days of testing, all 7 showed this novelty effect on our replication measure. Furthermore, 6 of the 7 subjects demonstrated increases in the magnitude of their novelty scores on the replication measures.

In this study, we also found a strikingly consistent pattern of correlational findings that indicated that individual differences in novelty discrimination were significantly related to differences in birth status and perinatal medical risk factors. Higher levels of HAS recovery to novel visual stimuli were positively correlated with weight and gestational age of the 16 subjects at birth. The reported significant negative correlations in this study indicated that preterms with higher mortality risk scores (Lubchenco, Searls, & Brazie, 1972), with more postnatal medical complications, and with longer periods of hospitalization showed lower levels of differential responsiveness to familiar and novel stimuli. While previous studies have reported significant differences in visual recognition performance between groups of preterm and full-term infants tested on PL tasks at later postnatal ages (e.g., Rose, Gottfried, & Bridger, 1979; Sigman & Parmelee, 1974), the findings in this study indicated that the within-group continuum of perinatal risk factors in preterm infants was related to quantitative differences in their visual recognition performance in the first days of postnatal life.

An important conclusion to be drawn from this study is that human newborns demonstrate a congenitally organized responsiveness to some classes of visual novelty. When adequate familiarization time is provided, and the stimulus features or attributes that can serve as a basis for differentiating familiar and novel stimuli do not exceed the visual discriminative and encoding capacities of the infant, novelty facilitates motivated visual exploration. Processing time as a locus of developmental change in infant recognition memory (e.g., Fagan, 1975) has not been the focus of interest in our studies. Rather, given that all subjects were equated on a performance measure of familiarization, differences in recognition performance as a function of type of recognition task can be attributed to developmental changes in the visual encoding abilities of infants as a function of maturation and/or experience. Although preterm newborns showed some capacity to differentiate between familiar and novel visual information, given the nature of the recognition task (i.e., to differentiate familiar and novel stimuli varying simultaneously on many stimulus dimensions), recognition may have been based on some rudimentary capacity to detect differences in the more gross sensory properties of these checkerboard patterns. To date, the research literature has failed to provide studies designed to determine what features and attributes of visual stimuli can serve as a basis for pattern recognition for infants prior to 1 month of postnatal age. The few habituation studies that have provided evidence of visual recognition with infants under 2 months of age (e.g., Friedman, 1975; Hunter & Ames, 1975) have been limited to assessments with patterns that differed simultaneously on multiple stimulus features and dimensions. However, based largely on the results of habituation and PL studies, there has been a consensus among the reviewers of this literature (Bond, 1972; Fantz *et al.,* 1975; Haith, 1976; Salapatek, 1975) that before 2 months of age infants show little evidence of discriminating between two-dimensional visual patterns that are equated for brightness, size, and amount and density of contour. In the area of pattern perception, a distinction has often been made between visual discriminations based on lower-order sensory variables (e.g., brightness, amount and density of contour) and higher-order structure (e.g., spatial configurations of elements, processing of patterns as a unified whole, and gestalt organizing principles). Results of HAS studies with full-term infants, beginning as early as 1 month of postnatal age, suggest that these estimates of the young infant's visual encoding capacities, based on the results of PL and habituation studies, may be quite conservative. HAS studies conducted in our laboratory have indicated that 1-month-old infants recognize differences between familiar and novel stimuli on the basis of (*a*) unidimensional changes in either color or form (Milewski & Siqueland, 1975; Siqueland; 1969); (*b*) changes in shapes of achromatic forms (Milewski & Siqueland, 1975); (*c*) changes in shapes of line drawings of geometric patterns equated for size and amount of contour (Milewski, 1976); and (*d*) changes in compound color–form stimuli that consisted of rearrangement of familiar form and color components into novel compounds (Siqueland & Osman, in preparation). The question of whether the visual discriminative capacities seen in these visual recognition studies with 1-month infants are also present at birth or emerge rapidly over the first weeks of postnatal development awaits further empirical studies.

Although these HAS studies provided findings indicating that some rudimentary capacity for form perception may be inherent in the organization of the immature visual system of infants as early as 4 weeks of postnatal age, Milewski (1976) has provided evidence of important subsequent developmental changes in the form recognition abilities of infants between 1 and 4 months. In his doctoral research, Milewski found evidence for developmental changes in the ability of infants to visual encode and recognize changes in the form elements of two-form-element patterns. The results obtained in Milewski's studies of infant form recognition converge with the findings of reported developmental changes in the visual scanning behavior of infants when they are presented with abstract geometric patterns (Salapatek, 1975) and also with more complex stimuli such as human faces (Bergman, Haith, & Mann, 1971; Donnee, 1973; Maurer, 1969). These visual scanning studies have shown that, before approximately 2 months of age, infants neither fixate or appear to attend to internal features of abstract forms or faces. Whereas younger infants principally fixate external features of adult faces, older infants fixate primarily the internal features, mostly the eyes (Maurer & Salapatek, 1976), and they fixate primarily the internal features of abstract forms. Milewski found that when presented with two-form-element patterns, with one element enclosed within the other, 1-month infants failed to recognize a change in the internal form elements. In contrast, 4-month infants experienced no such difficulties and recognized changes in the contours of both the external and internal form elements. In the next section of this chapter, we will briefly present the major findings of these form recognition studies with full-term infants, which have shown that, dependent on the nature of the form recognition task, stimulus novelty effects were either invariant with age differences beginning at 1 month or varied as a function of age. These studies provided the necessary baseline findings of developmental changes in form recognition with full-term infants, and based on these findings, subsequent studies were conducted with preterm infants to assess the role of maturational factors and visual experience in the development of these form recognition abilities.

Developmental Changes in the Visual Recognition of Form Contours

Milewski (1976) presented infants with two-form-element geometric patterns, where the elements consisted of line drawings of circles, triangles, and squares, one centered within the other. During the novelty test phase, independent groups of 1- and 4-month infants were presented either with a change in the shape of the smaller internal form, the external form, or both the internal and external forms, or with no change in the shapes of the initial form elements. Whereas 4-month infants demonstrated visual recognition (i.e., HAS recovery) for all three of the form change conditions, 1-month infants failed to detect changes in the internal forms but discriminated changes in the other two form change conditions. A series of control experiments by Milewski indicated that the failure of 1-month infants to recognize changes in the internal form elements was not attributable to visual acuity limitations or to the amount of angular separation between the external and internal forms.

In two subsequent experiments, using Milewski's experimental design and stimuli, we extended our analysis of early developmental constraints on the form processing abilities of full-term infants. In one experiment, 2- and 3-month-old infants were presented with Milewski's stimuli. During the novelty test phase, groups of infants ($N = 8$) were presented with either a change in the shape of the internal or the external form or no change in the familiar stimuli. This experiment was conducted to determine more precisely the chronological age at which full-term infants discriminate changes in the internal form elements. In a second experiment, 1-, 2-, 3-, and 4-month infants were presented with two-form-element patterns, but with the smaller of the two forms positioned adjacent to and outside the borders of the larger forms. The sizes and shapes of the two form elements were identical to Milewski's, with the center of the smaller form positioned parallel to and 29° from the center of the larger form. This second experiment was designed to determine whether differences in relative size of the two forms constrained detection of changes in the smaller forms, independent of their spatial location within the borders of the larger external form. During the novelty test phase, independent groups of infants at each age level ($N = 8$) were presented with either a change in the smaller adjacently positioned forms or no change in the familiar forms. The result from these two experiments are summarized in Figure 15.2, which shows the mean HAS recovery scores for each of the experimental groups during the novelty posttest minutes. Figure 15.2a shows the results for the first experiment, where 2- and 3-month infants were presented with external and internal form element changes. For comparative purposes we have also included Milewski's data from 1- and 4-month infants on these recognition tasks. Figure 15.2b summarizes the results from the second experiment,

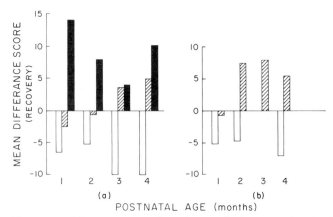

FIGURE 15.2. *Mean group difference scores collapsed across the 5-min novelty test phase. Scores for internal and external novel form conditions are presented in Figure 15.2a. Open bars show control; lined bars, internal form change; shaded bars, external form change. Scores for small adjacent novel form conditions are presented in Figure 15.2b. Open bars show control; lined bars, small adjacent form change.*

where infants were presented with changes in the adjacently positioned smaller forms.

The findings of these two experiments can be summarized briefly. Based on statistical comparisons between the HAS recovery scores for the novelty stimulus groups relative to their no-shift controls at each age level, the following effects are statistically reliable ($p < .05$ or less; nondirectional t tests). Infants at 3 months of age, like 4-month infants, showed reliable recognition of changes in both the external and the internal form elements. In contrast, 2-month infants, similar to 1-month infants, discriminated the external form changes but not the internal form changes. In the second experiment (see Figure 15.2b), where the four age groups were presented with the task of recognizing changes in the smaller adjacent positioned forms, only 1-month infants failed to provide evidence of discriminating changes in the smaller forms. In a subsequent experiment, when a group of 1-month subjects ($N = 8$) were presented with changes in the larger adjacently positioned form during the novelty test phase, reliable recovery of HAS was found.

Given the results of these experiments, we can conclude that both relative size and spatial positioning of form elements place constraints on the processing of form for infants under 2 months of age. For 1-month infants, failure to process change in the smaller form was not dependent upon its position within the boundaries of the larger form. Size differences were sufficient to preclude detection of changes in the smaller of the two forms. By 2 months of age, stimulus size placed no constraints on the processing of form elements, but failure to detect changes in the smaller forms was dependent on its internal spatial position. By 3 months, neither relative size nor position within the boundaries of the larger forms placed constraints on ability of infants to recognize changes in the smaller forms.

The finding that overall stimulus size exerts less control in constraining processing of form information as the infant matures is consistent with the findings of a number of previous studies (Cohen, 1972; Fantz et al., 1975; Maisel & Karmel, 1978; Ruff & Turkewitz, 1975). In accounting for developmental changes in the ability of infants to process internal form elements, Salapatek (1975) and Milewski (1976) based their explanation on a view of perceptual development originally proposed by Hebb (1949). They assumed an innate capacity for the detection of a primitive, sensory, figure–ground organization of the visual field, with form discrimination and recognition being learned subsequently. An emphasis upon hypothesized developmental changes in the neurophysiological components of vision are seen in Salapatek's theoretical account of the changes that occur in form perception in the second month of postnatal development. Following the reasoning of Bronson (1974), the early visual perception of infants is seen as controlled by subcortical mechanisms involved in the spatial localization and detection of luminous flux until 8 weeks of age, when the cortical or primary visual system, which is capable of processing pattern detail and visual form, becomes functional. However, this dichotomy between cortical and subcortical neural mechanisms to account for age shifts in the perceptual development of infants has been criticized as too simplistic in light of neuroanatomical, physiological, and behavioral findings (Haith & Campos, 1977; Maisel & Karmel, 1978; Vaughan, 1975; Weiskrantz, 1974). Even at 1 month of age, infants in our studies demonstrated form recognition based on an ability to detect differences between forms equated for amount of contour (i.e., external form discrimination task). Given that an ability for discrimination of patterns where contour density is held constant has not been found as a residual visual capacity in decorticostriate primates (Humphrey, 1974; Weiskrantz, Cowey, & Darlington, 1973), the ability of infants to recognize changes in the external form contours would suggest significant involvement of the primary visual system as early as 1 month of postnatal age. It may be more accurate to consider cortical and subcortical systems functioning in an immature state in the early form processing of younger infants. Despite limitations imposed by immaturity of the infant's visual system and by limited visual experience, form perception appears to be inherent in the organization of the infant's visual system as early as 1 month. At this age, however, external contours of form appear to define figure–ground relationships through dominant size and enclosure such that the contours of smaller internal forms are not processed. The differences seen in the form recognition performance of 2- and 3-month full-term infants on the internal form recognition task indicate a relatively rapid developmental change in the form processing abilities of infants between 8 and 12 weeks of postnatal age. Age differences in the form recognition performance of full-term infants depended solely on the nature of the two form recognition tasks. With these findings providing evidence of reliable developmental changes in the form processing abilities of infants, we have subsequently conducted a series of experiments to assess the recognition performance of preterm infants on these two types of form recognition tasks: one where performance with full-term infants was invariant with age differences beginning at 4 weeks (i.e., external form changes) and the other where performance was reliably influenced by age differences (i.e., internal form changes).

Our studies on the development of form recognition with preterm infants reflect an attempt to address two important questions:

1. What do differences in maturational levels contribute to the form recognition performance of preterm infants, and are developmental changes a function of age from birth (postnatal age) or a function of both prenatal and postnatal development levels (conceptional age)?

2. Are deficits or developmental lags in form recognition performance associated with preterm birth status and perinatal risk factors when preterm infants are equated for differences in maturational levels at time of testing?

Although the research literature has provided a small number of previous studies focusing on these issues with preterm infants (e.g., Fagan, Fantz, &

Miranda, 1971; Fantz *et al.,* 1975; Rose *et al.,* 1979; Sigman & Parmelee, 1974), they have been limited to comparisons between populations of full-term and preterm infants on PL measures of visual recognition. Collectively, the results of these PL studies have shown that visual experience, prior to an age when birth normally occurs, does not appear to facilitate the developmental onset of visual recognition for preterm infants. However, they have provided somewhat contrasting findings with respect to the question of whether preterm birth status has a deleterious effect on the developmental onset of visual recognition in preterm infants.

In contrast to these previous studies, our research strategy has been one of focusing on assessments of form recognition performance in preterm infants as a function of differences in developmental factors within our populations of preterm infants. Although the findings previously obtained with full-term infants provided a basis for descriptive comparisons with the performance of preterm infants, statistical comparisons between full-term and preterm infants were not performed.

Development of Form Recognition in Preterm Infants

In these form recognition studies with preterm infants, the experimental procedures, the visual stimuli, and the measure of individual subject's novelty discrimination were identical to those employed with full-term infants. Although studies with full-term infants began at 4 weeks of postnatal age, preterm infants were not available for testing in our Brown University laboratories until 8 weeks of postnatal age. With this restriction, the goal in our assessments with preterm infants was to obtain measures of form recognition performance over a range of postnatal and conceptional ages that was comparable to those of the full-term infants previously tested.

In the first experiment, a group of 42 preterm infants, ranging from 40 to 48 weeks in conceptional age, were tested on the external form discrimination task at 8 weeks of postnatal age. With postnatal age held constant, differences in visual recognition performance were studied as a function of conceptional age at time of testing. In a second experiment, designed to provide some initial estimates of the relative contributions of differences in maturational levels and postnatal visual experience on the later-developing ability to process internal form change, 60 preterm infants were tested beginning at 12 weeks of postnatal age, or 45 weeks of conceptional age. In this second experiment, infants differed in both their postnatal and conceptional ages at time of testing and assessments were made to determine whether the onset of form recognition was simply a function of age from birth alone (postnatal age) or a function of prenatal plus postnatal development (conceptional age).

The 42 subjects tested on the external form discrimination task at 8 weeks of postnatal age had a mean birthweight of 2136 gm (SD = 298) and a mean gestational age of 35 weeks (SD = 2.66) and ranged from 40 to 48 weeks in conceptional age at testing. The 60 preterm subjects tested on the internal form discrimination task had a mean birthweight of 2070 gm (SD = 325) and a mean gestational age of 36 weeks (SD = 2.39). They ranged from 12 to 25 weeks in postnatal age and from 45 to 60 weeks in conceptional age at time of testing. As in our previous studies with full-term infants, HAS recovery scores during the 5-min posttest novelty phase provided the measure of visual recognition for each subject.

Figure 15.3 shows the mean HAS novelty scores for infants tested on these two form recognition tasks as a function of their conceptional age at time of testing. This figure shows the means for equal size samples of 14 subjects tested at each of the three conceptional age levels on the external form change task and for 15 subjects at each of the four conceptional age levels on the internal form change task.

We found no evidence for statistically reliable differences in the visual recognition performance for the three conceptional age groups on the external form discrimination task, and for the total sample of 42 subjects, no relationship was found between HAS novelty scores and conceptional age at testing ($r = -.01$, Pearson r). Although 7 of the 14 subjects in the youngest conceptional age group, as compared to 11 of the 14 subjects in each of the two older conceptional age groups, showed increased rates of HAS during the novelty phase (i.e., positive HAS recovery scores), performance differences between the three groups were not statistically reliable. Correlated t tests applied to the HAS recovery scores for each of the three conceptional age groups indicated reliable recovery for the two older groups ($p < .05$, one-tailed tests). Thus, these findings suggest that preterm infants show evidence of a developmental onset in form recognition, based on an ability to discriminate changes in the contours of the external forms, as early as 44 weeks of conceptional age.

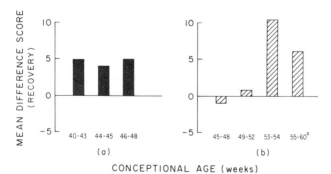

FIGURE 15.3. *Mean group difference scores collapsed across the 5-min novelty test phase. Scores for external form novelty condition, 2 months postnatal age, are presented in Figure 15.3a. Scores for internal form novelty condition, 3-4 months postnatal age, are presented in Figure 15.3b.* [a] *Five months postnatal age.*

Although visual comparisons of mean HAS scores obtained by preterm infants in this study with the HAS scores obtained by full-term infants in our previous study (see Figure 15.2a) suggest attenuated performance by preterm relative to full-term infants, statistical comparisons were not performed. Although we failed to show any evidence of a relationship between visual recognition performance as a function of conceptional age, a finding of a significant negative correlation between HAS novelty scores and frequency of maternal birth complications ($r = -.35$; $t[40] = 2.38$; $p < .05$) indicated that infants with more maternal birth complications showed attenuated levels of visual recognition on this task.

In contrast to our findings of no relationship between visual recognition performance and conceptional age of preterm infants on the external form task, the mean differences seen in HAS performance for the four conceptional age groups in Figure 15.3b were statistically reliable ($F[3,56] = 3.98$; $p < .05$). Subsequent t tests indicated that while both the 53–54- and the 55–60-week-old groups differed reliably from the 45–48-week group ($p < .05$, two-tailed tests), none of the other group differences were statistically reliable. In the two youngest conceptional age groups, only 6 of 15 and 7 of 15 infants, respectively, showed positive HAS novelty scores. In contrast, 12 of 15 subjects in each of the two older age groups showed positive HAS novelty scores. Correlated t tests applied to the HAS scores for each of the four conceptional age groups provided evidence of reliable stimulus novelty effects beginning at 53–54 weeks of conceptional age ($p < .05$ or less).

Given that the 60 preterm infants tested on the internal form discrimination task also varied in their postnatal ages at time of testing, comparable statistical tests were performed based on groupings by postnatal age. A grouping based on differences in postnatal age provided equal size samples of 15 subjects tested at 12–13, 14–15, 17–19, and 20–25 weeks. Briefly, although no reliable between-group differences were found in performance as a function of postnatal age, when correlated t tests were applied to the HAS scores for each of the four postnatal groups, reliable stimulus novelty effects were found beginning at 17–19 weeks of age ($p < .05$ or less). When correlational analyses were performed to assess the effects of postnatal and conceptional age differences on visual recognition performance, the results obtained were consistent with our findings of group differences as a function of conceptional rather than of postnatal age. For the total sample of 60 subjects, a significant positive correlation was found between HAS novelty scores and conceptional age at testing ($r = .32$; $t[58] = 2.52$; $p < .05$), whereas no relationship between novelty scores and postnatal age at testing was found ($r = .05$). When comparisons are made between full-term and preterm infants with respect to the developmental onset of form recognition, based on processing of internal form elements, somewhat contrasting developmental pictures are seen, depending upon whether comparisons are made using postnatal or conceptional age. While our previous studies with full-term infants provided evidence of reliable form recognition by 12 weeks of postnatal age, preterm infants did not show clear evidence of visual recognition prior to 17–19 weeks of postnatal age, a delay of at least 5 weeks. When comparisons between these groups of infants were made using conceptional age, both full-term and preterm infants demonstrated visual recognition around 52–53 weeks. The results of our studies with preterm infants indicated that the developmental onset of this internal form processing ability was not dependent upon age from birth alone but rather was a function of both prenatal and postnatal factors.

Although the results of these initial form recognition experiments with full-term and preterm infants permit only a general descriptive comparison, they provide some evidence for the important role of maturational factors in the developing form processing abilities of infants and indicate a similar developmental pattern for both full-term and preterm infants when differences in maturational levels at time of testing are taken into consideration. The available empirical findings from these studies suggest that some rudimentary capacities for processing form may be inherent in the visual system of infants. Although we do not know the earliest age at which full-term infants are capable of processing changes in the contours of external forms that are equated for amount of contour, this form processing ability is evidenced as early as 4 weeks of postnatal age, or 44 weeks of conceptional age. For preterm infants tested at 8 weeks of postnatal age, evidence of reliable visual recognition was seen as early as 44 weeks of conceptional age, and performance was not found to be reliably correlated with individual differences in conceptional ages ranging from 40 to 48 weeks at time of testing. Although both preterm and full-term infants were tested on the internal form discrimination task beginning at 12 weeks of postnatal age, comparable durations of postnatal visual experience did not result in comparable levels of visual recognition performance. Reliable visual recognition performance was not found in preterm infants prior to 53 weeks of conceptional age. This finding does not mean that visual experience was unimportant for the development of higher-order form abilities of infants, but it does suggest that some level of neural maturation is necessary for the assimilation of visual experiences. With these findings providing the necessary baseline developmental data on the changing form processing abilities of preterm infants, the subsequent experiments with preterm infants were conducted to determine whether deficits in these form processing abilities are associated with differences in birth status, perinatal risk factors, and duration of postnatal visual experience when preterm infants are equated for their levels of maturational development at time of testing. For this purpose, we tested independent samples of preterm infants on the external form discrimination task at 44 weeks of conceptional age, and on the internal form discrimination task at 52 weeks of conceptional age.

Differences in Form Recognition Performance among Preterm Infants

Using experimental procedures identical to those employed in the previous experiments with preterm infants, 23 subjects were tested on the external form discrimination task at 44 weeks of conceptional age, and 22 subjects were tested on the internal form task at 52 weeks of conceptional age. The 23 infants tested at 44 weeks had a mean birthweight of 2048 gm (SD 288) and a mean gestational age at birth of 34.45 weeks (SD 1.76) and ranged from 56 to 91 days (Median, 69 days) in postnatal age at testing. The 22 infants tested at 52 weeks had a mean birthweight of 2138 gm (SD 305) and a mean gestational age at birth of 34.86 weeks (SD 2.10) and ranged from 91 to 157 days (Median, 128 days) in postnatal age at testing.

For the 23 subjects tested on the external form task at 44 weeks of conceptional age, evidence of reliable recovery of HAS rate was found during the 5-min novelty test phase of the experiment. Nineteen of the 23 subjects demonstrated recovery in their HAS rates, with a mean increase of 6.32 HAS responses per minute (t [22] $= 3.10; p < .01$). Although none of the following correlational findings were statistically reliable, they represent an interesting pattern. Higher novelty HAS recovery scores were positively correlated with birthweight ($r = .24; t[21] = 1.15$) and gestational age at birth ($r = .27; t[21] = 1.32$) but negatively correlated with postnatal age at testing ($r = -.26; t[21] = 1.23$). The findings of reliable form recognition in preterm infants at 44 weeks of conceptional age replicates the findings obtained in our previous study. This experiment provided no evidence that postnatal visual experience, prior to an age when birth normally occurs, facilitated visual recognition performance. Rather, the obtained pattern of correlational findings indicated that, even when preterm infants are equated for differences in maturational levels at time of testing, poorer visual recognition performance was associated with indexes of immature birth status.

An examination of the visual recognition scores for the 22 preterm infants tested at 52 weeks of conceptional age indicated that 15 of the 22 subjects demonstrated recovery in their HAS rates during the novelty test phase, and a mean increase of 5.90 HAS response per minute was obtained for this group ($t[21] = 1.96; p < .05$, one-tailed test). Although our previous study had shown highly reliable stimulus novelty effects for preterm infants tested at 53 weeks of conceptional age, the marginally significant novelty effects obtained in this study are consistent with our previous findings. More importantly, the results of this experiment indicated that, when preterm infants were equated for maturational levels at time of testing, higher levels of HAS recovery to stimulus novelty were positively correlated with birthweight ($r = .39; t[20] = 1.92; p < .05$, one-tailed test) and gestational age at birth ($r = .44; t[20] = 2.20; p < .05$, two-tailed test) but tended to be negatively correlated with postnatal age at testing ($r = -.36; t[20] = 1.70$; nonsignificant).

The patterns of correlational findings obtained in these two experiments were strikingly similar. They failed to provide any evidence that visual experience, prior to a conceptional age when birth usually occurs, had any beneficial effects on the development of these form discrimination abilities in preterm infants. On both of these form recognition tasks, poorer novelty scores were associated with premature birth status (i.e., smaller weights and younger gestational ages at birth). Although the same pattern of correlation findings was found in both experiments, it was only on the internal form discrimination task that immature birth status was reliably associated with delays or deficits in visual recognition performance. While our previous studies indicated that preterm and full-term infants show comparable developmental onsets in their ability to process form changes when their performance was compared as a function of conceptional age, the results of the present experiments provide important additional findings. When preterm infants were matched for maturational levels at time of testing, depending on the visual encoding requirements of the recognition task, differences in birth status were reliably associated with quantitative differences in form recognition performance.

The question of whether these differences in visual recognition performance associated with preterm birth status reflect temporary delays or longer term deficits is one of both theoretical and clinical significance. Significant differences in performance as a function of birth status may be obtained only when assessments are made at a point in development when these perceptual processing abilities are initially emerging. In an attempt to provide some additional preliminary empirical findings related to this issue, we tested 20 preterm infants on the internal form discrimination task at 56 weeks of conceptional age, 4 weeks later than our prior study with preterm infants. Infants ranged from 112 to 160 days of postnatal age at time of testing. Correlational analyses revealed similar but statistically nonsignificant relationships between HAS novelty scores and birth status variables. Higher levels of HAS recovery were positively correlated with birthweight ($r = .28$; $t[18] = 1.25$; nonsignificant) and gestational age at birth ($r = .36$; $t[18] = 1.46$; nonsignificant). However, visual recognition scores showed significant negative correlations with postnatal age at testing ($r = -.50$; $t[18] = 2.45$; $p < .05$, two-tailed test), with frequency of postnatal complications ($r = -.50$; $t[18] = 2.46$; $p < .05$), and with number of days in hospital prior to discharge ($r = -.47$; $t[18] = 2.29$; $p < .05$). Despite the preliminary nature of these later findings, they suggest that perinatal medical risk factors were reliably associated with poorer visual form recognition performance at 56 weeks of conceptional age.

These HAS studies of visual pattern recognition have provided us with a number of findings to indicate the potential usefulness of our laboratory procedures in providing assessments of early similarities and differences in the ontogeny of visual processing and recognition memory abilities in full-term and preterm infants. It is important to note that our populations of preterm infants did not represent a particularly high-risk group of preterm infants. In our respective populations of preterm infants, fewer than 20% of the subjects had birthweights under 1800 gm and infants with birthweights of less than 1500 gm were minimally represented (i.e., less than 5%). Despite the moderate-risk characteristics of our preterm infants, some evidence of developmental delays and deficits were found to be associated with birth status and perinatal risk factors. Our long-term clinical objective is to explore relations between clinical morbidity factors commonly seen in very low birthweight preterm infants and developmental deficits on these early measures of visual recognition behavior. These initial findings with full-term and moderate-risk preterm infants have provided us with reliable findings with respect to some of the important developmental factors underlying changes in the rapidly emerging visual recognition abilities of infants. Subsequent longitudinal assessments of impairments in visuospatial functioning and intellectual competence in later childhood will allow us to evaluate the clinical significance of performance differences on these laboratory measures of visual recognition during the first weeks of postnatal age.

Acknowledgments

I gratefully acknowledge the contributions of William Oh, director of perinatal medicine, at the Women and Infants Hospital of Rhode Island, Providence, Rhode Island.

References

Bergman, T., Haith, M. M., & Mann, L. Development of eye contact and facial scanning in infants. Paper presented at the meeting of the Society for Research in Child Development, Minneapolis, April 1971.

Bond, E. K. Perception of form by the human infant. *Psychological Bulletin,* 1972, *77,* 225–245.

Bronson, G. The postnatal growth of visual capacity. *Child Development,* 1974, *45,* 873–890.

Cohen, L. B. Attention-getting and attention-holding processes of infant visual preferences. Child Development, 1972, *43,* 869–879.

Cohen, L. B. Habituation of infant visual attention. In T. J. Tighe & N. Leaton (Eds.). *Habituation: Perspectives from child development, animal behavior, and neurophysiology.* Hillsdale, N.J.: Erlbaum, 1976.

Cohen, L. B., & Gelber, E. R. Infant visual memory. In L. B. Cohen & P. Salapatek (Eds.), *Infant perception: From sensation to cognition* (Vol. 1). New York: Academic Press, 1975.

Donnee, L. H. Infants' developmental scanning patterns to face and nonface stimuli under various auditory conditions. Paper presented at meeting of the Society for Research in Child Development, Philadelphia, March 1973.

Fagan, J. F. Infant recognition memory as a present and future index of cognitive abilities. In N. R. Ellis (Ed.), *Aberrant development in infancy: Human and animal studies.* Hillsdale, N.J.: Erlbaum, 1975.

Fagan, J. F., Fantz, R. L., & Miranda, S. B. *Infant's attention to novel stimuli as a function of postnatal and conceptional age.* Paper presented at the meetings of the Society for Research in Child Development, Minneapolis, 1971.

Fantz, R. L., Fagan, J. F., & Miranda, S. B. Early visual selectivity as a function of pattern variables, previous exposure, age from birth and conception, and expected cognitive deficit. In L. B. Cohen & P. Salapatek (Eds.), *Infant perception: From sensation to cognition* (Vol. 1). New York: Academic Press, 1975.

Friedman, S. Infant habituation: Processes, problems and possibilities. In N. R. Ellis (Ed.), *Aberrant development in infancy: Human and animal studies.* Hillsdale, N.J.: Erlbaum, 1975.

Haith, M. M. Visual competence in early infancy. In R. Held, H. Leibowitz, & H. L. Teuber (Eds.), *Handbook of sensory physiology* (Vol. 8). Berlin: Springer-Verlag, 1976.

Haith, M. M., & Campos, J. Human infancy. *Annual Review of Psychology.* Palo Alto, Calif.: Annual Reviews Inc., 1977.

Hebb, D. O. *The organization of behavior.* New York: Wiley, 1949.

Humphrey, N. K. Vision in a monkey without striate cortex: A case study. *Perception,* 1974, *3,* 241–255.

Hunter, M. A., & Ames, E. W. Visual habituation and preference for novelty in five-week-old infants. Paper presented at the meetings of the Society for Research in Child Development, Denver, 1975.

Lubchenco, L. O., Searls, D. T., & Brazie, J. V. Neonatal mortality rate: Relationship to birth weight and gestational age. *Journal of Pediatrics,* 1972, *81,* 814–820.

Maisel, E. B., & Karmel, B. Z. Contour density and pattern configuration in visual preferences of infants. *Infants Behavior and Development,* 1978, *1,* 127–140.

Maurer, D. The scanning of faces by infants. Unpublished manuscript, 1969.

Maurer, D., & Salapatek, P. Developmental changes in the scanning of faces by infants. *Child Development,* 1976, *47,* 523–527.

Milewski, A. E. Infant's discrimination of internal and external pattern elements. *Journal of Experimental Child Psychology,* 1976, *22,* 229–246.

Milewski, A. E., & Siqueland, E. R. Discrimination of color and pattern novelty in one-month infants. *Journal of Experimental Child Psychology,* 1975, *19,* 122–136.

Olson, G. M. An information processing analysis of visual memory and habituation in infants. In T. J. Tighe & N. Leaton (Eds.), *Habituation: Perspectives from child development, animal behavior, and neurophysiology.* Hillsdale, N.J.: Erlbaum, 1976.

Rose, S. A., Gottfried, A. W., & Bridger, W. H. Effects of haptic cues on visual recognition memory in fullterm and preterm infants. *Infant Behavior and Development,* 1979, *2,* 55–67.

Ruff, H., & Turkewitz, G. Developmental changes in the effectiveness of stimulus intensity on infant visual attention. *Developmental Psychology,* 1975, *11,* 705–710.

Salapatek, P. Pattern perception in early infancy. In L. B. Cohen and P. Salapatek (Eds.), *Infant perception: From sensation to cognition* (Vol. 1). New York: Academic Press, 1975.

Sigman, M., & Parmelee, A. H. Visual preferences of four-month-old premature and full-term infants. *Child Development,* 1974, *45,* 959–965.

Siqueland, E. R. Further developments in infant learning. Paper presented at the 19th International Congress of Psychology, London, 1969.

Siqueland, E. R., & DeLucia, C. A. Visual reinforcement of nonnutritive sucking in human infants. *Science,* 1969, *165,* 1144–1146.

Siqueland, E. R., & Osman, N. B. Perception of color-form compounds in infants. In preparation.

Vaughan, H. G. Electrophysiologic analysis of regional cortical maturation. *Biological Psychiatry,* 1975, *10,* 513–526.

Weiskrantz, L. The interaction between occipital and temporal cortex in vision: An overview. In F. O. Schmitt & F. G. Worden (Eds.), *The neurosciences third study program.* Cambridge, Mass.: MIT Press, 1974.

Weiskrantz, L., Cowey, A., & Darlington, C. Spatial responses by destriated monkeys to brief flashes of light. *Brain Research,* 1973, *66,* 360.

Werner, J. S., & Siqueland, E. R. Visual recognition memory in the preterm infants. *Infant behavior and Development,* 1978, *1,* 79–94.

16

Visual Development in Pre- and Full-Term Infants: A Review of Chapters 12-15

KEITH D. WHITE
YVONNE BRACKBILL

The four projects reported in this section all capitalize on the infant's well-known tendency to look longer at novel stimuli than at familiar stimuli. Differential responsiveness to familiar versus novel patterns implicates memory (or a memory-like process) as a determinant of experimental outcome. Some faculty for retaining information about stimulus events is necessary for a stimulus to become familiar through repeated or prolonged exposure. Thus, when infants respond in a reliably different manner to novel and familiar stimulus patterns, one can infer that (*a*) the sensory–perceptual systems were capable of dectecting a difference between the old and new patterns; *and* (*b*) information about the familiarized patterns was retained over time; *and* (*c*) the detection of a difference between familiar and novel patterns was capable of altering the observed responses.

The processes of detection, retention, and response generation must all operate in concert for the infant to demonstrate a familiar versus novel discrimination. This in turn complicates the task of interpreting negative experimental outcomes, that is, those that fail to find evidence of discrimination. Failure to detect or to retain or to respond can all individually or jointly lead to negative findings, and their relative contributions are thus confounded.

As Cohen (Chapter 13, this volume) points out, research with normal infants has shown the habituation–dishabituation paradigm to be a useful device for exploring the development of visual attention, recognition memory, and information-processing ability. It is a natural extension to question whether preterm infants differ from full-term infants along these dimensions.

Cohen compared 23 "severely" preterm infants (mean gestational age

PRETERM BIRTH AND
PSYCHOLOGICAL DEVELOPMENT

about 30 weeks) to full-term infants matched at corrected chronological ages 20, 33, and 49 weeks. All subjects were drawn from lower socioeconomic status families. The babies were habituated to a photograph of a human face and subsequently tested for dishabituation with photographs of the same face, a different face, a lion's face, and a nonface stimulus. There were no marked differences between preterm and full-term infants in mean fixation times to the dishabituating stimulus. (Neither were there differences between full-terms and only moderately preterm subjects, Cohen notes, although he does not present these data.) There were differences, however, between both lower-class groups and an additional control group drawn from middle-socioeconomic-class families.

Rose (Chapter 14, this volume) expanded the habituation paradigm to study the development of cross-modal transfer, with stimuli presented either tactually or orally during familiarization trials and visually during dishabituation trials. Subjects were older full-term and preterm infants (mean gestational age, 33 weeks), matched for conceptional age[1] and socioeconomic status. Middle-class full-term infants were able to transfer across modalities, whereas lower-class full-term infants, middle-class preterm infants, and lower-class preterm infants were not able to do so. On an easier, intramodal habituation task (visual familiarization stimulus followed by novel visual stimulus), all three groups performed with equal efficiency.

In a second study, Rose pitted a visual-only habituation condition against a condition in which 6-month- and 12-month-old preterm and full-term infants engaged in both visual and haptic (touch and manipulation) familiarization. The pattern of response for 12-month-old preterms was similar to that for 6-month-old full-terms: Significant evidence of memory appeared only in the visual-only condition. In addition, and without regard to significance level, evidence indicated that the visual–motor task was more difficult than the visual-only task. Additional studies suggested that this result largely reflects differences in speed of processing visual information and that prematures show particular deficits in speed of encoding visual information about shape.

Caron and Caron (Chapter 12, this volume) used the habituation paradigm to study the infant's developing ability to process categorical information and relational concepts. These investigators devised a series of stimuli whose features changed in some respects but remained invariant in others. Substantively, these perceptual problems sampled a variety of concepts: spatial (above–below), qualitative (same–different), and naturalistic configuration ("faceness"). Each stimulus could be encoded on habituation trials in either absolute or relational terms. Stimuli presented on dishabituation trials

---

[1] In this discussion, *conceptional age matching* means that full-term and preterm infants were conceived on approximately the same date, so that full-terms have longer gestational ages but shorter postnatal ages than do preterms in the comparison group.

tested for differences in fixation times to absolute or relative components. An additional treatment condition varied the number of different exemplars presented during habituation trials. The subjects, all from middle-class families, were full-term and preterm infants with a median gestational age of 33 weeks.

Results showed that preterm infants did not respond to change in the relative or invariant component (change in configuration) but did respond to the absolute perceptual feature (change in detail), whereas their full-term counterparts did respond to stimulus change in relational or categorical terms.

Siqueland (Chapt. 15, this volume) has adapted the habituation paradigm to an operant response methodology; his procedure makes use of the selective viewing tendency by allowing it to serve as a reinforcing agent in an operant setting. The infant's opportunity to view a pattern is contingent on its rate of high-amplitude nonnutritive sucking. As long as the stimulus is novel enough, the infant sucks to keep it visible. Both studies reported by Siqueland used a correlational design in which preterm infants of varying conceptional ages served as subjects. In the first experiment, a group of preterms with a mean gestational age of 35 weeks and conceptional ages ranging from 40 to 50 weeks were tested for responsiveness to external form changes in the visual display. Responsiveness to internal form changes was the focus of a second experiment, in which the preterm subjects had a mean gestational age of 36 weeks and ranged in conceptional age from 45 to 60 weeks.

There were no significant differences in external form recognition performance as a function of differences in conceptional age, although there was a significant negative correlation between dishabituation scores and number of perinatal complications. The second experiment, on the other hand, revealed a significant positive correlation between internal form recognition and conceptional age.

Despite the kernel of commonality in their methodology conferred by the fact that all these investigators used an habituation paradigm, the four projects differ considerably in the extent to which they found reliable differences in visual behavior between full-term and preterm infants. These differences in outcome are not attributable to differences in subjects' ages, since Cohen's group of preterms had a mean gestational age of 3–4 weeks less than that of any other group in the four projects, yet the similarities in preterm–full-term performance reported by Cohen were greater than in any of the other projects.

Rather, a more likely reason for this difference in outcome is a considerable difference in the difficulty of the tasks used by the investigators. Caron and Caron, who found highly significant differences between full-terms and preterms, employed complicated stimuli and a demanding task, one that is less readily related to the sensory capabilities of the visual modality than it is to the cognitive capacities that presumably extend across sensory modalities.

Rose added difficulty as a dimension by requiring the infant to integrate information from more than one sensory modality and by making the task a perceptual–motor one rather than perceptual only. Under these conditions, she found full-term performance clearly superior to preterm performance. The superiority disappeared, however, when the two groups were compared in their response to an easier, visual-only task.

By way of contrast to the demanding tasks used by Caron and Caron and by Rose, the tasks used by Siqueland and by Cohen were much easier. Both investigators used visual displays that are relatively simple and responses that infants are well equipped to make.[2] Neither investigator found marked differences in dishabituation between groups.

That the probability of finding intergroup differences is functionally related to task difficulty has been pointed out for another at-risk infant population: those whose mothers have received drugs during labor and delivery (Brackbill, 1979).[3] Also in this connection, note that Siqueland found a strong negative correlation between the number of medical complications and visual form recognition scores. In fact, the correlation was as high ($r < .50$) as that between the scores and postnatal age. Unfortunately, there are no comparable data analyses in the other investigations reported in this section.

In addition to the psychological and medical variables, the sociological variable, socioeconomic status, appears to be of prime importance, with middle-class babies performing better than lower-class babies. In commenting on his own results, Cohen notes, "Perhaps the influence of the lower-social-class environment is so crucial that it may mask the effects of high-risk factors in the newborn [p. 252]" and points to the National Institute of Neurological and Communicative Disorders and Stroke Collaborative Perinatal Project finding that class-related variables were better predictors of later IQ than were prenatal or perinatal variables. Rose's data also show that a low socioeconomic status, like low gestational age, depresses performances. In the Caron and Caron project, socioeconomic status was held constant, in that experimental and control subjects were drawn from the same (middle) class. Siqueland does not report on the socioeconomic status of his subjects.

A basic theoretical question these chapters raise concerns the relative im-

[2] An interested reader could verify differences in difficulty of two-dimensional stimuli by comparing the Fourier power spectra of familiar versus novel patterns (see, e.g., Tieger & Ganz, 1979).

[3] Although none of the authors presents information about the prenatal, perinatal, and postnatal medication to which their subjects were exposed, it may be the case that preterm infants in each of these four projects have received more drugs than full-term controls. Three reasons for so suspecting are (a) infants receive inadvertent medication at the maternal dose, and the milligrams per kilogram bodyweight is higher for smaller babies; (b) a greater proportion of preterms than full-terms are delivered by cesarean section, which generally entails greater variety and quantity of drugs than does vaginal delivery; and (c) postnatal medication is higher on average in the intensive care unit than in the normal newborn nursery.

portance of experience[4] and maturation in determining visual development. Preterm infants have had a longer period of visual experience than full-terms of the same conceptional age. To the extent that deprivation paradigms are applicable in the present context, the literature suggests that this additional experience could result in superior visual development in preterms. Contributing to this supposition is a large body of anatomical and physiological studies on neural development showing that the visual nervous system is strikingly plastic and subject to the influences of experience. Deprivation of normal visual experience serves to alter the organization of the visual system, whether it is full deprivation by means of dark rearing, deprivation of one of the eyes by occlusion, or exposure only to selected or to degraded contours (e.g., Hirsch & Spinelli, 1971; Mitchell, Freeman, Millodot, & Haegerstrom, 1973; Wiesel & Hubel, 1963; but see Sherk & Stryker, 1976).

Additionally, behavioral studies of normal, institutionalized infants show that the quality of the visual surroundings influences the development of visually guided motor behaviors. Institutionalized infants often are limited to the bland visual surroundings of white sheets, brief contacts with personnel, few toys, etc; however, such minor enrichments as multicolored sheets or a mobile suspended above the crib can accelerate the development of accurate reaching and other aspects of eye–hand coordination (White, 1971; White, Castle, & Held, 1964; White & Held, 1966). Also, recent findings on the visual acuity of preterm and full-term infants show that preterms are the superior if the groups are compared on conceptional (i.e., maturational) age although the inferior when matched on postnatal age (Sokol & Jones, 1979).

Nevertheless, all four present chapters find either no difference or differences in favor of the full-terms on the visual tasks examined. Why have the supposed benefits of "extra" visual experience, enjoyed by the preterms between their time of birth and the normal due date, not been revealed here?

One possibility is that this extra postnatal experience may not be particularly visually enriched, because the infants' visual capacities are probably quite limited. Specific data for visual acuity of preterms between birth and due date (i.e., less than 40 weeks postmenstrual age) are virtually nonexistent, but if one considers the biological maturation of visual structures during the last trimester *in utero* and (cautiously) extrapolates backward the findings for full-term neonates and infants, one can only conclude that vision must be severely limited. Even in full-term neonates, the ability to focus crisp optical images on the retina from objects located at various distances (i.e., accommodation) is apparently absent, and good focus is only achieved for objects within a few centimeters of the eye (cf. Haynes, White, & Held, 1965). In some preterms, incomplete resorption of the hyaloid artery would further com-

---

[4] Postnatal age is a better index of the duration of experiences in toto regarding the visual versus other sense modalities. This is because the intrauterine environment is more devoid of things to see than it is of sounds (e.g., mother's heartbeat), tastes (amniotic fluid), pressure on the skin, gravitational effects on the vestibular organs, etc.

promise optical quality. Further, the incidence and severity of ocular astigmatism (meridional optical defocusing) is as much as five to ten times higher for infants below 6 months postnatal age than for older children or adults (Howland, Atkinson, Braddick, & French, 1978; Mohindra, Held, Gwiazda, & Brill, 1978). These factors as well as incomplete retinal differentiation, myelinization of the optic nerve, etc., lead to the poor visual acuity evidenced by full-term neonates.[5] Our best guess is that during the extra experience of preterms between birth and due date their view of the world is extremely blurred, particularly for objects more distant than several inches from the eyes.

A second possibility is that the present paradigms simply fail to reveal the supposed advantage of preterms due to their extra experience. These studies have indeed made clever use of the visual familiarization paradigm and have contributed to our understanding of ways that birth status may influence later maturational competence. However, one must give serious consideration to the possiblility that familiarization procedures are not sensitive to certain effects (e.g., the visual control of locomotion or posture; see Dichgans & Brandt, 1978; Held & Hein, 1963) or may not be the optimal choice for certain theoretical purposes (see, e.g., Dobson & Teller, 1978). Also, the visual tasks utilized in the present studies require different levels of complexity in visual information processing. Within the present results, there is a trend such that the advantage of full-terms over preterms correlates with task complexity. The visual actuity results of Sokol and Jones (1979) in finding preterms the superior also fit this trend, as their task was simply passive observation during the recording of the visually evoked components of EEG. It may be that some of these tasks rely on a level of visual information processing that is unimproved by the extra experience of preterms. One cannot easily reject an alternative explanation, however, that the nature of certain tasks might tend to obscure true behavioral differences that are due to experience by the unwanted, overpowering influences of other factors (such as wandering attention).[6]

Even allowing for these possible reasons why the expected benefits of extra

[5] A recent review of infant visual acuity studies (Dobson & Teller, 1978) reports, for full-term neonates, estimated Snellen-equivalent acuity scores ranging from 20/350 to 20/1600. For comparison, consider as an illustration that an adult whose best vision is assessed at 20/200 is considered "legally blind," and this adult's acuity is roughly two to eight times better than the neonate's. Even this relatively limited visual experience seems essential to avoid such disorders as amblyopia ex anopsia, though it may contribute rather little to "higher order" perceptual processes.

[6] Researchers on infant behavior soon realize that their subjects are more inarticulate and vulnerable, and less collaborative with experimental needs, than the older subjects for other kinds of psychological research. Seemingly simple studies may prove to be devilishly difficult, and to devise and validate new procedures will surely exercise the ingenuity of developmental scientists. The payoff to be expected, though, is to bring our presently foggy view of visual development in infants into the crisp focus necessary for achieving theoretical and practical advancements.

visual experience were not revealed here as advantageous to preterms one must now ask, "Wouldn't the equivalent visual performance be expected from preterms and full-terms on the basis of equal maturation?" Yet, when the preterms were neither maturationally nor experientially disadvantaged relative to the full-terms, their performance was nevertheless inferior on the more complex tasks. We should also be reminded that preterm birth status predicts educational lags and deficits in the later school years (Taub, Goldstein, & Caputo, 1977), when preterm and full-term experience and maturation have virtually the same durations. How then do the preterms become disadvantaged? At present, we do not know.

The present studies reflect an increasing awareness in the scientific community that it is essential to study the various factors accompanying birth status, as well as the ways in which these factors influence development and competence in the later childhood and adult years. Several studies indicate that the factors impinging upon the infant around the time of birth may mold the future course of development. It is especially important to establish which particular perinatal risks contribute to the learning disabilities or other handicaps that may be evidenced at later stages of life. Likewise, it is important to identify any early signs that predict the onset of a future handicap. Armed with this knowledge, it might prove possible to minimize or to avoid the special perinatal risk factors that most strongly jeopardize future psychological development. As an added benefit, the ability to predict impending handicap via its early signs might enable us to devise remedial treatments that, through sufficiently early application, could ameliorate or even avert disability.

References

Brackbill, Y. Obstetrical medication and infant behavior. In J. D. Osofsky (Ed.), *Handbook of infant development*. New York: Wiley, 1979.

Dichgans, J., & Brandt, T. Visual–vestibular interaction: Effects on self-motion perception and postural control. In R. Held, H. Leibowitz, & H. Teuber, (Eds.), *Handbook of sensory physiology* (Vol. 8). New York: Springer Verlag, 1978.

Dobson, V., & Teller, D. Visual acuity in human infants: A review and comparison of behavioral and electrophysiological studies. *Vision Research*, 1978, *18*, 1469–1484.

Haynes, H., White, B., & Held, R. Visual accomodation in human infants. *Science*, 1965, *148*, 528–530.

Held, R., & Hein, A. Movement produced stimulation in the development of visually-guided behavior. *Journal of Comparative and Physiological Psychology*, 1963, *56*, 872–876.

Hirsch, H., & Spinelli, D. Modification of the distribution of receptive field orientation in cats by selective visual exposure during development. *Experimental Brain Research*, 1971, *13*, 509–527.

Howland, H., Atkinson, J., Braddick, O., & French, J. Infant astigmatism measured by photorefraction, *Science*, 1978, *202*, 331–333.

Mitchell, D., Freeman, R., Millodot, M., & Haegerstrom, G. Meridional amblyopia: Evidence for modification of the human visual system by early visual experience. *Vision Research,* 1973, *13,* 535–558.

Mohindra, I., Held, R., Gwiazda, J., & Brill, S. Astigmatism in infants. *Science,* 1978, *202,* 329–330.

Sherk, H., & Stryker, M. Quantitative study of cortical orientation selectivity in visually deprived kittens. *Journal of Neurophysiology,* 1976, *39,* 63–70.

Sokol, S., & Jones, K. Implicit time of pattern evoked potentials in infants: An index of maturation of spatial vision. *Vision Research,* 1979, *19,* 747–756.

Taub, H., Goldstein, K., & Caputo, D. Indices of neonatal prematurity as discriminators of development in middle childhood. *Child Development,* 1977, *48,* 797–805.

Tieger, T., & Ganz, L. Recognition of faces in the presence of two-dimensional sinusoidal masks. *Perception and Psychophysics,* 1979, *26,* 163–167.

White, B. *Human infants: Experience and psychological development.* Englewood Cliffs, N.J.: Prentice-Hall, 1971.

White, B., Castle, P., & Held, R. Observations on the development of visually directed reaching. *Child Development,* 1964, *35,* 349–365.

White, B., & Held, R. Plasticity of sensorimotor development. In J. Resenblith & W. Allinsmith, (Eds.), *The causes of behavior: Readings in child development and educational psychology* (2nd ed.). Boston: Allyn & Bacon, 1966.

Wiesel, T. N., & Hubel, D. H. Single-cell responses in striate cortex of kittens deprived of vision in one eye. *Journal of Neurophysiology,* 1963, *26,* 1003–1017.

V

Longitudinal Follow-up: Two Years and Above

17

Developmental Follow-up of Pre- and Postterm Infants[1]

TIFFANY MARTINI FIELD
JEAN RYDBERG DEMPSEY
H. H. SHUMAN

Most babies are born at term, thanks to mother nature and modern medicine. Those who are not born at term, namely, pre- and postterm babies, are fewer in number but constitute a large sample of infants born at risk. Shortened or prolonged gestations per se are not necessarily risk factors if the maternal, fetal, and placental systems have been functioning optimally and if the neonate does not experience perinatal or postnatal complications. Unfortunately, a nonterm delivery is often symptomatic of dysfunction in these systems, and the infant is thus vulnerable to complications.

A number of investigators have suggested that the preterm infant is not necessarily at risk for developmental delays or deficits if he does not experience the postnatal complications often associated with immaturity, such as metabolic disorders, central nervous system (CNS) dysfunction, or respiratory distress syndrome (RDS) (DiVitto & Goldberg, 1979; Sostek, Quinn, & Davitt, 1979). Similarly, a number of studies on the postterm infant have suggested that postterm gestations are typically not a problem unless the placenta has deteriorated and the infant manifests the postmaturity syndrome (Clifford, 1954). The most common complication experienced by the immature preterm infant is RDS, and the most frequent complication of the postterm infant is the postmaturity syndrome.

A range of developmental outcomes has been reported for both preterm RDS and postterm postmaturity syndrome infants. Studies of infants surviving mild RDS with respiratory assistance suggest that they experience early developmental delays (Fisch, Gravem, & Engel, 1968) but by age 4 years

The study reported in this chapter was supported in part by grants from the Public Health Department of Massachusetts and the March of Dimes/National Foundation.

receive normal IQ scores (Ambrus, Weintraub, Niswander, Fischer, Fleishman, Bross, & Ambrus, 1970; Fisch, Bilek, Miller, & Engel, 1975). However, despite their normal IQ scores, these children appear to have an increased incidence of language production delays and hyperactivity (Field, Dempsey, & Shuman, 1979). Survivors of more severe RDS treated by mechanical ventilation experience a greater incidence of developmental deficits (Harrod, L'Heureaux, Wangensteen, & Hunt, 1974; Johnson, Malachowski, Grobstein, Daily, & Sunshine, 1974; Outerbridge & Stern, 1972; Stahlman, Hedwall, Dolanski, Foxelius, Burko, & Kirk, 1973).

Developmental outcomes reported for the postterm postmaturity syndrome infant range from no problems to delayed social development (Lovell, 1973), severe illnesses and sleep disturbances (Zwerdling, 1967), reading disabilities (Butler & Alberman, 1969), neurological handicaps (Wagner & Arndt, 1968), and cerebral palsy (Drillien, 1968). Although postmature infants often do not experience medical complications at birth, we have classified them as being at risk because of their questionable developmental outcomes. The variability of outcomes for both these risk groups suggests the importance of finding early assessment scales or predictor variables that might identify those preterm RDS infants continuing at risk and those postterm postmaturity syndrome infants developing deficits.

The purpose of the present study was to describe the developmental course of the preterm and postterm infant who had experienced the most common complications associated with preterm and postterm delivery, namely, RDS and postmaturity syndrome. The development of these nonterm infants was compared to that of term infants, and an attempt was made to identify early measures that might predict their continuing developmental delays.

Study Method

Subjects

Subjects were 151 infants born during the period of February 1975 to November 1976 at the Baystate Medical Center, Springfield, Massachusetts. They were assigned to the study groups according to the neonatal status of healthy term, preterm with respiratory distress syndrome, or postterm with postmaturity syndrome. The preterm RDS group comprised 46 infants (25 females, 21 males). They averaged 1600 gm birthweight, 32 weeks gestation, 3 days mechanical ventilation, and 32 days intensive care. The postterm postmaturity syndrome group comprised 46 infants (25 females, 21 males) who averaged 3600 gm birthweight, 42 weeks gestation, and two postmaturity symptoms (e.g., meconium-stained, parchment-like skin; a long thin body; and a wizened look, Clifford, 1954). The normal term group comprised 59 infants (30 females, 29 males) who averaged 3300 gm birthweight and 40 weeks gestation. The preterm RDS group alone was designated medically at risk because of the combined factors of short gestation, low birthweight, minimum of 12 hours mechanical ventilation, and 3–4 weeks intensive care. Both the preterm RDS and postterm postmaturity syndrome groups were considered behaviorally at risk because of nonoptimal performance on the Brazelton neonatal scale. The infants were born to white, middle-class, high-school-educated mothers averaging 25 years of age, and most of the infants were later born.

A random selection of normal term and postterm postmaturity syndrome infants were entered into the study at 2–3 days postdelivery. All of the preterm RDS infants who were cared for in our intensive care nursery during 1975–1976 and received a minimum of 12 hours mechanical ventilation were enrolled in the study just prior to discharge.

Procedure

Several assessments were made at 4-month intervals during the first year and at 1-year intervals thereafter; at the time of writing, the infants were currently receiving their 3-year assessments. A number of assessments were selected in order to describe the early behavioral, mental, and motor development of these infants. Assessment dates were calculated from the mother's expected date of delivery rather than from the infant's real birth date as an adjustment for gestational age differences.

Prior to the analyses, log transformations were made on those variables that were not normally distributed. Multivariate and univariate analyses and subsequent multiple comparisons were performed to determine differences between the term and nonterm groups. Since there were multiple dependent measures from each assessment period, multivariate analyses were performed to determine whether there were group differences on these measures. Univariate analyses of variance were performed to determine the particular assessments of each period for which the groups showed differences.

Data were first subjected to multivariate analyses of variance (MANOVAs). One-way MANOVAs were performed on variables grouped according to assessment periods (i.e., perinatal, 4-month, 8-month, and 1- and 2-year variables). The test of significance employed was Wilk's λ criterion, and the approximate F cited was derived statistically using Rao's approximation (Morrison, 1967; Rao, 1973).

Since several ANOVAs were performed to determine the specific variables on which the groups differed, an error rate, or p level, per comparison was set at .001 in order to maintain an error rate of .05 for the experiment as a whole. The Bonferroni t table based on the experiment error rate divided by the number of comparisons was used to determine levels of significance for univariate t tests (Myers, 1972).

Assessments and Results

Perinatal Assessments

Perinatal and obstetric histories were assessed, since prenatal and obstetric complications have been reported for both the postmature (Clifford, 1954) and RDS groups (Outerbridge & Stern, 1972). The Obstetric Complications Scale (OCS) adapted from the Prechtl scale (1968) by Littman and Parmelee (1978) was used for this assessment. This scale consists of a list of events that can be defined as optimal or nonoptimal, including such pregnancy events as infection, bleeding, hypertension, toxemia, and diabetes, and such birth events as gestational age, birth measurements, and Apgar scores. The data for this index derive from the obstetric history and delivery record.

The neonatal variables included the Postnatal Complications Scale (PNCS) (Littman & Parmelee, 1978) and the Brazelton Neonatal Behavioral Assessment Scale (NBAS) (Brazelton, 1973). The PNCS assesses the infant's postnatal course, including conditions that reflect an increased risk of mortality and morbidity, such as respiratory distress, hyperbilirubinemia, and metabolic and temperature disturbances. This scale was used since at least the RDS infants often experience a number of postnatal complications in addition to their respiratory distress (e.g., hyperbilirubinemia and metabolic disturbances).

The Brazelton scale includes responses to visual and auditory stimulation, attention to faces and voices, arousability, reflex behavior, muscle tonus, motor maturity, cuddliness, consolability, and self-quieting ability. These are then summarized by four a priori scoring dimensions, labeled interactive processes, motoric processes, organizational processes–state control, and organizational processes–physiological response to stress (Als, Tronick, Lester, & Brazelton, 1977). Brazelton assessments of the preterm RDS infants were made prior to discharge, when the infants averaged 37 weeks conceptional age (gestational age plus age from birth). Since Brazelton (1975) and his colleagues have questioned the validity of their instrument for use with preterm infants, we decided to make these assessments when the preterm infants approximated term gestational age. Differences relating to this broad age range might still be expected. Nonetheless, we wanted to assess the newborn as he might present himself to his parents, and the Brazelton scale was considered the most adequate measure of the newborn's interaction skills.

As can be seen in Table 17.1:

1. Both nonterm groups experienced obstetric complications. That is, the scores on the OCS were more optimal for the term than the nonterm groups. An item analysis of the OCS suggested that common pregnancy problems were hypertension, toxemia, and bleeding. Low birthweight, gestational age, and Apgar scores were frequent complications for the RDS infant, and fetal heart rate variability was a problem for both nonterm groups.

TABLE 17.1

Means for Perinatal Assessments that Yielded Significant Group Differences at p < .001

| | Group means | | |
| | | | |
Variable	Preterm RDS	Normal term	Postterm postmature
Obstetric Complications Scale	78	117	102
Birth measurements			
Weight (gm)	1597	3338	3581
Length (cm)	41	54	58
Head circumference (cm)	28	34	—
5-min Apgar	7	9	—
Brazelton interactive process [a]	2.30	1.70	2.21
Brazelton motoric process [a]	2.63	1.88	2.25
Postnatal Complications Scale	71	152	—

[a] Lower scores are optimal.

2. Birth measurements were higher for the postterm than the term group and lower for the preterm than the term group.

3. Five-minute Apgar scores were similar for the term and postterm groups, whose scores in turn were higher than those of the preterm group.

4. Both nonterm groups received inferior Brazelton interactive and motoric process scores, but for different reasons. The RDS babies were typically floppy, hypotonic and difficult to arouse and alert and had weak reflexes, a flat affect, and a long-latency–short-duration raspy cry, although they rarely cried. Conversely, the postmatures tended to be hyperirritable, extremely labile, hypertonic and difficult to pacify, and they frequently emitted short-latency cry sounds much like a "donkey's bray." The Brazelton behaviors of the RDS and postmature infants were very different, the RDS being hypo-active and the postmature hyperactive. These extremes in neonatal behavior made it difficult for the Brazelton testers to elicit optimal performance and may present problems for the parents during feeding and other early interactions. The strange cries of both the RDS and postmature infants—the weak respiratory cry of the RDS and the braying-like cry of the postmature infants—may contribute to early interaction disturbances (Lester & Zeskind, 1979), and the additional motoric weakness exhibited by the RDS infants may enhance their parents' view of them as "fragile" infants and elicit different kinds of early caretaking responses.

5. Postnatal complications of the RDS group, particularly hyperbilirubinemia and respiratory and metabolic disturbances, were relatively severe, resulting in significantly lower scores on the Postnatal Complications Scale. These additional complications of hyperbilirubinemia and metabolic disturbances for the RDS infant are consistent with those reported by other RDS investigators (Fitzhardinge, Pape, Arstikaitis, Boyle, Ashby, Rowley, Netley, &

Swyer, 1976; Stahlman *et al.*, 1973). It is not surprising that the postmature infants did not experience postnatal complications, since only extreme or more advanced cases of postmaturity reportedly exhibit postnatal complications (Clifford, 1954). However, since many postmature infants experienced prenatal complications, their perinatal course might be more closely monitored.

Four-Month Assessments

The 4-month assessments, which took place in the hospital's video studio, included growth measurements (weight, length, and head circumference), a standard pediatric examination, the Denver Developmental Screening Test (Frankenburg & Dodds, 1967), the Infant Temperament Questionnaire (Carey, 1970), and filmed mother–infant feeding (Field, 1977b) and face-to-face play interactions (Field, 1977a). The Denver was used at this time instead of the Bayley scales (Bayley, 1969), since the pediatricians on our team were more familiar with the Denver. Mother–infant feeding and face-to-face interactions were assessed, since previous studies from this longitudinal follow-up suggested some disturbed interactions among these nonterm infants (Field, 1977a, 1977b). Interactions were coded for the amount of infant gaze aversion and fussiness and the amount of mother attentiveness and stimulation. The temperament questionnaire was used since a recent study on normal infants reported relationships between Brazelton, temperament, and Bayley measures (Sostek & Anders, 1977). The Infant temperament questionnaire is a mother's assessment of her infant's temperament based on the Thomas, Chess, and Birch (1968) interview and includes questions related to the infant's rhythmicity, intensity, adaptability, activity, mood, distractability, and threshold to stimulation. A summary score categorizes the infant as having a "difficult" or "easy" temperament.

As can be seen in Table 17.2:

1. Four-month weight measures were significantly lower for the RDS than the term infants, and significantly higher for the postterm infants.

2. Both nonterm groups received inferior ratings on the Denver Developmental Screening Test. An examination of the subscales of the Denver suggested that the postmature infants received inferior ratings on personal–social items and the RDS infants received inferior ratings on personal–social as well as fine- and gross-motor items. These inferior social and motor ratings were consistent with those of the Brazelton neonatal and the later Bayley developmental scales.

3. The mothers of both nonterm groups viewed their infants as having "difficult" temperaments, as evidenced by their less optimal temperament scores. The most striking area of difficult temperament related to the distractability items. The mothers' responses to these items suggested that the infants were difficult to distract from such ongoing activities as fussiness or crying.

TABLE 17.2
Means for 4-Month Assessments that Yielded Significant Group Differences at p < .001

	Group means		
Variable	Preterm RDS	Normal term	Postterm postmature
Weight (gm)	5872	6428	6603
Denver developmental [a]	1.83	1.14	1.52
Infant temperament [a]	2.89	1.83	2.66
Interaction ratings [a]			
Face-to-face	2.20	1.71	2.28
Feeding	2.38	1.45	—

[a] Lower scores are optimal.

4. Both nonterm groups received less optimal ratings than the term group on face-to-face interactions at 4 months. Ratings of the interaction tapes suggested that both groups of nonterm infants were more fussy and gaze averted more often or were less attentive than term infants, and their mothers were more active in their attempts to elicit attention and responses from their infants. Most of the nonterm infants and their mothers appeared to experience difficult interactions. In view of this finding, it is not surprising that the mothers rated their infants as having "difficult" temperaments on the Carey questionnaire.

5. The preterm group alone received less optimal ratings on feeding interactions, which related to the preterm infants being slow feeders and their mothers being overstimulating in their attempts to encourage ingestion of milk.

These inferior temperament and interaction ratings at 4 months combine to suggest that the social interaction problems of the nonterm infants were not confined to the newborn period.

Eight-Month Assessments

Eight-month assessments were made in the homes of the infants. These included the Bayley Mental, Motor, and Behavioral Developmental Scales (Bayley, 1969), the Infant Temperament Questionnaire, and the Caldwell Home Stimulation Inventory (Caldwell, Heider & Kaplan, 1966). The Bayley assessments were chosen since they are standardized and widely used, enabling comparisons with other longitudinal studies. The Caldwell inventory assesses among other things the amount of contact the infant has with adults and the availability of age-appropriate play materials in the home. Although our groups came from comparable socioeconomic backgrounds, we were concerned that the nonterm infants might differ on the Caldwell measure if

TABLE 17.3

Means for 8-Month Assessments that Yielded Significant Group Differences at p < .001

Variable	Group means		
	Preterm RDS	Normal term	Postterm postmature
Bayley mental	88	104	82
Bayley motor	77	106	—
Carey temperament [a]	2.72	1.57	2.48

[a] Lower scores are optimal.

parents were treating them differently and/or were not adapting environments to the developmental delays exhibited by their risk infants.

As can be seen in Table 17.3:

1. The RDS infants received lower scores on both the Bayley mental and motor scales, although their scores were considerably lower on the motor than the mental scale, and the postmatures received Lower Bayley mental scores. Despite a correction for gestational age differences, the RDS infants were continuing to show developmental delays at this period. The discrepancy between their motor and mental scores is consistent with findings on other RDS samples. Ambrus *et al.* (1970) and Fitzhardinge *et al.* (1976), for example, reported considerably lower motor than mental scores for RDS infants. A continuing motoric weakness of the RDS infants seemed to contribute to their lower Bayley motor scores. In addition, an item analysis of the Bayley mental scale suggested that many of the items failed by the RDS infants required fine motor skills. Often the infants appeared to have the requisite cognitive abilities (e.g., object permanence and awareness of object displacements) but failed to complete the tasks successfully because of a lack of coordination and fine motor dexterity. The lower mental scores for the postmature infant are more difficult to understand, although limited attention span and restlessness noted on their Bayley behavioral records may have contributed to their low mental scores.

2. There were no group differences on the Caldwell home stimulation assessment.

3. The mothers of the nonterm groups again at 8 months rated their infants as having difficult temperaments, suggesting some stability of infant temperament and/or stability of the mother's assessment of infant temperament during early infancy.

One-Year Assessments

One-year assessments occurred in a hospital lab and included growth measurements, a pediatric examination, the Pediatric Complications Scale (Littman & Parmelee, 1978), the Ainsworth "strange-situation" procedure

TABLE 17.4
Means for 1-Year Assessments that Yielded Significant Group Differences at p < .001

	Group means		
Variable	Preterm RDS	Normal term	Postterm postmature
Weight (gm)	9280	10,208	—
Head circumference (cm)	—	46	47
Pediatric Complications Scale	91	118	—
Bayley mental	90	110	86
Bayley motor	80	105	—
Bayley behavioral	45	52	46

(Ainsworth & Wittig, 1969), and the Bayley mental, motor, and behavioral scales. The Pediatric Complications Scale is a pediatrician's checklist of abnormal rates of growth and occurrences of illness, injury or hospitalization, physical anomalies, neurological abnormalities, and hearing and visual deficits. The Ainsworth strange-situation procedure was used to determine whether the nonterm infants were exhibiting any attachment disturbances (Main, 1975).

As can be seen in Table 17.4:

1. The RDS babies averaged lower weight and height and the postmatures greater head circumference measurements than the term infants.
2. The term infants experienced the least number of pediatric complications, for example, illnesses and hospitalizations, and the preterm infants the greatest number.
3. Both nonterm groups again received lower Bayley mental and motor scores, particularly the preterm group.
4. Both nonterm groups received less optimal ratings on the Bayley behavioral record.
5. There were no group differences on the Ainsworth strange-situation procedure.

Two-Year Assessments

Two-year assessments occurred in a hospital lab and included growth measurements, a pediatric examination, the Pediatric Complications Scale (PCS), the Bayley mental, motor and behavioral scales, the Behavior Problem Checklist (Quay & Peterson, 1975), the Vineland Social Maturity Scale (Doll, 1965), and a mother–infant play interaction. The Behavior Problem Checklist is a mother's assessment of her child's problematic behaviors, including hyperactivity, distractability, short attention span, irritability, impulsiveness, specific fears, and unclear speech. The Vineland Social Maturity Scale assesses such social milestones as dressing self and helping with household tasks. An assessment of mother–infant interaction occurred during a spontaneous floor play situation. The procedure and toys were similar to those used in another study of 2-year-old child–mother language patterns (Ringler, Kennell, Jarvella, Navojosky, & Klaus, 1975). The mother was told that we wanted to record a sample of the child's language during his free play with her and with the toys. The mother and infant were then left in a room with a selection of toys, and 10 min of infant and mother language were recorded and coded for the following language features: (*a*) the number of questions, statements, and imperatives used by the mother; and (*b*) the infant's working vocabulary (total number of novel words), mean length of utterance, and verbosity (total number of words per 10-min language recording).

As can be seen in Table 17.5:

1. The RDS infants continued to weigh less than the term infants, although their length and head circumference no longer differed, while the postmature infants continued to weigh more, were longer, and had larger head circumferences than the term infants.
2. Pediatric complications of the RDS group were greater than those of the term and postmature groups.
3. Both nonterm groups again received lower Bayley mental and motor

TABLE 17.5
Means for 2-Year Assessments that Yielded Significant Group Differences at p < .001

| | Group means | | |
| | Preterm RDS | Normal term | Postterm postmature |
Variable			
Weight (gm)	11,413	12,231	12,987
Length (cm)	—	86	89
Head circumference (cm)	—	48	51
Pediatric Complications Scale	99	123	—
Bayley mental	95	118	104
Bayley motor	92	115	102
Behavioral Problem Checklist [a]	31	26	—
Vineland Social Maturity Scale	110	123	—
Language ratings			
Mother			
Imperatives [a]	20	17	—
Questions	55	48	—
Statements	25	32	—
Infant			
Verbosity	82	155	—
Working vocabulary	30	54	—
MLU	1.3	1.8	—

[a] Lower scores are optimal.

scores than the term infants, although the differences between RDS and term infants were greater than differences between postmature and term infants.

4. The RDS infants manifested more behavioral problems, such as hyperactivity, irritability, unclear speech, and short attention span on the Behavior Problem Checklist

5. The RDS infants received lower social quotients than did the term and postmature infants on the Vineland Social Maturity Scale.

6. The language recordings of free floor play between infants and mothers suggested that mothers of RDS infants issued more imperatives and questions and fewer statements than the mothers of the term infants. The RDS infants emitted fewer words and exhibited a smaller working vocabulary and a shorter mean length of utterance.

Discussion

Using various assessment scales throughout the first 2 years of life, we were able to identify consistent differences (though the differences were of lesser magnitude by the end of the second year of development) between term and nonterm infants in the areas of medical, physical, mental, motor and behavioral development. The RDS infants had more obstetric and postnatal complications, lower 5-min Apgar scores, and more pediatric complications throughout the first 2 years of life. They were also consistently smaller than the normal term infants, whereas the postterm postmature infants were larger. Delays in mental and motor development (especially the latter) were identified in the RDS infants as early as the newborn period and continuing throughout the 2 years. By 2 years, additional delays were noted in social maturity and language production. The postterm postmature infants also showed developmental delays particularly on the Bayley mental scale assessments. In terms of their behavioral development, both groups of nonterm infants were difficult to test as newborns and received inferior interaction scores on the Brazelton. At 4 months, they performed less optimally on the personal–social items of the Denver, received less optimal interaction ratings during face-to-face interactions with their mothers, and were described by their mothers as having "difficult" temperaments. At 2 years of age, the RDS group alone was showing behavioral problems.

Despite these medical, physical, mental, motor, and behavioral differences, the home environments of term and nonterm infants did not differ. Although this may indicate that the parents were not treating their nonterm infants differently and were sensitive to the importance of developmentally appropriate play material and experiences, the Caldwell scale may be less sensitive to differences within an homogenous social class (i.e., the middle class of our term and nonterm infants). The Caldwell also failed to discriminate preterm infants within another homogenous social class, the lower class (Bakeman, 1978), suggesting that it may be a better discriminator of home environments across rather than within social class.

The continuing developmental delays shown by our RDS infants suggest that RDS may contribute to the effects of prematurity or that gestational age adjustments do not compensate for differences between preterm and term groups. Other investigators of prematurity have also suggested that even after gestational age corrections have been made preterm infants continue to show developmental delays (Caputo, Goldstein, & Taub, 1979). As suggested by Hunt (Chapter 19), even small delays at this age may be important. Not having a preterm control group (without RDS) in this study obviates any definitive statement on the degree to which RDS contributes to prematurity.

It should also be noted that despite significant differences those differences between our preterm RDS and term groups are considerably diminished by 2 years. The Bayley scores of the RDS group (95 for mental and 92 for motor) are closer to the mean for this scale than they were at 1 year (90 for mental and 80 for motor). The scores of the term infants are considerably higher than Bayley mean scores at both 1 and 2 years (110 and 105 at 1 year and 118 and 115 at 2 years), suggesting that the norms for the Bayley scale may be shifting or the term infants may be testing at the ceiling for the Bayley on many items at 2 years. Thus, it is not clear whether the preterm infants are only delayed in comparison with this superior performance of full-term infants or whether the norms shifted such that the high scores of the term infants constitute average performance and the scores of the preterms RDS group relatively delayed performance.

A study of earlier survivors of RDS by our group suggests that by 4 years the language delays and behavioral problems of the RDS group are more pronounced (Field et al., 1979) than they were at 2 years in the present study. Thus, the 2-year indicators of these potential developmental problems probably suggest early intervention efforts.

Just as the neonatal problems of the postmature infant are more subtle, an interpretation of their continuing developmental delays is more difficult. It is not clear whether intrauterine stress due to placental deterioration or large birth size or other factors contributed to these delays. The long-term effects of placental deterioration and associated fetal hypoxia are largely unknown. Although there is some evidence that large-for-date infants are at risk for developmental deficits (Lubchenco & Little, 1977), it is not clear whether the postterm postmaturity syndrome infants of this study can be compared to a large-for-date group. Nonetheless, despite the absence of neonatal complications in the postterm infants, their perinatal complications and deflated Brazelton and Bayley scores suggest that the development of postterm postmaturity syndrome infants, like that of preterm RDS infants, should be closely monitored. Being born not at term is not necessarily a risk factor, but when compounded by such syndromes as respiratory distress or postmaturity, the risk for developmental delays appears to be more pronounced.

Acknowledgments

We would like to thank the mothers and infants who participated in this study. For assistance with data collection, additional thanks go to Catherine Benson, Cyrus Dabiri, Norma Hallock, Judith Hatch, Sally Leeds, Catherine Larned, and George Ting.

References

Ainsworth, M., & Wittig, B. Attachment and exploratory behavior of one-year-olds in a strange situation. In B. M. Foss (Ed.), *Determinants of infant behavior*. London: Methuen, 1969.

Als, H., Tronick, E, Lester, B. M., & Brazelton, T. B. The Brazelton Neonatal Behavioral Assessment Scale (BNBAS). *Journal of Abnormal Child Psychology*, 1977, *5*, 205–213.

Ambrus, C., Weintraub, D., Niswander, K., Fischer, L., Fleishman, J., Bross, I., & Ambrus, J. Evaluation of survivors of the respiratory distress syndrome. *Journal of Pediatrics*, 1970, *120*, 296–302.

Bakeman, R. Personal Communication; 1978.

Bayley, N. *Manual for the Bayley Scales of Infant Development*. New York: Psychological Corp., 1969.

Brazelton, T. B. *Neonatal Behavioral Assessment Scale*. London: Spastics International Medical Publications, 1973.

Brazelton, T. B. Working session on the Brazelton supplement for premature infants at the biennial meeting of the Society for Research in Child Development, Denver, March 1975.

Butler, N. R., & Alberman, E. D. *Perinatal problems: The second report of 1958 British perinatal mortality survey*. London: Livingston, 1969.

Caldwell, B. M., Heider, J., & Kaplan, B. The inventory of home stimulation. Paper presented at the meeting of the American Psychological Association, New York, September 1966. (Available from Center for Early Development and Education, 814 Sherman, Little Rock, Arkansas 72202.)

Caputo, D. V., Goldstein, K. M., & Taub, H. B. The development of prematurely born children through middle childhood. In T. Field, A. Sostek, S. Goldberg & H. H. Shuman (Eds.), *Infants born at risk*. New York: Spectrum 1979.

Carey, W. B. A simplified method of measuring infant temperament. *Journal of Pediatrics*, 1970, *77*, 188–194.

Clifford, S. H. Postmaturity—with placental dysfunction: Clinical syndrome and pathological findings. *Journal of Pediatrics*, 1954, *44*, 1–13.

DiVitto, B., & Goldberg, S. The effects of newborn medical status on early parent–infant interaction. In T. Field, A. Sostek, S. Goldberg, & H. H. Shuman (Eds.), *Infants born at risk*. New York: Spectrum, 1979.

Doll, E. A. *Vineland Social Maturity Scale*. Minnesota: American Guidance Service, Inc. 1965.

Drillien, C. M. Studies in mental handicap, II: Some obstetric factors of possible aetiological significance. *Archives of Disease in Childhood*, 1968, *43*, 283–288.

Field, T. Effects of early separation, interactive deficits, and experimental manipulations on infant–mother face-to-face interaction. *Child Development*, 1977, *48*, 763–771. (a)

Field, T. Maternal stimulation during infant feeding. *Developmental Psychology*, 1977, *13*, 339–540. (b)

Field, T., Dempsey, J., & Shuman, H. H. Developmental assessments of infants surviving the respiratory distress syndrom. In T. Field, A. Sostek, S. Goldberg, & H. H. Shuman (Eds.), *Infants born at risk*. New York: Spectrum, 1979.

Fisch, R., Bilek, M., Miller, L., & Engel, R. Physical and mental status at 4 years of age of survivors of the respiratory distress syndrome. *Journal of Pediatrics*, 1975, *86*, 497–503.

Fisch, R. O., Gravem, H. J., & Engel, R. R. Neurological status of survivors of neonatal respiratory distress syndrome. *Journal of Pediatrics,* 1968, *73,* 395.

Fitzhardinge, P. M., Pape, K., Arstikaitis, M., Boyle, M., Ashby, S., Rowley, A., Netley, C., & Swyer, P. R. Mechanical ventilation of infants of less than 1,50l grams birth weight: Health, growth and neurological sequelae. *Journal of Pediatrics,* 1976, *88,* 531.

Frankenburg, W. K., & Dodds, J. B. The Denver Developmental Screening Test. *Journal of Pediatrics,* 1967, *71,* 181–191.

Harrod, J. R., L'Heureaux, P., Wangensteen, D. O., & Hunt, C. D. Long-term follow-up of severe respiratory distress syndrome treated with IPPV. *Journal of Pediatrics,* 1974, *84,* 277.

Johnson, J. D., Malachowski, N. C., Grobstein, R., Daily, W. J. R., & Sunshine, P. Prognosis of children surviving with the aid of mechanical ventilation in the newborn period. *Journal of Pediatrics,* 1974, *84,* 272.

Lester, B. M., & Zeskind, P. S. The organization of crying in the infant at risk. In T. M. Field, A. M. Sostek, S. Goldberg, & H. H. Shuman (Eds.), *Infants born at risk.* New York: Spectrum, 1979.

Littman, B. & Parmelee, A. H. Medical correlates of infant development. *Pediatrics,* 1978, *61,* 470–474.

Lovell, K. E. The effect of postmaturity on the developing child. *Medical Journal of Australia,* 1973, *1,* 13–17.

Lubchenco, L. O., & Little, G. A. The outcome of large, preterm infants: An unexpected high-risk population. *Pediatric Research,* 1977, *11,* 421.

Main, M. Autism and adaptation. Paper presented to the International Society for the Study of havioral Development, University of Surrey, Guildford, July 1975.

Morrison, D. F. *Multivariate statistical methods.* New York: McGraw-Hill, 1967.

Myers, J. L. *Fundamentals of experimental design.* Boston: Allyn & Bacon, 1972.

Outerbridge, E. W., & Stern, L. Developmental follow-up of artificially ventilated infants with neonatal respiratory failure. *Pediatric Research,* 1972, *6,* 412.

Prechtl, H. F. R. Neurological findings in newborn infants after pre and paranatal complications. In J. H. P. Jonxis, H. D. Vissez, & J. A. Troelstra (Eds.), *Dysmaturity and prematurity.* Leiden: Droese, 1968.

Quay, H., & Peterson, D. R. Manual for the behavior problem checklist. Unpublished manuscript, 1975. (Available from first author, Mailman Center for Child Development, Miami Florida 33152.)

Rao, C. R. *Linear statistical inference and its applications.* New York: Wiley, 1973.

Ringler, N. M., Kennell, J. H., Jarvella, R., Navojosky, B. J., & Klaus, M. H. Mother-to-child speech at 2 years—effects of early postnatal contact. *Journal of Pediatrics,* 1975, *1,* 141.

Sostek, A. M., & Anders, T. F. Relationships among the Brazelton neonatal scale, Bayley infant scales, and early temperament. *Child Development,* 1977, *48,* 320–323.

Sostek, A., Quinn, P., & Davitt, M. K. Behavior, development and neurologic status of premature and full-term infants with varying medical complications. In T. Field, A. Sostek, S. Goldberg, & H. H. Shuman (Eds.) *Infants born at risk.* New York: Spectrum, 1979.

Stahlman, M., Hedwall, G., Dolanski, E., Foxelius, G., Burko, H., & Kirk, V. A six-year follow-up of clinical hyaline membrane disease. *Pediatric Clinics of North America,* 1973, *20,* 433.

Thomas, A., Chess, S., & Birch, H. G. *Temperament and behavior disorders in children.* New York: New York Univ. Press, 1968.

Wagner, M. G., & Arndt, R. Postmaturity as an aetiological factor in 124 cases of neurologically handicapped children. In R. C. MacKeith & M. C. O. Bax (Eds.), *Studies in infancy.* London: Heinemann, 1968.

Zwerdling, M. A. Factors pertaining to prolonged pregnancy and its outcome. *Pediatrics,* 1967, *40,* 202–212.

The Relation of
Early Infant Measures to
Later Development[1]

MARIAN SIGMAN

SARALE E. COHEN

ALAN B. FORSYTHE

Consistency in the rate of behavioral development from birth through the first years of life has not been demonstrated with any power. In addition, prediction from early medical complications to later mental performance is poor. Some authors have suggested that qualitative change in the infant's behaviors and skills is responsible for the lack of prediction from one age period to another (McCall, Hogarty, & Hurlburt, 1972). According to this viewpoint, infant development is not a steady progression but a series of stages that can be negotiated with varying degrees of success.

There is another possible explanation for both the lack of consistency in the infant's developmental progress as well as the restricted effects of early trauma. Of all periods of life, infancy may represent a time of special responsiveness between organism and caregiving environment. Because of primitive adaptive mechanisms, the neonate is particularly dependent on the responses of the caregiver. Furthermore, caregivers may be primed to respond in specific ways to the characteristics of the infant, whether in an adaptive fashion that facilitates optimal development or a maladaptive fashion that limits it.

With both systems changing rapidly, there is more plasticity in each. Because the relationship between the two is evolving, a measure of either system may not accurately reflect the other. In contrast, later in childhood, the relationship between child and caregiving environment is more stabilized, so that an assessment of one provides substantial information about the other and it is quite difficult to bring about change in either alone. Thus, the iden-

[1] This research was supported by National Institute of Child Health Development Contract 1–HD–3–2776 and by a grant from the William T. Grant Foundation.

tification of continuity from early infancy may depend on frequent assessments of the transactions between child and environment.

These assessments must focus on the interaction between caregiver and child. For most infants, the relationship between infant and caregiving environment is reflected predominantly in this interaction. The principal caregiver provides most of the infant's early learning experiences. Furthermore, the infant's own behaviors have a substantial impact on this interaction. We are suggesting that predictions of developmental level from events and observations in the first few months of life to early childhood outcomes may be misleading unless the nature of the caregiver–infant interactions is considered. This suggestion is based on conclusions from our longitudinal study of preterm infants carried out at the University of California, Los Angeles.

In predicting developmental status at age 2 years from a battery of diagnostic assessments carried out in the first year of life as part of this longitudinal study, the major predictors were behavioral and developmental measures at 8–9 months of age (Sigman & Parmelee, 1979). Most notable about the best subsets of effective predictor variables was the absense of early medical and behavioral factors. We have attempted to understand the underlying basis for the absence and presence of predicted relationships between the early measures and outcome. The aim of this chapter is to review these findings. Our tentative conclusion is that for the most part it was the early measures related to caregiver–infant interaction that were subsequently tied to developmental outcome. Furthermore, the predictive relationship between early measures and outcome may have been mediated by the caregiver–infant interaction. Consistency in early development may derive from the stability maintained in the interaction of caregiver and child despite the variability in early medical and behavioral factors.

For purposes of illustrating our evidence, three separate data sources will be discussed in detail. First, we will concentrate on the complex relationship between early medical complications and outcome. In this analysis, we have employed the overall risk scores, since the extent of medical complications was most meaningfully reflected in total scores. Second, the data from one type of behavioral measure, assessments of visual attention, will be discussed. In the final section, an integrated model for relating all the first-year risk scores is presented.

Infant Assessments in the First 2 Years of Life

To review our longitudinal study briefly, a risk-assessment system was developed that included measures of the infants at term through 9 months, with outcome assessment at 2 and 5 years. Only the 2-year outcome measures have been administered to the entire sample to date, so discussion will be restricted to the 18-month Bayley mental score and 24-month Gesell score.

Assessments and outcome measures included in the original risk score

TABLE 18.1

Correlations between Individual Diagnostic Measures and Outcome Assessments

Meaures	Age at administration in months[a]	18-month Bayley	24-month Gesell
Obstetric Complications Scale	Birth		
Postnatal Complications Scale	First month of life		
Sleep polygraph	Term		
Newborn neurological	Term		
Visual attention	Term	− .27*	
Caregiver–infant interaction	1	.21*	.21*
Sleep polygraph	3		
Pediatric Complications Scale	4	.23*	.23*
Gesell Developmental Scale	4	.38*	.29*
Visual attention	4		
Caregiver–infant interaction	8	.27*	.35*
Manipulative schemas	8	.21*	.26*
Exploratory behavior	8	.24*	.20*
Casati–Lezine	9	.36*	.39*
Gesell Developmental Scale	9	.60*	.48*
Pediatric Complications Scale	9	.23*	

* $p < .05$

[a] All ages are calculated from expected date of birth.

system (see Table 18.1) have been described in detail in Parmelee, Kopp, and Sigman (1976) and in Sigman and Parmelee (1979). The set of caregiver–infant assessments were not included in the original risk score system but were obtained to understand the process of early development. These assessments were based on home observations and have been discussed in Beckwith, Cohen, Kopp, Parmelee, and Marcy (1976). As our data indicated the importance of including the caregiving environment in predicting development, a summary home visit risk score was derived from a subset of reciprocal behaviors (Beckwith, in press).

Study Sample

Subjects were 126 preterm infants with a gestational age at birth of 37 weeks or less and a birthweight of 2500 gm or less. All were cared for in the UCLA newborn nursery. Gestational age was calculated according to maternal report. All testing was carried out at conceptional ages with correction for the length of prematurity. A breakdown of the distribution of subjects according to sex, language background, socioeconomic status, and birth order is shown in Table 18.2. Socioeconomic status (SES) was determined using a weighting system that combined the duration of maternal education with a rating of paternal occupation. The sample cells of high SES, Spanish-speaking infants were virtually empty, so that the language and SES variables were confounded.

TABLE 18.2
Distribution of Subjects

	Male (N)		Female (N)	
	First born	Later born	First born	Later born
High SES				
English	9	13	12	10
Spanish	1	0	0	0
Bilingual	2	1	0	0
Other	6	0	0	0
Low SES				
English	11	9	6	5
Spanish	10	11	6	9
Bilingual	3	0	1	1
Other	0	0	0	0

Medical Complications and Outcome

Medical complications were measured with several separate scales, one assessing obstetrical complications and the others recording illness and medical events throughout the first 2 years (see Table 18.1). As mentioned above, obstetrical and postnatal medical complications were not individually related to outcome (see Table 18.1), nor did they contribute significantly to best subsets generated from the measures in relation to Gesell developmental scores at 2 years. Example of two best subsets are shown in Tables 18.3 and 18.4. For the total sample, the only medical event scales that centered into the regression equation were the assessments of pediatric complications at 4 and 9 months. For the female sample, the group for whom prediction was most accurate, there was some contribution by postnatal and obstetrical complications, but the amount of the variance accounted for by these measures was small (see Table 18.4).

Furthermore, a division of the sample into high-risk and low-risk groups based on cumulative performance on the 14 original assessments did not differentiate the infants significantly at 2 years unless the two caregiver–infant measures were also included in the risk assessment. The explanation seemed to be that early medical and behavioral measures were classifying infants incorrectly, and only the inclusion of environmental measure rectified this misclassification. Partial suppport for this hypothesis comes from the finding that caregivers interacted more with infants suffering postnatal medical complications than with healthy infants (Beckwith & Cohen, 1978). Since caregiver–infant interaction at 1 and 8 months is related to developmental outcome at 2 years (Cohen & Beckwith, 1979), remediation by the environment may have diminished the effects of early illness.

TABLE 18.3

Best Subset Regression of the Diagnostic Measures to the 2-Year Gesell Examination for Total Sample[a]

Diagnostic measure	Cumulative adjusted R^2
Gesell examination, 9 months	.20
Manipulative schema, 8 months	.24
Caregiver–infant interaction, 8 months	.26
Casati-Lezine, 9 months	.27
Visual attention, term	.28
Pediatric Complications Scale, 4 months	.29
Visual attention, 4 months	.30
Sleep polygraph, 3 months	.30
Pediatric Complications Scale, 9 months	.30
Exploratory behavior, 8 months	.30
	$(F = 6.37, p < .001)$
All measures	.28
	$(F = 4.0, p < .001)$

[a] $N = 126$.

Outcome at 9 Months

We postulated that early medical complications might be related to later development in several complex ways. First, infants who were sick early in life might continue to suffer pediatric complications that would affect their overall development. A negative association between the number of pediatric complications suffered from 4 to 9 months of age and the 9-month Gesell

TABLE 18.4

Best Subset Regression of the Diagnostic Measures to the 2-Year Gesell Examination for the Female Sample[a]

Diagnostic measure	Cumulative adjusted R^2
Caregiver–infant interaction, 8 months	.31
Exploratory behavior, 8 months	.37
Caregiver–infant interaction, 1 month	.49
Postnatal factors, 1 month	
Pediatric Complications Scale, 9 months	.51
Obstetrical Complications Scale, term	.59
Casati–Lezine Scale, 9 months	.63
Manipulative schema, 8 months	.65
Sleep polygraph, term	.66
	$(F = 11.7, p < .001)$
All measures	.62
	$(F = 5.9, p < .001)$

[a] $N = 50$.

score has been identified for this sample (Littman & Parmelee, 1978). An indirect way in which the early complications suffered by the infant might have been linked to subsequent development would be through the environment. The model, then, allows for medical complications to have both direct and indirect influences on development.

In order to test this hypothesized model, path analysis of the data from the entire sample was carried out. Path analysis is a method for relating variables to each other, both directly and indirectly, and assessing the degree of association between variables with standardized regression coefficients. Like other forms of analysis, the possibility exists that other, stronger associations may never be disclosed since all possible relationships between variables are not tested. For this hypothetical model, the variables used were the risk scores of caregiver–infant interaction, and the Gesell score at 9 months. In all cases, a higher score represents more optimal conditions.

The path model and standardized regression coefficients (*R*s) are shown in Figure 18.1. Almost all the regression coefficients were significant. The indirect path from postnatal complications through caregiver interaction to out- However, there was some influence by medical complications, so that illness did deflate developmental progress to some extent. Thus, the results showed two different and opposing links between early illness and later performance. One reflected the remediation effect by the environment; the caregivers of sick babies interacted more than the caregivers of healthy babies, and the level of care did relate to the infant's later performance. On the other hand, sickness did tend to continue and finally depressed development to some degree. Early illness had no direct association with outcome because the two paths had opposite effects that cancelled each other out.

To illustrate these results, the data can be shown for a single case. In Figure 18.2, the scores for one infant are presented with values standardized using the means and standard deviations of the entire sample for each measure. As the figure shows, even with a low postnatal complications scale score, the income was much stronger than the direct path through medical complications.

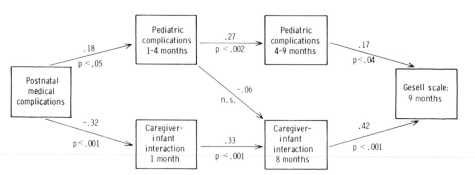

FIGURE 18.1. *Path model and standardized regression coefficients for the sample of preterm infants to 9-month Gesell score.*

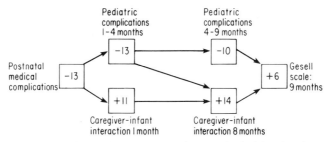

FIGURE 18.2. *Standardized risk scores for an individual female infant.*

fant performed better than the mean on the Gesell at 9 months. She did not perform as well as one expect given the level of interaction nor as poorly as might be suggested by the nature of her pediatric complications.

In order to understand the effects of early illness on subsequent development, the environmental transactions between the infant and caregiver had to be considered not only for this infant but for the sample as a whole. Of course, there were infants for whom the developmental score was more strongly influenced by pediatric problems. Several children with serious physical complications, including three with moderate cerebral palsy, were included in the sample. An example of the path diagram for one infant with cerebral palsy is shown in Fig. 18.3. For these infants, Gesell scores at 9 months tended to be more highly associated with the pediatric events scale than with caregiver–infant interaction. This may not be so true at 5 years, when the outcome measure involves fewer motor skills and more cognitive abilities. In other words, there were children whose physical problems dominated their development. Subsequent outcome measures may show that the nature of the environmental response to such problems remains important.

Sex Differences

Analyses were carried out separately for males and females because of the significant sex differences reported for the overall cumulative risk score system (Sigman & Parmelee, 1979). With the overall system, prediction to out-

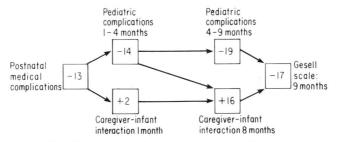

FIGURE 18.3. *Standardized risk scores for an infant with cerebral palsy.*

come was significant for females but not for males. Furthermore, the regression of the 16 measures to outcome was significantly greater for females than males ($F = 2.50$, $p < .01$).

The separate path analyses showed one notable difference. As measured by the overall risk score, caregiver–infant interaction at 1 month was not linked significantly to postnatal complications for males. On the other hand, boys who were less healthy through the first 4 months did engage in more reciprocal interactions with their caregivers ($r = -.23$, $p < .05$) by 8 months of age. It appears that caregivers were slower to differentiate between males on the basis of health status. We have found other sex differences in the relationship between infant variables and subsequent caregiver–infant interactions, although the variables themselves were distributed similarly for males and females (Sigman & Beckwith, 1980).

Two-Year Outcome

Similar path analyses to 24-month Gesell showed that the pediatric events path had decreasing effects on infant outcome (see Figure 18.4). Neither complications assessed at 9 months nor complications assessed at 24 months related significantly to Gesell score at 24 months, although 4-month pediatric complications score did. It may be that early illness has a more profound effect on behavioral development than does later illness.

There was also a major sex difference in the relationship of caregiver–infant interaction to 24-month Gesell score. While caregiver–infant interaction at 8 months was significantly associated with 24-month Gesell score for the females ($r = .52$, $p < .01$), the relationship was insignificant for the males ($r = .13$). The influence of the caregiver–infant interaction on the infant's development was more sustained for female than for male infants.

These sex differences appear when the risk scores are used. In analyses of individual factor scores, there were no overall gender differences. However,

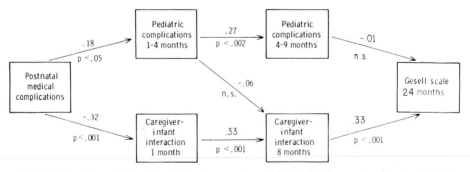

FIGURE 18.4. *Path model and standardized regression coefficients for the sample of preterm infants to 24-month Gesell score.*

there were more separate significant relationships for females than for males (Cohen & Beckwith, 1979).

Visual Attention and Outcome

Just as the early medical factors were uncorrelated with outcome, so the risk scores from the early behavioral measures contributed very little to accurate prediction (see Table 18.1). The only term measure to enter into the best-subset regression was the visual attention measure (see Table 18.3). Based on our findings with medical complications, we postulated that the term visual attention measure might have had some stability because of its relationship to subsequent caregiver–infant interaction. Analyses were carried out to determine if total attentiveness was associated with outcome and caregiver–infant interaction.

Attentiveness at Term

The purpose of this assessment was to measure the responsiveness of the infant to visual stimuli. Attentiveness was measured with a two-dimensional, black and white 2 × 2 checkerboard chosen for its demonstrated salience to newborns. The matrix was shown for three trials of 60-sec duration and illuminated with alternating flashling lights on the second trial. The infants' visual responses were observed, and total fixation times in sec were recorded for each trial.

In developing the measure, we postulated that attentive infants had behavioral states that were in better control, so that they could make maximum contact with the external environment. Although this seems true for full-term infants (Sigman, Kopp, Parmelee, & Jeffrey, 1973), many preterm infants, tested at matched conceptional age, showed extremely long durations of visual attention (Sigman, Kopp, Littman, & Parmelee, 1977). The long fixations shown by many preterm infants seem to stem from a failure to show appropriate response decrement (Sigman & Beckwith, 1980).

The data from the longitudinal study show an inverse relation between total fixation time at term and outcome at age 2 years. The correlations between total fixation time and Bayley mental score ($r = -.23$, $df = 117$, $p < .05$) and 24-month Gesell ($r = -.19$, $df = 121$, $p < .05$) were negative and low but significant. The associations were significant for the females ($r = -.36$, $df = 47$, $p < .05$ for 18-month Bayley; $r = -.27$, $df = 46$, $p < .05$ for 24-month Gesell) and not for the males ($rs = -.13$ and $-.07$).

In order to assess whether caregivers varied their interactions according to attentiveness as measured in the laboratory, the sample was divided equally according to total attentiveness on all three trials. All low-attentiveness infants, whether male or female, were held more by their caregivers 1 month later in the home. Low-attentiveness females were involved in greater verbal and visual interaction with their caregivers than the other three groups of infants; caregivers did not differentiate between high- and low-attentiveness males in terms of their verbal interactions.

Thus, the data revealed that preterm infants, particularly females, who fixated the laboratory stimuli for sizeable lengths of time were interacted with less at home 1 month later. The direction of effects cannot be specified. Since these preterm infants went home from the hospital at about 36 weeks conceptional age, most had been home for at least 1 month before the laboratory assessment. Some infants may have been interested in inanimate stimulation because of a dearth of social stimulation at home. On the other hand, preterm infants who showed prolonged engagement with inanimate stimuli in the laboratory may have acted similarly at home, thereby eliciting fewer caregiver responses.

In any case, visual attentiveness was related to both outcomes and to caregiver–infant interaction. The link between these measures seems to have been the home interaction. Path analysis suggests that the association is, in fact, an indirect one through the caregiver–infant interaction. Standard regression coefficients from total fixation time to the caregiver–infant interaction risk score ($R = .26$, $df = 111$, $p < .006$) and from caregiver–infant interaction to 24-month Gesell score ($R = +.27$, $df = 111$, $p < .004$) were significant, but the direct path was no longer significant when this indirect link was considered. The tie between the attentiveness of the preterm infant and later developmental competence seems to derive from the caregiver's response to the infant's behaviors.

Visual Discrimination at 4 Months

At four months, differentiation and recognition was studied using a variety of stimulus comparisons (Sigman & Parmelee, 1974). A paired comparison technique was employed with 10-sec trials. The infant was first shown a photograph of a woman's face paired with a 12 × 12 checkerboard matrix. The following sequence of eight trials paired checkerboards varying in number of squares with the position of the simple and complex checkerboards counterbalanced over trials. The following four trials paired drawings and photographs of faces with features in regular and scrambled arrangements. The final sequence showed the infant the same 12 × 12 checkerboard for four trials, followed by the paired presentation of familiar and novel representations with the position of novel and familiar stimuli varying over trials.

The infant's attention to each stimulus was observed and recorded. For each infant, then, there was a measure of initial preference for a representation of an animate or inanimate stimuli, a measure of preference for complexity, a measure of attentiveness to social stimuli, and a measure of preference for novel over familiar stimuli.

In a previous publication (Sigman & Parmelee, 1974), we reported that preterm infants were less likely to show preferences for novel stimuli then were full-term infants. However, analysis of the data from the longitudinal study indicated that about two-thirds of the preterm infants did look longer at the novel stimulus. Infants who showed a preference for novel stimuli differed from the infants who did not show this preference on the early risk measures (Hotelling's $T^2 = 3.47$, $p < .01$). The small group of preterm infants who did not show a novelty preference had suffered more obstetrical complications. In other words, preterm infants who looked longer at familiar stimuli tended to have had more complicated births.

Furthermore, for the females, the strength of novelty preference was significantly related to social and verbal interaction at home 3 months earlier (see Table 18.5). Girls who looked longer at novel rather than familiar stimuli had been given more social attention by their caretakers at 1 month of age. In addition, females who looked longer at all the representations of social stimuli had been more involved with their caretakers in mutual visual regard at 1 month of age (see Table 18.5). This result is similar to findings reported by Moss and Robson (1968) with a full-term sample. Although mean fixation time was greater to the 12×12 checkerboard than to the paired photograph of a woman's face for the entire sample, those female infants who showed a greater preference for the woman's face had been more involved in mutual visual regard. Preference for the woman's face over the geometric form was also related to 24-month Gesell score for the females. Preference for social stimuli was the only part of this assessment that showed any predictive validity.

TABLE 18.5

Correlations between the Caregiver–Infant Interaction Factors and 4-Month Visual Preference Measures for the Female Infants [a]

Interaction factors	Preference for novel stimuli	Preference for photographed face	Total fixation–faces
Socal	.28*	—	—
Responsive holding		—	—
Verbal	.31*	—	—
Mutual gazing		.29*	.36*
Stressful holding		—	—
Gesell score, 24 months		.32*	—

[a] $N = 50$.

* $p < .05$

The strength of novelty preference did not relate to outcome for either males or females. A comparison of the Gesell scores of the 67 infants who showed a novelty preference with the scores of the 23 infants who did not show such preferences was not significant. The ability to recognize visual stimuli did not predict to 2-year outcome for this sample of infants.

In summary, the only component that did relate to outcome was a measure of responsiveness to social representations that also related to social interaction 3 months previously. In terms of our overall statement regarding prediction, the results from the 4-month visual attention measure substantiate our previous results. Only in those cases where the behavioral measures were correlated with the earlier interaction was there any predictive significance. However, behavior could be related to interaction without having any link to outcome.

A Conceptualization of Early Relations

In order to understand the processes of development, we formulated a developmental model of the relation between our diagnostic assessments and outcome. For the purposes of this initial formulation, the 9-month Gesell score was used as an outcome variable and the 9-month cognitive measure was omitted from consideration. All the other assessments were included, as were the demographic factors of sex, socioeconomic status, birth order, and language background.

The model is presented in Figure 18.5, along with the standardized regression coefficients derived from the data on the 126 preterm infants. As can be seen, we hypothesized three general paths. The first path, shown at the top of the figure, represents medical complications assessed over time. The middle section of the figure is the path representing the relationships between behavioral, neurological, and developmental assessments of the infant. The lower section of the figure presents the hypothesized link between the environmental variables, including observations of caregiver–infant interaction and demographic factors.

Obviously, numerous other path models can be formulated. However, path analysis is most effective if one suggests a limited number of theoretically justified alternatives. The avoidance of overfitting requires a commitment to a limited number of hypothetical models. We based our path model on certain assumptions about the nature of relationships between variables. We present the results of our postulated model with the caveat that this is not the only possible model and that stronger coefficients might have been obtained.

The data presented in Figure 18.5 suggest that the environmental path is most critical in determining outcome. To the extent that status on the 9-month Gesell is predicted by the earlier measures, the strongest earlier assessments are the 8-month caregiver–infant interaction measure and the 4-month Gesell

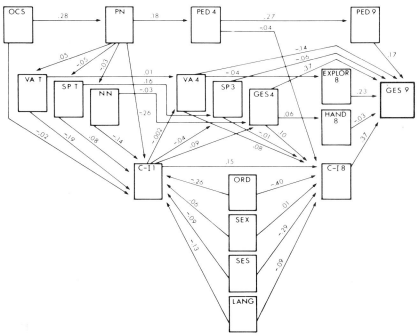

FIGURE 18.5. *Path model for all the diagnostic measures. The age of administration is indicated by the numeral or letter following the abbreviation, with T representing term date. OCS, Obstetric Complications Scale; PN, Postnatal Complications Scale; PED, Pediatric Complications Scale; VA, visual attention; SP, sleep polygraph; NN, newborn neurological examination; GES, Gesell scale; EXPLOR, exploratory behavior; HAND, manipulative schemas; C-I, caregiver-infant interaction. Demographic factors are included with ORD representing birth order and LANG representing language background.*

scale. The latter is related to the 9-month Gesell although not associated with the interaction measure. Thus, the path data indicate that certain 4-month assessments do have associations with outcome independent of the interaction measures. The approach to data analysis illustrated here is now being extended to the 2-year outcome measures.

Discussion

In summary, analyses of the relationships between early measures and outcome were carried out because of previous indications that early measures had little direct impact on outcome. These analyses have shown that neonatal condition is related to outcome in complex ways. We have hypothesized that the interaction of child and caregiver is a mediating link between the early events and behaviors and future competence.

While the evidence for this hypothesis is fairly strong for the term assessments, the results are less clear by 4 and 8 months. Some of the 4- and 8-month measures were individually related to outcome even when they did not tie into the caregiver–infant interaction. Other measures, such as the visual attention assessment, were not predictive except for the component associated with earlier social interaction. On the other hand, O'Connor (1980) has found a strong relationship between a 4-month measure of auditory discrimination and Bayley score at 18 months for a portion of the females in this same sample. This relationship was significant even when demographic factors were considered. However, no significant relationship existed for the male sample.

The sex differences reported by O'Connor have emerged from all our analyses of the larger sample. Relationships between early measures and outcome have frequently been significant for females and insignificant for males. Yang and Moss (1978) suggest that endogenous factors are more stable for males, whereas environmental factors have more influence on females. Our data corroborate the second part of this statement.

Several other studies have demonstrated significant relationships between early behavioral measures and subsequent outcome for full-term infants. Roe (1978) found that differential vocal response to an interactive mother versus an interactive stranger was highly related to Stanford-Binet scale score at age 3 years for a small sample of males. Fagan (1979) reported a significant association between degree of novelty preference in early infancy and verbal intelligence at 4 and 6 years of age.

Of course, the relationship between the infant characteristic and outcome in Fagan's study may be attributable to environmental factors. The predictive relationship between preference for novelty and outcome may be due to the environment's role in fostering this preference. We have presented evidence, at least for females, that preference for novelty is greater among infants who previously had more social attention from their caregivers. Cohen (Chapter 13, this volume) has shown that preference for novelty is partly a function of socioeconomic status. Rose and Bridger (1979) have found that early stimulation can enhance preference for novelty in preterm infants. Thus, the consistencies that have been identified may result from some environmental pattern of stimulation or interaction.

While the identification of diagnostic predictors is critical for selecting truly high-risk infants who need intervention, the planning of treatment depends on an understanding of the processes of development. Even though "marker" variables may be critical for diagnosis, treatment may need to focus not on these markers but on the conditions that maintain the marker variables or give them significance. Intervention will have to focus on the environmental factors that limit or enhance the child's cognitive problems. In this chapter, we have attempted to move from an identification of marker variables to an understanding of developmental processes.

In summary, the data from our longitudinal study indicate that infant characteristics in the first few months of life do not relate directly to outcome on developmental examinations at 2 years of age but do have some indirect effect. We have argued that the significance of early medical events and infant behaviors must be assessed in the light of the caregiver–infant interaction. Even in those studies where predictive relationships have been identified, we may need to understand developmental processes in order to plan intervention.

References

Beckwith, L. The influence of caregiver–infant interaction on development. In E. J. Sell (Ed.), *Follow-up of the high-risk newborn: A practical approach*. Springfield, Ill.: Thomas, in press.

Beckwith, L., & Cohen, S. E. Preterm birth: Hazardous obstetrical and postnatal events as related to caregiver–infant behavior. *Infant Behavior and Development*, 1978, *1*, 403–411.

Beckwith, L., Cohen, S. E., Kopp, C. B., Parmelee, A. H., & Marcy, T. G. Caregiver–infant interaction and early cognitive development in preterm infants. *Child Development*, 1976, *47*, 579–587.

Cohen, S. E., & Beckwith, L. Preterm infant interaction with the caregiver in the first year of life and competence at age two. *Child Development*, 1979, *50*, 767–776.

Fagan, J. F. Infant recognition memory and later intelligence. Paper presented at the Bienniel Meeting of the Society for Research in Child Development, San Francisco, March 1979.

Littman, B., & Parmelee, A.H. Medical correlates of infant development. *Pediatrics*, 1978, *61*, 470–474.

McCall, R. B., Hogarty, P. S., & Hurlburt, N. Transitions in infant sensorimotor development and the prediction of childhood IQ. *American Psychologist*, 1972, *27*, 728–748.

Moss, H. A., & Robson, K. S. Maternal influences in early social visual behavior. *Child Development*, 1968, *39*, 401–408.

O'Connor, M. J. A comparison of preterm and full-term infants on 4-month auditory discrimination and 18-month Bayley. *Child Development*, 1980, *51*, 81–88.

Parmelee, A. H., Kopp, C. B., & Sigman, M. Selection of developmental assessment techniques for infants at risk. *Merril-Palmer Quarterly*, 1976, *22*, 177–199.

Roe, K. V. Infants' mother–stranger discrimination at 3 months as a predictor of cognitive development at 3 and 5 years. *Developmental Psychology*, 1978, *14*, 191–192.

Rose, S. A., & Bridger, W. H. Enhancing visual recognition memory in preterm infants. Paper presented at the Biennial Meeting of the Society for Research in Child Development, San Francisco, March 1979.

Sigman, M., & Beckwith, L. Infant visual attentiveness in relation to caregiver–infant interaction and developmental outcome. *Infant Behavior and Development*, 1980, *3*, 141–154.

Sigman, M., Kopp, C. B., Littman, B., & Parmelee, A.H. Infant visual attentiveness in relation to birth condition. *Developmental Psychology*, 1977, *13*, 431–437.

Sigman, M., Kopp, C. B., Parmelee, A. H., & Jeffrey, W. Visual attention and neurological organization in neonates. *Child Development*, 1973, *44*, 461–466.

Sigman, M., & Parmelee, A. H. Visual preferences of four-month-old premature and full-term infants. *Child Development*, 1974, *10*, 687–695.

Sigman, M., & Parmelee, A. H. Longitudinal evaluation of the high-risk infant. In T. M. Field, A. M. Sostak, S. Goldberg, & H. H. Shuman (Eds.), *Infants born at risk*. New York: Spectrum, 1979.

Yang, R. K., & Moss, H. A. Neonatal precursors of infant behavior. *Developmental Psychology*, 1978, *14*, 607–613.

___19___

Predicting Intellectual Disorders in Childhood for Preterm Infants with Birthweights below 1501 gm[1]

JANE V. HUNT

The pediatric specialty of neonatology, introduced in the early 1960s, provides intensive care for the sick newborn infant. In centers providing such care, decreases in mortality rates for very small preterm infants have been dramatic. For example, Schlesinger (1973) reported deaths per live births at the Johns Hopkins Hospital, Baltimore, Maryland, for infants weighing less than 1001 gm at birth (less than 2.2 lb.) as decreased from 100% in 1961–1962 to 85% in 1967–1968 and deaths for infants weighing 1001–1500 gm (2.2–3.3 lb.) as decreased from 48% to 18% during the same period. Continuing improvements in the medical management of the fetus and newborn preterm infant contributed to a continuing decrease in mortality during the 1970s. For infants born at the University of California in San Francisco with birthweights of 750–1500 gm, mortality decreased from approximately 50% in 1965–1968 to 25% in 1973–1974 (Tooley & Phibbs, 1976).

The regionalization of neonatal intensive care has increased its availability to infants born outside specialized centers. Stewart and coworkers (Stewart, Turcan, Rawlings, & Reynolds, 1977) reported the survival of infants weighing less than 1000 gm for two time periods, 1966–1970 and 1971–1975. For those born alive at the University College Hospital in London, England, survival remained about the same (20%), but there was an increase in survival from 29% to 49% for those born elsewhere and transferred to that hospital. Presumably the quality of intensive care after initial survival elsewhere contributed to the improvement noted in the outborn group. Similar results have been reported by Fitzhardinge and coworkers in Toronto, Canada (Fitzhardinge, Kalman, Ashby, & Pape, 1978). For 250 infants with birthweights

[1] This research was supported in part by Pulmonary SCOR Grant HL19185.

PRETERM BIRTH AND
PSYCHOLOGICAL DEVELOPMENT

under 1501 gm born elsewhere and transferred to their care in 1974, 66% survived; survival was 51% for those weighing under 1000 gm.

We can conclude that, although many of the smallest premature infants still die in the first hours or days of life, the number of survivors is increasing. These infants constitute a new population, in that many of them have overcome illnesses that previously proved fatal. Hyaline membrane disease is a conspicuous example of a disease that now is frequently survived, whereas formerly this complication, associated with lung immaturity, often resulted in death.

Infants born as early as 3 weeks before term are considered premature. Those with birthweights of 1500 gm are, on average, born 9 weeks before term, with a gestational age of 31 weeks (as compared with 40 weeks for the full-term infant). Gestational age for those weighing 1000 gm is likely to be approximately 27 weeks, or 3 months premature. Survivors have been reported as young as 25 weeks of gestational age or with birthweights below 800 gm (below 1.8 lb.). These fragile preterm infants, whose survival usually depends upon sophisticated perinatal care and medical technology, are at risk not only of dying but of surviving with some handicaps that will diminish their potential for a normal life. Both medical and ethical concerns have prompted a number of centers providing neonatal intensive care to study the subsequent intellectual and physical development of these very premature survivors, who, it should be emphasized, constitute only a fraction of all preterm births.

Comparisons across studies are somewhat difficult because of differences in the socioeconomic characteristics of populations, differences associated with inborn versus outborn status as noted above, variations in age of assessment and kinds of developmental measurements used, and even differences in definitions of handicapped and normal outcome. In general, the outlook for the small preterm infants has changed over the years since intensive neonatal care was introduced. Data from early follow-up studies such as that of Drillien (1967) were not encouraging, but the prognosis improved greatly as children born into improved treatment programs became old enough for evaluations (Stewart & Reynolds, 1974). The incidence of such severe handicaps as blindness, deafness, cerebral palsy, and severe mental retardation has steadily diminished in published reports across the years (see review by Thompson & Reynolds, 1977). These handicaps are detectable relatively early in life. Other handicaps, such as language and learning disabilities and even moderate and mild mental retardation, may not be apparent until childhood. Where thay have been looked for, such handicaps have been found with unusual frequency in very low birthweight populations (Fitzhardinge & Ramsay, 1973; Francis-Williams & Davies, 1974). The relatively high incidence of these less devastating handicaps (now being detected in childhood) attests to the continuing high-risk status of very small preterm infants. However, not all infants have developed handicaps, and the causes of differences in outcome are of great interest and concern.

If the very small infant is born without congenital abnormalities or primary diseases, the likelihood of handicaps (like that of mortality) may depend primarily on the quality of perinatal care. Drillien (1972) has suggested that such infants are delivered prematurely "by accident" and are potentially normal at birth, although we cannot discount the possibility that the unknown etiology of prematurity may also contribute to the etiology of handicaps. We know (from discrete laboratory studies of animals) that some medical problems present distinct threats to the integrity of subsequent brain development. These problems are more likely to occur in small preterm infants. They include abnormal physiologic states before and immediately after birth, difficulties encountered during resuscitation and the first hours of postnatal life, and the occurrence of various complications associated with extreme prematurity during the first days and weeks following birth. Any of these problems may raise the spectre of brain damage, but the fate of an individual surviving infant is usually difficult to predict at the time that the problems are being identified and treated.

Some preterm infants survive severe physiologic stresses and neonatal complications without subsequent developmental handicaps. Our concern increases if the stressed neonate exhibits neurologic or behavioral abnormalities, but in some cases these symptoms prove to be transient. As the medical crises are overcome, we observe the infants for indications of developmental problems. Some severe handicaps can be determined early in infancy. However, as noted, other serious problems are less obvious in infancy and may go undetected until childhood. Many intellectual disabilities fall into this category.

Intellectual handicaps range in severity from those that limit the child in a serious way through those that merely present obstacles to normal progress in the usual educational setting. The severity of the disorders in childhood surely depends not only upon the extent of initial brain damage but also upon the child's inherent potentialities and the effects of subsequent life experiences, but the dynamics of the interaction between initial deficit, genetic potential, environmental effects, and intellectual outcome are not well understood. Remediation and improved function may occur naturally in a supportive environment or through specific intervention; preterm infants reared in poverty, a condition that is already high risk for intellectual problems, not surprisingly have an added risk for handicaps (Birch & Gussow, 1970; Drillien, 1964). Better prediction of significant intellectual handicaps in childhood has obvious practical benefits. Improvements in perinatal medical care are producing an increasing population of these high-risk survivors, and we want earlier estimates of the long-term effects of such changes in treatment. Improved prediction could also result in earlier appropriate remedial efforts for children with potential problems, thus reducing the magnitude of childhood hand-icaps.

In studying high-risk infants, we are therefore concerned with two major issues: identifying important developmental problems as early as possible and, searching out the conditions that cause the problems. Although these issues seem reasonably straightforward, they are in fact exceedingly complex. First, we want to identify problems before they happen. We would like to know in advance which of today's infants will have learning or language disorders 5 years from now—intellectual problems almost totally unrelated to the infant's current repertoire of abilities. Also, we look for causes of problems by using methods that are necessarily largely correlational. The methods give us information about associations between selected variables and outcome, but determining cause is likely to be a complex and elusive goal.

The longitudinal research design is appropriate to study the prediction of intellectual disabilities in childhood. By following the mental development of children from birth into childhood, we can examine the immediate and delayed consequences of perinatal events, the relations among earlier and later behavioral deficits, and the interactions among perinatal events, environmental circumstances, and the subsequent expression of intellectual disorders. Longitudinal studies of normal infants and children have suggested some of the problems and limitations of this method. In unselected groups of normal infants, IQ-type scores determined in infancy did not correlate with intelligence test scores at older ages (Bayley, 1940, 1949; Honzik, Macfarlane, & Allen, 1948). That is, relative precocity or delay below 2 years of age did not predict later intelligence. Correlations with school-age scores did not become robust in these normal groups until age 4 years. Even at older ages where high correlations were found, individual developmental rates that did not conform to normative expectations were frequently noted; developmental spurts and lags in mental growth were apparent in many normal children. These fluctuations in rate of gain on the tests resulted in some large IQ fluctuations across age, changes that were often not readily explained by obvious factors in the child's life, such as health factors or family events. Therefore, some IQ changes are considered normal and may be expected in any longitudinal study.

Some special problems for the prediction of abnormalities in development have been reported in follow-up studies of medically high-risk infants. Neonatal neurological abnormalities are not necessarily predictive of later intellectual problems (cf. Amiel-Tison, 1969). Group prediction may be improved when additional neonatal behavioral data are included in the analysis (Tronick & Brazelton, 1975), but prediction for any individual is far from reliable. Also, marked behavioral delays during the first several months of life, as evidenced by abnormally low developmental test scores, may not be predictive of future performance. For example, although many retarded children have a history of delayed development in infancy, other children with equally low infant scores may function normally at older ages (Holden, 1972).

Such a lack of prediction despite demonstrable abnormalities in infancy suggests transient functional disruptions that do not reflect permanent damage in all cases. Even beyond infancy, specific deficits, such as language disabilities, may be observed at one age but not at a later age (Corah, Anthony, Painter, Stern & Thurston, 1965; Phibbs, Harvin, Jones, Talbot, Cohen, Crowther, & Tooley, 1971). Presumably, environmental factors may exert important remedial effects in childhood (Sameroff & Chandler, 1975), but more research is needed before we can say that such delayed effects are not predictive of any future problem in high-risk groups.

To study the antecedents of childhood disabilities, our procedure is to follow a defined group of high-risk infants in a prospective study by consistent repeated tests and measurements of mental development to identify those individuals with developmental problems at successive ages. Once the problem and nonproblem groups are determined, we can then search for discriminating predictors in our antecedent data. This procedure is being used to follow the intellectual development of a group of small preterm infants (birthweights at or below 1500 gm) born at the University of California in San Francisco.

The University of California (San Francisco) Longitudinal Study

Background and Characteristics of the Preterm Group

Since 1965, certain categories of infants who required intensive neonatal care have been enrolled in a prospective developmental study at the University of California in San Francisco. Categories have included infants with hyaline membrane disease, small preterm infants, and other groups representing special regimens of treatment or specific complications of the newborn. Of these categories of survivors, the small preterm infant appears to be at greatest risk for intellectual handicaps. Those who were born at the university hospital (rather than born elsewhere and transferred) are an important subgroup for study because of the availability of consistent, detailed perinatal data.

Infants born in our hospital with birthweights at or below 1500 gm are routinely enrolled in the follow-up study as they leave the intensive care nursery, and strenuous efforts are made to enlist the participation of their parents in the program and to maintain contact with them. From 1965 through mid-1978, we enrolled 173 such infants, representing 88% of the survivors. Once participation in the study has been established, we have had good success in maintaining the group, and 94% of the children are still being followed.

Data have been examined for 114 children in the study who were born between 1965 and 1975 (all who were at least 2 years of age). General characteristics of this group are shown in Table 19.1. Approximately one-half the group had birthweights below 1250 gm, and one-tenth were below 1000 gm

TABLE 19.1

Characteristics of 114 Infants with Birthweights below 1501 gm Born at the University of California in San Francisco, 1965–1975

Characteristic	Percentage	Characteristic	Percentage
Birthweight (gm)		Gestational age (weeks)	
< 1000	10.6	25–27	9.6
1000–1250	38.9	28–30	43.9
1251–1500	50.5	31–33	36.9
		34–37	9.6
Mid-parent education		Maternal age (years)	
Less than high school (1)	18.6	15–19	19.8
High school graduate (2)	41.2	20–24	32.1
Some college (3)	18.6	25–29	28.3
College graduate (4), or		30–34	8.5
higher (5)	21.6	35–40	11.3
Race		Apgar scores, 1 min	
Caucasian	57.0	1–3	43.4
Black	23.2	4–6	37.2
Spanish	11.6	7–9	19.4
Other	8.2		
Males	46.5	Apgar scores, 5 min	
Hyaline membrane	39.5	1–3	7.3
Multiple births	17.5	4–6	29.4
Small for dates (< 3 S.D.)	9.6	7–10	63.3

at birth. Gestational age, determined from mothers' menstrual histories and expected dates of delivery, ranged from 25 to 37 weeks, but most infants fell within 28–33 weeks.

Mid-parent educational levels were determined by averaging the ratings for both parents on a five-point scale. The modal educational level was high school graduate, but a substantial number of parent sets (approximately 40%) had higher average ratings. Maternal age was most commonly in the range from 20 through 29 years, with approximately 20% above and 20% below this age range. The children were predominantly Caucasian, and the next largest racial group was black. There were relatively few Spanish-speaking families, and many of these were bilingual. Other racial groups, including Asian families, were also largely bilingual. Generally, bilingual parents (including those of European extraction) were not teaching English as a first language to their children.

Apgar scores (reflecting the condition of the infant on a scale from 0–10) were low at 1 min of age, with a modal value of 1–3. By 5 min of age the modal value was closer to normal (scores of 7–10). This shift in Apgar scores suggests the vigorous resuscitation efforts of the intensive care team who typically were alerted and were standing by at the time of delivery. Slightly less than half the group were males. Almost 40% of the children had experienced and survived neonatal hyaline membrane disease.

In summary, Table 19.1 suggests a group from predominantly middle-class Caucasian families but with a broad range of racial and educational backgrounds. The medical risk status of the group is suggested not only by the major variable of birthweight but also by gestational age, initial Apgar scores, and the high incidence of hyaline membrane disease.

Trends related to year of birth were investigated for the 114 children described in Table 19.1. Children born in three time periods—1965–1969, 1969–1972, and 1973–1975—were compared on a number of variables. No significant changes across the years were found for average birthweight, gestational age, Apgar scores at 1 and 5 min of age, or maternal age. The midparent educational level was slightly but significantly lower for those born in 1965–1968 compared with those born in 1969–1972. Our sample appears to be relatively constant in these measurements across the first 10 years of enrollment in the longitudinal study.

The longitudinal protocol calls for assessments at 6 and 12 months and yearly through age 8. The children are also seen at 11 and 14 years. Assessments include medical, psychological, neurological, and social evaluations. General assessments of intellectual ability include scores from the Cattell Test of the Infant Intelligence at 6, 12, and 24 months (scores adjusted for prematurity), the Stanford-Binet Intelligence Scale at ages 3, 4, 5, and 6 years, and the Wechsler Intelligence Scale for Children (WISC) at 8 and 11 years. Other tests are given at specific ages to assess such special abilities as visual–motor integration, language, and academic skills. In addition, ratings are assigned (normal, suspect, or abnormal) for a number of specific functional abilities at each test age, and a composite rating is determined on a seven-point scale. Thus, if a child is definitely abnormal on one or more dimensions considered critical to intellectual performance at that age, his composite rating will reflect this condition. These ratings are essentially clinical judgments. For example, if an infant or very young child is hyperactive, he may be rated as normal or suspect; but if the hyperactivity and accompanying distractibility persist into later childhood, his global rating will drop to the abnormal range. The clinical ratings are particularly useful in detecting children with developmental problems who have test scores in the normal range. Medical, neurological, and social assessments contribute to this general assessment of development.

Outcome in Early Childhood (4–6 years)

As the children approached school age, many intellectual problems could be identified with some certainty. The Stanford-Binet IQ has clinical validity at this age in predicting both school success and future scores, although, as noted, prediction for any individual may be imperfect. The supplementary tests of language ability and visual–motor integration available for this age assessed abilities similar to those measured at older ages.

We have examined intellectual status at 4–6 years for 72 children (born 1965–1974) who have been tested one or more times at these ages. The Stanford-Binet IQs at 4, 5, and 6 years were highly intercorrelated (4 × 5, .77; 4 × 6, .82; 5 × 6, .88), and, where applicable, scores were averaged for the individual to give a composite IQ for early childhood. The distribution of these averaged scores for the 72 children is shown in Figure 19.1. Those children with definite intellectual or sensorimotor disabilities that were expected to interfere with subsequent school progress are indicated. Those who survived the serious neonatal complication of hyaline membrane disease are also shown in the figure.

Disabilities in this group occurred across much of the IQ range, including the normal range (IQ 84 and above). There were 10 children (14%) with IQs below 68; these scores fall more than 2 standard deviations below the expected average, conventionally accepted as the range of mental retardation. Another 10 children with scores in the borderline range (IQ 68–83) had definite

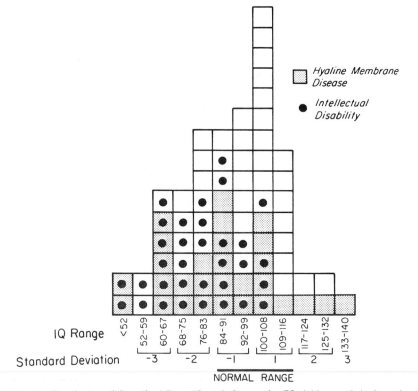

FIGURE 19.1. *Distribution of Standford-Binet IQ at 4–6 years for 72 children with birthweights ≤ 1500 gm.*

disabilities (5 others in this range were rated "suspect"). An additional 13 children (18%) had definite disabilities even though IQs were in the normal range, bringing the total with some evidence for disabilities in early childhood to 46%. The 4 children with scores below 60 were born before 1969, attesting to the decline in the most devastating intellectual handicaps. However, moderate and mild handicaps continued to appear in more recently born children. Of the 17 tested children who were born in 1973-1974, 8 had handicaps and 2 of these had scores in the retarded range (below IQ 68). The continuing high-risk status of this very low birthweight group is evident.

COMPARISONS BETWEEN NORMAL AND ABNORMAL OUTCOME GROUPS

The 33 children with definite developmental problems at 4–6 years were compared with all others (12 rated normal and 27 rated suspect). The large suspect group reflected the concerns of the examiners for children with immaturities and low-normal specific skills, but these children could not be described as having true disabilities at this age. Comparisons between the two outcome groups are shown in Table 19.2. Tendencies were generally in the expected direction (more favorable values for the group without definite intellectual problems), but the differences were not significant, and the two groups were remarkably similar in average birthweight, gestational age, and Apgar scores.

The values for mid-parent education represent some education beyond high school in each group, but less than a college degree.

As indicated in Figure 19.1, children who had neonatal hyaline membrane disease were overrepresented in the group with disabilities. Of the 29 children with hyaline membrane disease, 19, or 65.5%, had handicaps; in contrast, 14 children, or 32.6% of those who did not have this disease, had handicaps in

TABLE 19.2

Comparisons between Children with Intellectual Problems at 4–6 Years of Age and All Others for 72 Children with Birthweights ≤ 1500 gm

Characteristic	Intellectual problems			All others		
	Average	SD	N^a	Average	SD	N^b
Birthweight (gm)	1203.3	223.9	33	1291.4	169.6	39
Gestational age (weeks)	29.8	2.8	33	30.4	2.8	39
Mid-parent education (1 = low)	2.5	1.2	33	3.0	1.1	34
Maternal age	25.9	6.8	32	24.9	6.2	35
Apgar score, 1 min	4.1	2.3	33	4.7	2.6	39
Apgar score, 5 min	6.7	1.9	33	7.2	1.8	37

[a] $N = 33.$

[b] $N = 39.$ Not all measures available for each child.

early childhood. The twofold increase in incidence of problems for those with hyaline membrane disease suggests the importance of examining neonatal conditions associated with the disease for predictors of disabilities.

Significant sex differences were not found in the incidence of handicaps. Of the 34 males, 17 (50%) had disabilities at 4–6 years; of the 38 females, 16 (42.1%) had disabilities. There were sex differences in the extremes of each comparison group, since 8 of the 10 children with IQs in the retarded range were males and 8 of the 12 who were considered entirely normal were females. These extremes were reflected in a significant IQ difference between the sexes: males, 87.0; females, 94.4. Our data suggest that the outcome for girls is more favorable in terms of the severity but not the incidence of handicap.

The association between sex and hyaline membrane disease was examined. The incidence of problems in those who had hyaline membrane disease was similar for each sex (64.7% for males, 66.7% for females), but fewer of the girl infants had developed this disease (50.0% for males, 31.6% for females). The sexes were not significantly different in either birthweight or gestational age, so it can be argued from our data that, in a comparison of survivors, males with birthweights below 1501 gm are at higher risk than females for hyaline membrane disease and associated intellectual disabilities in early childhood.

COMPARISONS OF TEST SCORES AT THREE AGES

Infant tests at 6 and/or 12 months of age were given to 62 of the 72 children tested at 4–6 years, and 65 of them were tested at 2 and/or 3 years. Infant tests were averaged for each child where applicable, as were the tests at 2 and 3 years of age. Averaging was done to increase the numbers available for comparisons at younger ages.

Average scores and correlations among the three composite ages are shown in Table 19.3; separate means and correlations are presented for the group of children with intellectual problems at 4–6 years and for all others.

IQ differences between the groups increased steadily across the ages, from 10 points at 6–12 months to 16 points at 2–3 years and 25 points at 4–6 years. IQ correlations between ages differed for the two groups. Only those with handicaps at 4–6 years showed significant correlations between scores at 6–12 months and scores at older ages. Correlations between 2–3 years and 4–6 years were highly significant for both groups, but the correlation was larger for the group with handicaps. The larger interage correlations for the handicapped group were probably caused by the broader distribution of scores in that group, as shown in Figure 19.1; the larger standard deviations reflect this greater dispersion of scores.

The decreasing average IQ across ages for the group with intellectual problems in early childhood suggested that infant scores failed to predict problems. Prediction was examined more directly for this group by examining shifts across ages in four diagnostic score categories: normal (IQ 100 or

TABLE 19.3
Mental Test Scores and Intercorrelations at Three Ages for Groups with and without Intellectual Problems at 4-6 Years of Age

Test	Test scores for group with intellectual problems			Intercorrelations by IQ score		Test scores for all others			Intercorrelations by IQ score	
	Average	SD	N	6-12 months	2-3 years	Average	SD	N	6-12 months	2-3 years
IQ 6-12 months	92.3	17.6	31			102.5	13.9	31		
IQ 2-3 years	80.3	13.3	32	.44**		96.2	12.0	33	.30	
IQ 4-6 years	77.0	18.6	33	.37*	.86***	102.7	14.3	39	-.11	.64***

* p < .05
** p < .01
*** p < .001

339

higher), low-normal (IQ 84–99), borderline (IQ 68–83), and retarded (IQ below 68). The distribution of scores in these categories at three ages is shown in Table 19.4.

The modal score category at 6–12 months for the group with intellectual problems was normal (IQ 100 or higher), with 41.9% of the group testing at that level, whereas only 12.1% of the group tested at that level at 4–6 years. If testing had been discontinued after 1 year, a large proportion of the group would have been considered normal. At the other extreme, 29.1% tested in the borderline and retarded ranges in infancy compared with 60.6% at 4–6 years, representing a twofold increase in scores low enough to cause concern. At 2–3 years, 56.3% of the group earned scores that were low enough to cause concern, and almost no children scored at or above IQ 100.

In contrast, the group without intellectual problems showed a more constant score distribution by IQ category across age. The modal value was for scores in the normal category at all ages, although a greater proportion had scores in the low-normal range at 2–3 years. This relative consistency suggests that scores from the Cattell test and the Stanford-Binet are not grossly divergent at the ages tested; the finding of comparable percentages in the borderline range at each age and the fact that no normal children scored at the retarded level at the younger ages tend to confirm the validity of the measures. Our data indicate that the average performance of a group in infancy was not predictive of the incidence of later intellectual problems in that group, and many infants with incipient disabilities had normal tests during the first year. Group prediction improved considerably at 2–3 years.

Prediction for the individual was even more uncertain. Changes in individual classifications (normal, low-normal, borderline, and retarded) were examined. For the group with intellectual problems, individual score shifts from infancy to 4–6 years reflected the downward IQ trend in the group. A

TABLE 19.4

Percentages of Children Scoring in Four IQ Categories at Three Test Ages for Groups with and Without Intellectual Problems at 4–6 Years of Age

		Percentage			
	N	Normal (IQ ≥ 100)	Low-Normal (IQ 84–99)	Borderline (IQ 68–83)	Retarded (IQ < 68)
Intellectual problems					
6–12 months	31	41.9	29.0	19.4	9.7
2–3 years	32	3.1	40.6	43.8	12.5
4–6 years	33	12.1	27.3	30.3	30.3
All others					
6–12 months	31	67.7	19.4	12.9	—
2–3 years	33	48.5	39.4	12.1	—
4–6 years	39	61.5	28.2	10.3	—

large proportion (61%) of individuals in this group had infant scores in a higher category than that determined at 4–6 years. In contrast, a greater percentage of individuals in the normal group showed stability in score category between these ages. Nevertheless, more than half of those in the non-problem group shifted either upward or downward in diagnostic IQ category between infancy and early childhood. Prediction from infancy to early childhood for the individual, even in gross diagnostic categories, was unreliable.

Of special concern were the 10 children with scores in the retarded range at 4–6 years of age. Of the eight tested at 6–12 months, two had scores above 100, one had a low-normal score, three had scores in the borderline range, and two had scores below 68. Thus, five of eight had scores low enough to cause concern during infancy. By contrast, for nine children tested in infancy who were considered entirely normal at 4–6 years, six had scores above 100 and three had scores in the borderline range; three of nine therefore had scores low enough to cause concern during infancy. Precise prediction from infant scores appears to be dubious even for extreme cases, with important errors of classification found in both directions.

At 2–3 years, the IQ correlation with 4–6 years for the group with problems was .86, and the average IQ changed only 3 points (see Table 19.3). However, individual shifts in diagnostic category for this group were found for 44% of individuals, with 25% still testing higher at the younger age. For the group with no intellectual problems, score category stability was found for 64% of individuals, although 24% tested in a lower category at 2–3 years than they did at 4–6 years. Considering all children in both groups, accurate diagnosis by IQ category for the individual improved from 34% at 6–12 months to 60% at 2–3 years. Better individual prediction at 2–3 years is not surprising. The comparison ages are closer together, and tests at 2–3 years measure abilities similar to those tested in early childhood. Despite this improved prediction, individual shifts in diagnostic score categtories were not unusual.

Nine of the 10 retarded children were tested at 2–3 years. None scored above 100, one had a low-normal score, four had scores in the borderline range, and four had scores below 68. Thus, at this age, eight of nine children had scores low enough to cause concern. Nine children who were entirely normal at 4–6 years were tested at 2–3 years. Seven of them had scores above 100, and two tested in the low-normal range; none was scoring low enough to cause concern. Prediction of extreme cases was much improved over infancy.

In summary, test scores at 6–12 months were not predictive of outcome in early childhood. Although a marginally significant correlation was found between test scores at these ages for the group with intellectual disabilities, the correlation appeared to be the result of greater score dispersion at 4–6 years in this group. In other ways, infant scores were less predictive for the group with disabilities; averaged IQs were more divergent between ages, a higher proportion of that group had normal IQs in infancy compared with later scores, and downward shifts in individual diagnostic score categories were more pronounced. Individual changes in diagnostic categories between infancy and early childhood were common in both groups, totaling 66% of all children.

Prediction to 4–6 years improved at 2–3 years. IQ correlations were highly significant, and the proportions in the diagnostic IQ categories were more constant. Individual shifts in IQ categories from this age to 4–6 years occurred less frequently than from infancy but were found in 40% of the children. Retardation was more obvious by 2–3 years although not clearly defined in all instances.

COMPARISONS OF CLINICAL RATINGS AT THREE AGES

Another source of information at each test age was the clinical impression of development based on all tests and observations. Ratings were assigned on the basis of written protocols for evaluations from 1965–1976. Since then, a more formal rating of specific developmental parameters has been used. The overall rating is based on the examiner's impression of disabilities that interfered with intellectual functioning at the age of evaluation. A rating of 1 or 2 was given to children who showed no evidence of disability; ratings of 3, 4, and 5 were used for children who were increasingly suspect for developmental problems; ratings of 6 and 7 were given to children with definite abnormalities at that age. All children assigned to the group with intellectual problems had a composite rating greater than 5 at 4–6 years. Comparisons between the group with intellectual problems and all others are presented in Table 19.5.

The average ratings at 6–12 months were higher for the group with subsequent intellectual problems and well within the suspect range, but the large standard deviation for that group suggests the wide spectrum of ratings assigned in infancy. By 2–3 years, the group with problems was better identified, and the average rating approached the level of definite disability. The group without disabilities established an average rating of mildly suspect at 2–3 years that persisted at 4–6 years. The intercorrelations among ratings indicated that ratings given at 6–12 months were significantly associated with ratings at 2–3 years and these correlations were more significant than the IQ correlations for the same ages (see Table 19.3). However, the correlations between infant ratings and ratings at 4–6 years were no more impressive than the IQ correlations between these ages. The correlations between ratings at 2–3 and 4–6 years were not so large as IQ correlations between those ages. Ratings and IQs at the same age showed high correlations, as would be expected, but infant ratings were no more predictive of IQ at older ages than were the infant IQs.

In summary, correlations using the global clinical ratings gave information similar to that derived from IQ correlations. There was some indication that ratings at infancy and 2–3 years were more closely associated than were the IQs at those ages, but in other respects, the ratings were similar to or less powerful than IQ comparisons.

TABLE 19.5
Ratings of Developmental Status and Intercorrelations at Three Ages; for Groups with and without Intellectual Problems at 4-6 Years of Age

m	Intellectual problems			Intercorrelations		All others			Intercorrelations	
	Average	SD	N	6-12 months	2-3 years	Average	SD	N	6-12 months	2-3 years
6-12 months	3.48	2.25	31			2.27	1.63	31		
2-3 years	5.77	1.54	32	.54***		3.33	2.11	33	.50**	
4-6 years	6.66	.52	33	.36*	.49**	3.11	1.38	39	-.04	.53***

* $p < .05$
** $P < .01$
*** $p < .001$

343

DISCUSSION OF SCORES AND RATINGS

Predicting intellectual disabilities in early childhood from infant developmental test scores appears unlikely, expect for infants scoring in the retarded range (IQ below 68). In our small group of children with problems, only 3 of 31 scored this low in infancy. By 2–3 years, a score in the borderline range (IQ 68–83) appeared to be reasonably predictive. When the group with disabilities was compared with the normal group, there was a nearly fourfold increase of scores in the borderline range.

The developmental ratings at each age did not provide much additional information for prediction, even though the definition of the handicapped group was based on such ratings and cut across a wide IQ range. The rating scale is statistically crude in comparison with the IQ variable, and a more continuous distribution of ratings might provide better information. However, the general rating used (a seven point scale) probably approached the limits of reliable clinical judgments. Specific criteria used to generate the ratings may eventually provide clues for better prediction. The significant correlation between ratings at infancy and 2–3 years is encouraging, considering the clinical tendency to "wait and see" that permeates infant evaluations.

The drop in IQs at 2–3 years for both groups (see Table 19.4) may be an artifact of prematurity. We have adjusted IQ for prematurity on the Cattell test at 6, 12, and 24 months with some confidence because of previous research (Hunt & Rhodes, 1977) but did not adjust scores at older ages. A study by Brandt (1979) reported the mental development of preterm infants studied at the University Clinic, Universitäts-Kinderklinik und Poliklinik in Bonn, Germany. Her data indicated that scores for premature infants should be adjusted through early childhood.

OTHER CORRELATIONS WITH IQ AT THREE AGES

The low IQ correlations between infancy and older ages suggested that major variables be examined for their correlations with IQ at each of the three ages. As in previously noted analyses, the two groups of handicapped and normal children were examined separately for comparative purposes. This procedure had the added statistical advantage of restricting the IQ range in each group so as to preclude inflated correlations.

As shown in Table 19.2, those children who did and did not develop intellectual problems in early childhood were not significantly different in average measures of birthweight, gestational age, Apgar scores at 1 and 5 min of age, maternal age, or mid-parent educational level. The correlations of these variables with IQ at three ages are shown in Table 19.6.

At 4–6 years, only mid-parent education was significantly correlated with IQ. For the group without intellectual problems, the correlation of .50 was similar to that found for other groups of normal children at that age. The same correlation was lower but still significant for the group with intellectual problems. Thus, although the occurrence of handicaps was found in children

TABLE 19.6
Correlations at Three Ages for Groups with and without Intellectual Problems at 4-6 Years of Age

	IQ scores for group with intellectual problems			IQ scores for all others		
Characteristic	6–12 months (N = 31)	2–3 years (N = 32)	4–6 years (N = 33)	6–12 months (N = 31)	2–3 years (N = 33)	4–6 years (N = 39)
Birthweight	.52***	.21	.10	−.32*	−.29	−.12
Gestational age	.15	.20	.07	−.56***	−.50***	−.08
SD BW/GA	.20	−.02	.10	.34*	.36*	−.03
Apgar score, 1 min	.20	.22	.13	−.08	−.36*	−.20
Apgar score, 5 min	.31*	.03	−.04	.01	−.37*	−.14
Maternal age	−.13	−.10	.01	−.24	.14	.05
Mid-parent education	.20	.24	.37*	−.12	.50**	.50***

* p < .05
** p < .01
*** p < .001

from all socioeducational levels, the extent of the handicap, as expressed by the IQ, was associated with familial circumstances. Birthweight, gestational age, and other variables examined were not correlated with IQ in early childhood for either group in this low-birthweight population.

In contrast, a different pattern of correlations was noted between the same variables and IQ at 6–12 months. Developmental status in infancy did not correlate with mid-parent education, a result similar to that noted in many longitudinal studies. Infant scores correlated with birthweight, but the direction of the correlation differed in the two comparison groups. A positive correlation was obtained for the group with childhood handicaps, but for the normal group, there was a significant negative correlation between infant IQ and both birthweight and, especially, gestational age. The negative correlations indicated that some of the most premature infants had the highest developmental scores in infancy, whereas more mature infants had some of the lower scores in the normal group. When relative size for gestational age was considered (SD BW/GA), based on Usher's normative data (Usher & McLean, 1969), a low positive correlation with infant IQ was found in the normal group. This result indicated that some of those in the normal group who were smaller for dates score lower in infancy. Some errors in determining gestational age may have contributed to this finding, because infant scores were adjusted for prematurity. It is possible that some of the relatively small-for-date infants may have been biologically younger than the assigned gestational ages. However, no such effect was found for the handicapped group.

At 2–3 years of age, no correlation was found for the handicapped group between IQ and any other variable in Table 19.6. In contrast, the normal group continued to show a negative correlation between IQ and gestational age. Mid-parent education also showed a substantial correlation with IQ at this age, attesting to the increasing importance of familial effects on normal IQ. An examination of the data revealed no correlation between mid-parent education and gestational age; the continuing relative success of some of the most premature infants in this group was apparent even though IQ adjustments for prematurity were discontinued at age 3 years. The low but significant negative correlations between IQ and Apgar scores were puzzling; Apgar scores showed no significant associations with gestational age.

The correlational data suggested that socioeducational influences may have overwhelmed and obscured associations with the major biological variables by early childhood, a finding noted in other studies (see review by Sameroff & Chandler, 1975). The association between birthweight and infant development in the handicapped group suggested some transient effects. The paradoxical negative association between gestational age and IQ in the normal group strongly suggested a dichotomous population; either intellectual damage is prevented or it is sustained, and when it is prevented the smallest and most premature infants may do well. Therefore, it is important to examine specific variables for their contribution to outcome in infants of very low birthweight;

predictions based only on comparative birthweight or gestational age in this group are not valid.

Outcome in Middle Childhood (8 years)

We have assumed that intellectual problems leading to educational disabilities could be detected by careful assessments at 4–6 years. High IQ correlations between early and middle childhood are expected, but the possibility remains that not all educational problems can be anticipated. A small number (30 children) who were tested at 4–6 years have also been evaluated at age 8 years. Some preliminary results have been examined.

The clinical ratings at 4–6 years were used to define the two outcome groups, abnormal and all others (normal and suspect)—that were compared previously. The consistency of those ratings into school age has been examined for the first 30 children tested at 8 years of age. Ratings at 4–6 years were: 12 with intellectual problems, 7 suspect, and 11 normal. The 12 children rated as having definite problems at 4–6 were also rated as having problems at 8 years. Of the 7 in the suspect category, 4 remained in that category, 2 were rated as normal at 8 years, and 1 was rated as having a disability. The 11 children rated normal at 4–6 years showed the greatest shift in ratings; only 4 remained in the normal category, 6 shifted to suspect, and 1 showed definite disabilities. Six of the 7 who slipped from the normal rating were also tested at 2–3 years, and only 1 of those was considered normal at that age (4 were suspect, 1 was abnormal). In contrast, the few children who remained in the normal category at 8 years were also rated normal at age 2–3 years. Thus, those who shifted out of the normal category at age 8 usually showed some evidence for concern at 2–3 years. It appears from our data that ratings at 2–3 years should not be regarded lightly.

Correlations between IQs at 4–6 years and 8 years were highly significant ($r = .81$, $p < .001$), a finding to be expected when the range of IQs being compared is broad. Half of the children had IQ shifts of 10 or more points, 6 increasing and 9 decreasing at 8 years. Six children had IQ changes of more than 15 points with 5 decreasing. The large IQ shifts were not usually accompanied by changes in ratings. Also, the changes in ratings were not always associated with shifts in IQ, and of the 7 children previously considered who slipped from normal ratings at 8 years, only 3 had IQ decreases of more than 10 points and 1 had an increase of 11 points.

At 4–6 years, the IQ was derived from the Stanford-Binet Intelligence Scale, and at 8 years, the Wechsler Intelligence Scale for Children (WISC) was given. (Two blind retarded children were given other tests at both ages.) The WISC generates a separate verbal IQ and performance IQ as well as a total IQ. In most instances, downward shifts in IQ were less when scores at 4–6 years were compared with verbal IQ, suggesting that the additional performance tasks of the WISC contributed to drops in score. A comparison of verbal and performance IQs at age 8 adds to this impression, for of the 23 children who had 5 or more points difference between verbal and performance IQs, 15 of these had lower performance IQs. An inspection of problems at age 8 showed a high incidence of children with visual–motor integration difficulties, often accompanied by reading difficulties or problems in writing and drawing. Because so few children have thus far been tested at 8 years, and because they were born into different practices of neonatal care than are now found, it is not possible to predict that this specific disorder will continue to be found with the same frequency as more children reach this age.

In summary, tests at 8 years of age reidentified the group with significant problems determined at 4–6 years, with no exceptions, across a broad IQ range. Those who were in the suspect category at 4–6 years generally remained so at 8 years, with exceptions occurring in either direction (normal or abnormal). Those who were considered normal at 4–6 years were often considered less than entirely normal at 8 years, and this finding was almost always associated with some concerns at 2–3 years. Rating changes and IQ changes were not closely associated. Decreases in IQ were generally less when Stanford-Binet scores at 4–6 years were compared only with the verbal IQ of the WISC. In this group of low-birthweight children, a high incidence of visual–motor integration problems was noted across the entire IQ spectrum.

Discussion

Many medical centers now actively encourage investigations of the intellectual oucome of very small preterm infants. The intense interest in and anxiety about these infants stems from two sources. First, the infants represent an unknown population in the sense that many would surely have died without modern methods of intensive neonatal care. Also, the methods used in treatment are often invasive and carry the potential for iatrogenic complications. Behavioral studies that focus on these infants are formulated in, or largely influenced by, pragmatic considerations and questions of medical ethics. This is not to imply that such studies are generally lacking in theoretical orientation, and theories of differential development are often explicitly delineated. However, if the investigators who study these infants have one foot in theory, the other is surely planted in the nursery, for today's theory may be tomorrow's practice. For this reason, broad generalizations and overinterpretations of data are dangerous. The definitive study cannot be done; knowledge is accrued by replication and by conservative interpretations of results.

To study this new population we need, first, a good understanding of normal premature development during the first months of life. The neurologic studies of Amiel-Tison (1969, 1976) and the behavioral studies of Brazelton and coworkers (Als, Lester, & Brazelton, 1979; Gorski, Davison, & Brazelton, 1979) exemplify the careful documentation that is needed. In both, there has been an emphasis on separating normal from abnormal characteristics and on providing a system for appreciating those changes associated with recovery from illness. The preterm infant is different in many ways from the full-term infant anticipated by his parents, and the effects of these differences on early reciprocal social experiences have been documented (Beckwith & Cohen, 1978; Osofsky & Danzger, 1974).

The anxiety that such an infant engenders is often justified. Our data suggest that 4 out of 10 infants with birthweights at or below 1500 gm will experience developmental problems in childhood that will be of consequence and may require special educational efforts. The extent of the handicap appears to be strongly influenced by environmental circumstances. In our study, the association between IQ in the handicapped population and mid-parent education is suggestive. Others, such as Sameroff and Chandler (1975), have emphasized the primacy of the caretaking environment for outcome. When we considered specific deficits without regard to IQ, they were found across environmental categories of socioeconomic status and parent education. We found specific disabilities in a small group of 8-year-old children that suggested neurologic damage. Others, such as Francis-Williams and Davies (1974), have reported similar findings. Considering the unusual hazards that accompany extremely premature birth (hazards that formerly greatly restricted survival), it is possible that some brain damage does occur in many cases, even though its expression may be very much modified by the subsequent life history of the individual and, very likely, by his original intellectual potential.

The possibility of brain damage directs us to the circumstances surrounding perinatal and neonatal life. Here we encounter a large number of potentially damaging conditions, so many that we may wonder how any small preterm infant survives without damage. It is highly unlikely that a single variable or a consistent cluster of variables will predict all cases (Hunt, 1976). It is much more likely that there are a number of routes to developmental problems. On the other hand, there are a limited number of direct ways in which the brain is compromised, notably by hemorrhage, ischemia, toxins, infections, and trauma. It is a common experience that two infants may have the same apparent history of perinatal complications yet differ radically in outcome. One critical difference must be the presence or absence of specific effects on the brain. Our data suggest that such effects cannot be predicted reliably from general conditions such as birthweight, even for the smallest surviving infants. In contrast, hyaline membrane disease, an illness associated with a number of specific complications, exerts a negative effect on outcome in our data and that of others, such as Lubchenco and coworkers (Lubchenco, Bard, Goldman, Coyer, McIntyer, & Smith, 1974). The measurement of discrete physiologic states in the neonate may bring us closer to identifying precursors of direct effects.

Developmental status in the first year of life is not a good predictor of developmental disabilities in childhood. Neurologic and behavioral deficits are often transient, attesting to the recovery of normal function in many infants. More worrisome is the appearance of disabilities at older ages that were not predicted in infancy. Our longitudinal data indicate that unexpected problems may continue to occur as late as 8 years of age. However, there is also evidence that such problems may be accompanied by some concerns about development at 2–3 years of age, followed by relatively normal development from 4 to 6 years. This finding suggests that we must look more closely at specific components of cognitive development across the longitudinal data. Functional discontinuities across ages have been noted for normal children (McCall, 1976; McCall, Eichorn, & Hogarty, 1977) and may be of special importance for children with potential handicaps. The childhood downward shift in intellectual status across age in our subgroup with handicaps was not confined to families of low socioeconomic status or low educational level. Those children did not progress normally in the normal (unmodified) environment, and a careful inspection of their individual histories of intellectual development may be helpful in guiding us to appropriate intervention and remediation for similar cases in the future.

References

Als, H., Lester, B., & Brazelton, T. B. Dynamics of the behavioral organization of the premature infant: A theoretical perspective. In T. M. Field, A. M. Sostek, S. Goldberg, & H. H. Shuman (Eds.) *Infants born at risk: Behavior and development.* New York: Spectrum, 1979.

Ameil-Tison, C. Cerebral factors, neonatal status, and long-term follow-up. *Biological Neonatorum,* 1969, *14,* 234–250.

Ameil-Tison, C. A method for neurologic evaluation within the first year of life. *Current Problems in Pediatrics,* 1976, *7,* 1–50.

Bayley, N. Factors influencing the growth of intelligence in young children. *Yearbook of the National Society for the Study of Education,* 1940, *39,* (Pt. 2) 49–79.

Bayley, N. Consistency and variability in the growth of intelligence from birth to eighteen years. *Journal of Genetic Psychology,* 1949, *75,* 165–196.

Beckwith, L., & Cohen, S. E. Preterm birth: Hazardous obstetrical and postnatal events as related to caregiver–infant behavior. *Infant Behavior and Development,* 1978, *1*(4), 403–411.

Birch, H., & Gussow, G. D. *Disadvantaged children.* New York: Grune & Stratton, 1970.

Brandt, I. Physical, neuomotor and intellectual development of preterm and fullterm infants from birth to five years. Address delivered at the biennial meeting of the Society for Research in Child Development, San Francisco, March 1979.

Corah, N. L., Anthony, E. J., Painter, P., Stern, J. A., & Thurston, D. L. Effects of perinatal anoxia after seven years. *Psychological Monographs,* 1965, *79,* (3, Whole No. 596).

Drillien, C. M. *The growth and development of the prematurely born infant.* Edinburgh: Livingstone, 1964.

Drillien, C. M. The long-term prospects of handicap in babies of low birth weight. *Hospital Medicine,* 1967, *1,* 937–944.

Drillien, C. M. Aetiology and outcome in low-birthweight infants. *Developmental Medicine and Child Neurology,* 1972, *14,* 563–574.

Fitzhardinge, P. M., Kalman, E., Ashby, S., & Pape, K. E. Present status of the infant of very low birth weight treated in a referral neonatal intensive care unit in 1974. In *Major mental handicap: Methods and costs of prevention* (Ciba Foundation Symposium 59) Amsterdam: Elsevier / Excerpta Medica / North-Holland, 1978.

Fitzhardinge, P. M., & Ramsay, M. The improving outlook for the small prematurely born infant. *Developmental Medicine and Child Neurology,* 1973, *15,* 447–459.

Francis-Williams, J., & Davies, P. A. Very low birthweight and later intelligence. *Developmental Medicine and Child Neurology,* 1974, *16,* 709–728.

Gorski, P. A., Davison, M. F., & Brazelton, T. B. Stages of behavioral organization in the high-risk neonate: Theoretical and clinical considerations. *Seminars in Perinatology,* 1979, *3*(1), 61–72.

Holden, R. H. Prediction of mental retardation in infancy. *Mental Retardation,* 1972, *10* (1)., 28–30.

Honzik, M. P., Macfarlane, J. W., & Allen, L. The stability of mental test performance between two and eighteen years. *Journal of Experimental Education,* 1948, *17,* 309–324.

Hunt, J. V. Environmental risk in fetal and neonatal life and measured infant intelligence. In M. Lewis (Ed.), *Origins of intelligence: Infancy and early childhood.* New York: Plenum, 1976.

Hunt, J. V., & Rhodes, L. Mental development of preterm infants during the first year. *Child Development,* 1977, *48,* 204–210.

Lubchenco, L. O., Bard, H., Goldman, A. L., Coyer, W. E., McIntyre, C., & Smith, D. M. Newborn intensive care and long-term prognosis. *Developmental Medicine and Child Neurology,* 1974, *16,* 421–431.

McCall, R. B. Toward an epigenetic conception of mental development in the first three years of life. In M. Lewis (Ed.), *Origins of intelligence: Infancy and early childhood.* New York: Plenum, 1976

McCall, R. B., Eichorn, D. H., & Hogarty, P. S. Transitions in early mental development. *Monograph of the Society for Research in Child Development,* 1977, *42,*(3, Serial No. 171).

Osofsky, J. D., & Danzger, B. Relationships between neonatal characteristics and mother–infant interaction. *Developmental Psychology,* 1974, *10,* 124–130.

Phibbs, R. H., Harvin, D., Jones, G., Talbot, C., Cohen, M., Crowther, D., & Tooley, W. H. Development of children who had received intra-uterine transfusions. *Pediatrics,* 1971, *47* (4), 689–697.

Sameroff, A. J., & Chandler, M. J. Reproductive risk and the continuum of caretaking casualty. In F. D. Horowitz (Ed.), *Review of Child Development Research* (Vol. 4). Chicago: Univ. of Chicago Press, 1975.

Schlesinger, E. R. Neonatal intensive care: Planning for services and outcomes following care. *Journal of Pediatrics,* 1973, *82*(6), 916–920.

Stewart, A. L., & Reynolds, E. O. R. Improved prognosis for infants of very low birthweight. *Pediatrics,* 1974, *54,* 724–735.

Stewart, A. L., Turcan, D. M., Rawlings, G., & Reynolds, E. O. R. Prognosis for infants weighing 1000 g or less at birth. *Archives of Disease in Childhood,* 1977, *52,* 97–104.

Thompson, T., & Reynolds, J. The results of intensive care therapy for neonates: I. Overall neonatal mortality rates. II. Neonatal mortality rates and long-term prognosis for low birth weight neonates. *Journal of Perinatal Medicine,* 1977, *5,* 59–92.

Tooley, W. H., & Phibbs, R. H. Neonatal intensive care: The state of the art. In A. R. Jonsen & M. J. Garland (Eds.), *Ethics of newborn intensive care.* Berkeley: Institute of Governmental Studies, University of California, 1976.

Tronick, E., & Brazelton, T. B. Clinical uses of the Brazelton neonatal behavioral assessment. In B. Z. Friedlander, G. M. Sterritt, & G. E. Kirk (Eds.), *Exceptional infant: Assessment and intervention* (Vol. 3). New York: Brunner / Mazel, 1975.

Usher, R., & McLean, R. Interuterine growth of live-born Caucasian infants at sea level: Standards obtained from measurements in 7 dimensions of infants born from 24 and 44 weeks of gestation. *Journal of Pediatrics,* 1969, *74* (6), 901–910.

20

Neonatal Compromise and Later Psychological Development: A 10-year Longitudinal Study

DANIEL V. CAPUTO
KENNETH M. GOLDSTEIN
HARVEY B. TAUB

This chapter reports on a longitudinal study assessing the long-term (7–9½ years) development of low-birthweight (≤ 2500 gm) and full-sized (> 2500 gm) babies.[1]

Measures relating to the functioning of these subjects during the first year of life and in middle childhood included the following predictor variables: (a) indexes of prematurity; (b) prenatal and perinatal status; (c) demographic status; (d) maternal childrearing attitudes; and (e) measures of 1-year infant status. Outcome variables assessed in this study included: (a) intellectual development (IQ); and (b) visuomotor performance.

Predictor Variables

Neonatal Status and Prematurity

Although prematurity has been defined in numerous ways in the literature, the prematurely born has been differentiated from the maturely born principally on the basis of birthweight (Broman, Nichols, & Kennedy, 1975; Caputo & Mandell, 1970; Caputo et al., 1974; Corrigan, Berger, Dienstbier, & Strok, 1967; Dann, Levine, & New, 1964; DeHirsch, Jansky, & Langford, 1966; Douglas, 1960; Drillien, 1958; Frances-Williams & Davies, 1974; Kang & Cho, 1976; Lasky et al., 1975; Lis, 1969; Lubchenco et al., 1963; Phillips,

---

[1] In this chapter we use the term *prematurity* generically to encompass a variety of indexes of neonatal immaturity, including low birthweight, gestational age, head circumference, and birth length. Although this is at variance with technical usage, the four indexes are highly intercorrelated and the usage of the term *prematurity* appears warranted.

PRETERM BIRTH AND
PSYCHOLOGICAL DEVELOPMENT

1968; Rabinovitch, Bibace, & Caplan, 1961; Rubin, Rosenblatt, & Balow, 1973; Stewart, Turcan, Rawlings, Hart, & Gregory, 1978; Taub, Caputo, & Goldstein, 1975; Taub, Goldstein, & Caputo, 1977; Wiener, Rider, Oppel, Fischer, & Harper, 1965; Wiener, Rider, Oppel, & Harper, 1968; World Health Organization, 1961; Wright *et al.*, 1972). In most studies, the prematurely born child was found to function significantly more poorly than the maturely born with respect to intellectual development.

The literature reveals that low birthweight is also associated with anomalies in visual functioning or visuomotor performance. Drillien (1958) reported that 50% of her subjects weighing 1.4 kg (3 lbs.) or less at birth had visual defects; in 33% of her subjects, the defect was severe enough to be considered a handicap. This finding was confirmed in the work of Lubchenco *et al.* (1963). These researchers reported that almost 70% of their subjects with birthweights of 1500 gm or less had central or peripheral visual handicaps. Wiener *et al.* (1965) and Wiener *et al.* (1968) tested visuomotor functioning using the Bender Gestalt test. At 6–7 and again at 8–10 years of age, the low-birthweight subjects were found to be impaired with respect to visuomotor development. Lis (1969) also used the Bender Gestalt test and found that 63% of his prematurely born subjects scored below the norm.

Prenatal and Perinatal Status

Status before birth, at birth, and immediately following birth have been extensively studied in relation to the development of the child from infancy through childhood. The major variables that have been isolated for study are discussed in the following sections.

OBSTETRICAL MEDICATION

Widely diverging results vis-à-vis the child have been obtained in studies of the administration of pain-relieving drugs to the mother during labor (see Brackbill, 1979). Aleksandrowicz and Aleksandrowicz (1974); Bowes, (1970); Brackbill, Kane, Manniello, and Abrahamson (1974); Conway and Brackbill (1970), and Standley, Soule, Copans, and Duchowny (1974) noted that obstetric medication depresses orienting behavior in neonates, increases behavioral irritability, and interferes with habituation to stimulation, up to the age of 1 month. However, studies by Horowitz, Ashton, Culp, Gaddis, Levin, and Reichmann (1977) and Muller *et al.*, (1971) found no discernible effects of drugs administered to the mother on behavioral functioning of the child at 3 months and 9 years, respectively. The use of drugs in pregnancy (tranquilizers, antimicrobial agents, insulin, hormones, and antidiuretics) was found by Bowes (1970) to have no negative effects on central nervous system development. Similarly, Friedman, Brackbill, Caron, and Caron (1978) found no consistent differences in visual attention attributable to perinatal medication in 4- and 5-month-old infants.

ANOXIA AND CYANOSIS

The effects of anoxia and cyanosis on the development of intelligence have been related to birthweight. For children born weighing more than 1250 gm, cyanosis and/or anoxia is not generally associated with limitations of intellectual development, even through 6 years of age (Ambrus *et al.,* 1970; Bacola, Behrle, deSchweinitz, Miller, & Ma, 1966b; Gottfried, 1973; Outerbridge, Ramsay, & Stern, 1974; Robertson & Crichton, 1969). However, for the very smallest survivors, that is, those weighing less than 1250 gm, impairment in intellectual development was evident when cyanosis and/or anoxia was present at birth (Bacola, Behrle, deSchweinitz, Miller , & Ma, 1966a).

TYPE OF DELIVERY

Muller *et al.* (1971) related breech delivery to scholastic achievement through the third grade. Approximately one-quarter of the breech children had repeated one or more grades by 9 years of age. Arithmetic achievement scores of these children were significantly poorer than those of a control group born in the nonbreech position. The studies of Churchill (1959) and Churchill and Colfelt (1963) documented the relationship between breech delivery and the occurrence of epilepsy and cerebral palsy. The relationship between twinning and morbidity has been discussed by Caputo *et al.* (1974), Van Den Daele (1974), and Willerman and Churchill (1967).

OTHER PRENATAL AND PERINATAL FACTORS

A number of other factors appear in the literature relating prenatal and perinatal experiences to later developmental compromise. Reproductive efficiency is often compromised when the mother is either too young, that is, less than 16 years, or too old, that is, more than 40 years. Osofsky (1968) reported that infants delivered to extremely young mothers have a high incidence of neurological and developmental problems in childhood. Broman (1978) found that at age 4, children of adolescent mothers had lower IQ scores, a higher frequency of scores in the retarded range, and less advanced motor development. On the other hand, Russell and Millar (1969) found that babies born to mothers at the end of their reproductive cycle, or to mothers with five or more pregnancies, had a high probability of developmental jeopardy.

Stott (1973) found that maternal stress was related to developmental morbidity in the form of ill health, neurological dysfunction, developmental lag, and behavioral disturbance. The studies previously cited, along with the pioneering work of Pasamanick, Constantinou, and Lilienfeld (1956) and Pasamanick and Lilienfeld (1956), demonstrate the significant association between complications of pregnancy and birth and the occurrence of such developmental anomalies as cerebral palsy, epilepsy, intellectual deficit, behavioral disorders, learning disabilities, visual and hearing disorders, and emotional problems.

Demographic Status

The category of demographic status involves a number of variables related to the quality of the environment in which a child is raised. Included are such elements as parental occupational status, education, parity, family size, and other family characteristics. These epigenetic variables have taken on increased importance over the last decade in light of the genetically oriented arguments of Jensen (1969) and Herrnstein (1973).

Research on the relationship between these variables and the occurrence of developmental anomalies tends to be inconsistent and somewhat inconclusive. Burton (1968), in a study of 43,000 American high school students, found no consistent birth order differences in intelligence test scores within socioeconomic categories or within family-size groupings. Conversely, Kellaghan and Macnamarra (1972) found that both socioeconomic status (SES) and family size made significant contributions to differences in verbal reasoning scores. Murray (1971) reported that after controlling for the effects of family size and SES there were no significant differences between first borns and later borns on verbal and nonverbal tests. In an extensive study, Belmont and Marolla (1973) found that, among 40,000 19-year-old Dutch males, birth order and family size had independent relationships with intellectual performance. The relationship between family size and intelligence was not found in all social-class groupings, however.

Zajonc and Markus (1975) and Zajonc (1976) offer a "confluence model" to describe the development of intelligence without relying on such variables as race, genetics, family income, or social class. The basic postulate of the model is that the intellectual environment of the family depends on the number of family members and their respective ages.

Maternal Childrearing Attitudes

There are a number of investigations relating the level of cognitive competency in children to parental behaviors. It is assumed there is some consistency between parental behaviors and parental attitudes. Bayley and Schaefer (1964), in a longitudinal study of the intellectual development of children, assessed a large number of maternal behaviors in relation to later IQ. Among the behaviors studied, a significant relationship was found for both control and hostility.

Elardo, Bradley, and Caldwell (1975) reported that the quality of the home environment at 6 months of age related only weakly to their subjects' 6-month and 12-month scores on the Bayley Mental Development Index. However, the same measures of home environment were strongly related to their 3-year Stanford-Binet IQ scores. The aspects of home quality that proved to be the strongest predictors of 3-year IQ were the availability of appropriate play material and mother's involvement with the child. Regardless of race or social class, the children of families who provided play materials and who spent time with them had higher 3-year IQs.

Measures of Infant Status

Numerous studies appear in the literature evaluating the effectiveness of infant developmental scales as predictors of later development. Generally, these infant tests have not been found valid in predicting intelligence (IQ) in later years, particularly for intact infants. Bayley (1943) found no relationship between the Bayley Mental and Motor Developmental Scales and scores on the Stanford-Binet at ages 6 and 7 years. Anderson (1939) found nonsignificant correlations between intelligence measured at 3 months and at 5 years, and between intelligence measured at 1 year and at 5 years. The results of these studies are confirmed by the more recent findings of Bayley (1955), Stott and Ball (1965), and Thomas (1970).

McCall, Applebaum, and Hogarty (1973) measured the stability of the IQ and its relationships to other variables. Their longitudinal study involved repeated administrations of IQ tests to the same subjects between the ages of 2½ and 17 years. Their results indicated that predictions of later IQ from tests given prior to age 3 were difficult and that predictions from test data prior to age 2 were impossible. At about age 3, correlations with later IQ began to rise and became significant.

Although Bayley (1943, 1955) reported the ineffectiveness of early measures for later prediction, Cameron, Livson, and Bayley (1967), in a cluster analysis of the Bayley test items, found a vocalization factor that was moderately predictive of IQ for females to 36 years of age. This factor was ineffective for predicting later IQ for males. Sex differences in the predictive value of infant tests were also reported by McCall *et al.* (1973). These researchers found that Gesell developmental scores at 6 months successfully predicted Stanford-Binet IQ at 3½ years, but only for girls. In a study involving more than 600 subjects, Goffeney, Henderson, and Butler (1971) reported that Bayley scores obtained at 8 months successfully predicted scores on the Wechsler Intelligence Scale for Children (WISC) at 7 years. Once again, correlations were significant only for the female subjects.

In a discussion of the predictive value of infant tests, Honzik (1976) concluded that, in neurologically intact infants, scores obtained during the first months of life are not predictive of later intelligence. However, she maintained that infant tests show moderate predictive value for low-scoring children suspected of "organicity."

Method

The data reported in this chapter are based on bivariate and multivariate relationships of perinatal and 1-year descriptors to descriptors of functioning in middle childhood. The study was conducted at the Louis M. Wakoff Research Center of the Staten Island Mental Health Society, Staten Island, New York.

Subjects

The 64 children in the present study consisted of a representative sample from a group of 233 neonates who had participated in a developmental study through the first year of life. The sample consisted of 38 children (14 boys and 24 girls) who had been of low birthweight (≤ 2500 gm) and 26 children (10 boys and 16 girls) who had been full sized at birth (> 2500 gm). Four of the low-birthweight subjects and one full-sized subject were black. The children, born between July 1965 and January 1969, ranged in age from 7 to 9½ years ' follow-up. Characteristics of the follow-up and original samples were reported in earlier publications (cf. Caputo *et al.,* 1974; Goldstein, Caputo, & Taub, 1976; Taub *et al.,* 1977), where it was noted that the group of largely white, middle-class children in the follow-up study were demographically representative of children in the original sample, of children in the 1-year follow-up sample, and in fact of all children born on Staten Island, New York, during the original intake period. (See Table 20.1.)

Procedure

Data used in the present analyses were collected at three time periods: during the perinatal period, at the age of 1 year, and between the ages of 7 and 9½ years. The variables that were considered in the study are described in the following paragraphs. Details regarding the factor analytic reduction of some of the variables are reported by Goldstein, Caputo, and Taub (1976). With the exception of the current factor analysis of the demographic data, the results of the previous factor analyses were used in the data analyses.

PERINATAL DATA

The following data were collected while the mothers and their infants were still in the hospital after the birth of the children.

Demographic variables. Data were collected on seven demographic variables: father's education, mother's education, religion, private versus clinic services, race, father's occupational status, and mother's age. These seven demographic variables were subjected to a principal-components factor analysis, and two of the three significant factors, accounting for 57% of the

TABLE 20.1
Descriptors for Premature and Nonpremature Samples [a][b]

	≤ 2500 gm			> 2500 gm			
	N	Mean	SD	N	Mean	SD	χ² or t
N girls in sample	24			16		n.s.	n.s.
Age of child at assessment (months)	38	99.7	7.8	26	95.3	10.6	
Mother's age at birth of study child (years)	38	26.3	4.1	26	27.5	4.8	n.s.
N children in family at time of birth of study child	38	1.3	1.2	26	1.7	1.8	n.s.
Single births	38	71%	—	26	100%	—	χ² = 9.09*
Mother's IQ (Ammons) at birth of child	32	98.4	16.6	26	105.6	8.9	n.s.
Father's age at birth of child (years)	35	29.5	6.2	21	29.0	4.5	n.s.
Cattell DQ at 1 year of age	38	94.8	14.6	26	110.5	15.7	t = 4.10**
Father's occupation at follow-up[c]	35	3.3	1.4	26	4.0	1.5	n.s.
Father's education at follow-up	38	81%[d]	—	26	85%[d]	—	n.s.
Mother's education at follow-up	38	92%[d]	—	26	100%[d]	—	n.s.
Marital status of parents at follow-up	38	11%[e]	—	26	8%[e]	—	n.s.
N siblings younger than study child	38	1.0	1.3	26	.8	1.0	n.s.

[a] Reproduced with the permission of the Society for Research in Child Development from Taub, H. B., Goldstein, K. M., & Caputo, D. V. Indices of neonatal prematurity as discriminators of development in middle childhood. *Child Development*, 1977, *48,* 797–805.

[b] $N = 64$.

[c] Hamburger's (1958) 7-point scale, 7 being the lowest social class.

[d] Twelfth grade or more.

[e] Separated, widowed, or divorced.

* $p < .005$.

** $p < .001$.

total variance, were rotated to a varimax criterion. Variables with major loadings on the first factor, Social Class, were father's occupation, father's education, and mother's education; a high score on the factor is associated with lower social class. Variables with major loadings on the second factor, Ethnicity, were Catholic versus non-Catholic, white versus nonwhite, and use of private versus clinic service; a high score on the factor is associated with being nonwhite, non-Catholic, and using a clinic service.

Birth and obstetric variables. Factor analysis indicated that the 19-variable set of birth and obstetric variables could be described by seven factors, the first three of which accounted for 32% of the total variance. The three factors were Obstetric History (parity, number of full-sized births living, number of premature births living), Delivery and Related Variables (vaginal versus caesarean delivery, Apgar score, use of critical drug during pregnancy, type of anesthesia, single versus multiple birth, breech birth), and Complications (days infant hospitalized, cyanosis, number of complicating obstetrical conditions, other complications). A high score on the Obstetric History factor was associated with a large number of previous births, on the Delivery and Related Variables factor with a difficult delivery, and on the Complications factor with the presence of complications.

Sex of the child. A score of 1 was used for boys; a score of 2 was used for girls.

Prematurity. The four prematurity (or immaturity) variables of birth-weight, birth (crown–heel) length, head circumference, and days of gestation were represented by a single factor, Prematurity, which accounted for 76% of their total variance. A high score was indicative of prematurity.

Mother's discomfort. The three variables of mother's reported discomfort during pregnancy, during delivery, and 48 hours after delivery, were represented by a single factor, Discomfort, which accounted for 42% of their variance. A high score was associated with less discomfort.

Mother's childrearing attitudes. In an earlier report, Goldstein, Taub, Caputo, and Silberstein (1976) described the use of Schaefer and Bell's (1958) Parent Attitude Research Instrument (PARI), as modified by Chorost (1962), to measure maternal childrearing attitudes. The PARI was administered to mothers with 48 hours of delivery; it yielded scores on the two factors of Control and Hostility.

Mother's IQ. The Full-Range Picture Vocabulary Test (Ammons & Ammons, 1948) was used to assess mother's IQ.

ONE-YEAR DATA

The following data were collected when the children were 1 year of age and were used as predictor variables.

Developmental tests. Two tests were administered to the children when they were 1 year of age: the Cattell Infant Intelligence Scale (Cattell, 1960) and the Gesell Developmental Schedules (Gesell & staff, 1949). The Cattell test yielded a developmental quotient (DQ); the DQ and a developmental quotient corrected for the effects of gestational age (corrected DQ) were employed in subsequent analyses. The gestational age correction was made on the basis of mother's last reported menstrual period. Two scores from the Gesell scales were used: the Gesell motor scale basal score (which was highly related to the motor ceiling score, $r = .77$, $df = 168$, $p < .0001$) and the Gesell personal–social scale basal score (which was highly related to the personal–social ceiling score, $r = .69$, $df = 166$, $p < .0001$).

Rating scores. Four variables reflecting the baby's status at 1 year were derived from rating data. One was a social development score, which consisted of a child psychiatrist's judgments of the baby's relatedness and sociability; a high score indicated poorer social development. A rating of sensorimotor development was based on a physician's evaluation of strabismus, other visual impairments, appearance and function of the extremities, strength of grip, tremors, and other abnormal movements; a high score indicated poorer development. The remaining two variables were ratings of baby by mother on semantic differential scales (cf. Osgood, Suci, & Tannenbaum, 1957) reflecting potency and activity.

DATA IN MIDDLE CHILDHOOD

The dependent or outcome variables assessed at follow-up when the children were between the ages of 7 and 9½ years, are described in the following paragraphs.

Wechsler Intelligence Scale for Children—Revised (WISC-R). The 10 standard subtests of the WISC-R (Weschsler, 1974) were administered by trained testers who were unaware of the birth status of the child. A summary of the scores for both the low-birthweight and control subjects is presented in Table 20.2.

Bender Gestalt test. The Visual Motor Gestalt Test (Bender, 1946) was administered and scored on the basis of the scoring system developed by Koppitz (1963, 1975); scores are summarized in Table 20.2. High scores were indicative of good visuomotor performance.

Results

This section presents and discusses the bivariate relationships involving the congeries of variables studied. In view of the complex interrelationships among the predictor variables, multiple regression analyses are included for clarification.

The following classes of variables were considered as predictors of performance in middle childhood: demographic variables, maternal childrearing attitudes, maternal discomfort, birth and obstetric complications, prematurity and immaturity variables, and measures of functioning at 1 year. The sections that follow do not consider the data of boys and girls separately, since sex of

TABLE 20.2
Summary of WISC-R and Bender Gestalt Data [a,b]

	Total sample		Means			
			≤ 2500 gm		> 2500 gm	
	Mean	SD	Male	Female	Male	Female
Information	10.6	3.0	10.6	10.2	11.1	11.0
Similarities	10.3	3.4	9.6	10.8	10.2	10.2
Arithmetic	9.9	3.5	9.1	9.5	11.1	10.4
Vocabulary	10.7	3.4	10.8	10.5	10.6	11.1
Comprehension	12.1	3.5	11.4	12.2	12.0	12.7
Picture completion	10.6	3.0	10.9	9.3	11.9	11.4
Picture arrangement	10.7	3.1	10.4	10.3	11.9	11.1
Block design	10.3	3.3	9.6	9.2	13.2	10.6
Object assembly	9.9	3.3	9.6	8.8	12.0	10.3
Coding	10.1	3.1	9.1	9.6	10.8	10.8
Verbal IQ	104.0	14.4	101.6	103.2	106.0	106.1
Performance IQ	101.7	15.9	99.7	96.0	112.4	105.2
Full-Scale IQ	103.5	14.6	100.6	100.2	110.0	106.8
Bender Gestalt	9.9	.9	9.6	9.6	10.5	10.2

[a] Reproduced with the permission of the Society for Research in Child Development, from Taub, H. B., Goldstein, K. M. & Caputo, D. V. Indices of neonatal prematurity as discriminators of development in middle childhood. *Child Development*, 1977, *48*, 797–805.
[b] $N = 64$.

child did not correlate significantly with any of the dependent variables considered (see Table 20.4). Because of the large number of analyses, the .02 level of probability was used to determine statistical significance. Findings with an associated probability level of .02–.05 were considered to be tending toward significance.

The intercorrelations between pairs of predictor variables are summarized in Table 20.3. The bivariate correlations between predictor variables or factors and both WISC-R IQ and Bender Gestalt (Koppitz) scores are summarized in Table 20.4

Demographic Variables

In the bivariate analyses involving the two factors derived from the demographic variables the Social Class factor was related to intelligence, while the Ethnicity factor was not. The Social Class factor was significantly related to verbal (V)-IQ ($r = -.43$), to performance (P)-IQ ($r = -.45$), and to full-scale (FS)-IQ ($r = -.50$). It related significantly to three of the five verbal subtests (information, $r = -.48$; similarities, $r = -.46$; and vocabulary, $r = -.40$) and to four of the five performance subtests (picture completion, $r = -.34$; picture arrangement, $r = -.36$; block design, $r = -.35$; and ob-

TABLE 20.3
Significant Intercorrelations between Pairs of Predictor Variables (r above Diagonal, N below Diagonal)

Predictor variables	1	2	3	4	5	6	7	8	9	10	11	12	13	14	15	16	17	18	19
1. Social Class factor	—												-.26*						-.49****
2. Ethnicity factor		—												-.42***	.34*	.34*			-.35****
3. Obstetric History factor			—	-.27*						.36***								-.35***	
4. Delivery and Related Variables factor			64	—			.27*				-.35***	-.29*						.28*	-.31*
5. Complications factor					—		.50*****				-.37***								
6. Sex of the child						—											-.54*****		
7. Prematurity factor					64		—				-.56*****					.35*			
8. Discomfort factor								—			.29*	.27*							
9. Childrearing: Control (PARI)	59	58	58	64	64		64	64	—	.37***				-.46***	.28*				-.50****
10. Childrearing: Hostility (PARI)								56	58	—									
11. Cattell DQ			58	64	64						—	.90*****	.31*	.54****		.51****			
12. Cattell DQ-corrected				56		58					56	—		.42***		-.45****			
13. Gesell motor (basal)						58			37	42	42	36	—	.38***		-.53*****			
14. Gesell personal-social (basal)			42		42				37	42	42	36	42	—		-.46***			
15. Social development	39	39			39				53					39	—				
16. Sensorimotor development		39					39		39	39	39	33	39	39		—			.34**
17. Rating of baby's potency			60	60													—	.51*****	.36**
18. Rating of baby's activity																	61	—	
19. Mother's IQ	55	55	55	55	55				54		55	49	37	37					—

* p < .05
** p < .02
*** p < .01
**** p < .001
***** p < .0001

TABLE 20.4

Significant Correlations between Predictor Variables and IQ and Bender Gestalt Scores

Predictor variables	N	WISC–R scales				
		Infor-mation	Simi-larities	Arith-metic	Vocabu-lary	Compre-hension
Social Class factor	64	−.48*****	−.46****		−.40****	
Ethnicity factor	64					
Obstetric History factor	64		−.26*			
Delivery and Related Variables factor	64					
Complications factor	64					
Sex of the child	64					
Prematurity factor	64					
Discomfort factor	64					
Childrearing: Control	55	−.42***	−.31**		−.46****	−.27*
Childrearing: Hostility	55					
Cattell DQ	64					
Cattell DQ–Corrected	56					
Gesell motor (basal)	42					
Gesell personal-social (basal)	42	.31*			.46***	
Social development	39		−.33*	−.33*		−.48***
Sensorimotor development	39					
Ratings of baby's potency	61					
Ratings of baby's activity	59				.33**	.26*
Mother's IQ	55	.52****	.30*		.45***	

* $p < .05$
** $p < .02$
*** $p < .01$
**** $p < .001$
***** $p < .0001$

ject assembly, $r = -.36$). Higher social class was associated with higher IQ scores. The Ethnicity factor was unrelated to any of the 13 WISC-R scores.

The single variable, mother's IQ, was subsumed in our earlier reports under the rubric of demographic variables. In view of its important relationships to the dependent (or outcome) variables in the present study, it was considered apart from the other demographic variables. Mother's IQ showed the strongest pattern of significant bivariate correlations with the child's IQ scores in middle childhood, relating significantly to V-IQ ($r = .38$), to P-IQ ($r = .54$), and to FS-IQ ($r = .55$). It related significantly to two verbal subtests (information, $r = .52$; and vocabulary, $r = .45$) and tended toward a significant relationship with a third (similarities, $r = .30$). In addition, mother's IQ related significantly to four performance subtests (picture completion, $r = .35$; block design, $r = .53$; object assembly, $r = 45$; and coding, $r = .41$) and tended toward a significant correlation with the fifth (picture arrangement. $r = .28$). Mother's IQ also related significantly to the Bender Gestalt (Koppitz) visuomotor score ($r = .37$), children of mothers with lower IQ having poorer visuomotor ability. There was only one other significant relationship in the bivariate analyses between a predictor variable and the Bender Gestalt score (that involving the Prematurity factor, as noted later).

				WISC–R scales				
Picture Com-pletion	Picture arrange-ment	Block design	Object assembly	Coding	Verbal IQ	Perfor-mance IQ	Full-scale IQ	Bender Gestalt visuo-motor
− .34***	− .36***	− .35***	− .36***		− .43****	− .45****	− .50*****	
					− .29**		− .26*	
− .32***		− .37***	− .35***			− .36***	− .27*	− .40***
− .41***		− .43****			− .43****	− .38***	− .46****	
.34***	.27*		.32***			.34***	.30**	
.33*								
					.38**	.33*	.39**	
					− .46***		− .36*	
.36**			.41****			.28*		
.35***	.28*	.53*****	.45****	.41***	.38***	.54*****	.55*****	.39***

A number of multiple regression analyses were computed in order to clarify the interrelationships among the demographic and outcome data.

The first multiple regression analysis used the single variable mother's IQ and the Social Class factor as predictors. The use of these variables represents an imperfect attempt to assay the relative contribution of nature and nurture to the child's intellectual and perceptuomotor functioning in middle childhood.

As may be seen in Table 20.5, significant multiple correlations were obtained when the two predictors were employed in four analyses involving the outcome variables of WISC-R V-IQ, P-IQ, FS-IQ, and the Koppitz scores for the Bender Gestalt. (In view of the large number of analyses that would have been required, multiple regression analyses involving WISC-R subtests were not computed.)

The pairing of mother's IQ and the Social Class factor in multiple regression analyses yielded Rs with WISC-R IQs ranging from $R = .47$ for V-IQ to $R = .61$ for FS-IQ, accounting for 22–37% of the variance of IQ scores in middle childhood. The multiple R of .37 indicated that mother's IQ and the Social Class factor also significantly predicted Bender Gestalt (Koppitz) scores, accounting for 14% of the variance of these scores.

TABLE 20.5
Summary of Multiple Regression Analyses Using Demographic Variables as Predictors

Predictor variables (sets)	WISC-R V-IQ		WISC-R P-IQ		WISC-R FS-IQ		Bender Gestalt	
	t	r	t	r	t	r	t	r
(a)								
Mother's IQ	—	—	3.22	.41***	3.18	.40***	2.54	.33**
Social Class factor	−2.28	−.30*	—	—	−2.44	−.32**	—	—
R (2/52)	.47***		.58****		.61****		.37**	
(b)								
Mother's IQ	—	—	3.38	.43***	3.24	.42***	2.96	.39***
Mother's education	—	—	—	—	—	—	—	—
Father's education	—	—	—	—	—	—	2.13	.29*
Father's occupation	—	—	—	—	—	—	—	—
R (4/50)	.48***		.57****		.61****		.47**	

Outcome variables

* $p < .05$
** $p < .02$
*** $p < .01$
**** $p < .001$

Mother's IQ made significant independent contributions to P-IQ, FS-IQ, and Bender Gestalt scores. The Social Class factor made a significant independent contribution to FS-IQ and tended toward a significant independent contribution to V-IQ.

In the second set of multivariate analyses summarized in Table 20.5, the three major components of the Social Class factor (father's occupation, father's education, mother's education) were included in multiple regression analyses, along with mother's IQ as a fourth predictor variable. The purpose of this analysis was to clarify the role of the specific components of the Social Class factor, in conjunction with mother's IQ, in predicting WISC-R and Bender Gestalt performance. Once again, all four of the Rs were statistically significant.

As before, mother's IQ made significant independent contributions to P-IQ, FS-IQ, and Bender Gestalt scores. Of the three components of the Social Class factor, none made significant independent contributions to the four outcome variables. However, father's education tended toward a significant independent contribution to the Bender Gestalt scores.

Mother's Childrearing Attitudes

In bivariate analyses, the PARI factor of Control was significantly related to V-IQ ($r = -.43$), to P-IQ ($r = -.38$), and to FS-IQ ($r = -.46$), greater control being associated with lower IQ scores (see Table 20.4). Control was significantly related to three of the verbal subtests (information, $r = -.42$; similarities, $r = -.31$; and vocabulary, $r = -.46$) and tended toward a significant correlation with a fourth (comprehension, $r = -.27$). It was significantly related to two of the performance subtests (picture completion, $r = -.41$; and block design, $r = -.43$). The PARI factor of Hostility was unrelated to any of the WISC-R scores.

In the multiple regression analyses summarized in Table 20.6 (Part A), the two PARI factors of Control and Hostility related significantly to the three WISC-R variables but not to the Bender Gestalt scores. In all three significant analyses, PARI Control made a significant independent contribution to the outcome variables.

In view of the PARI's strong relationship to socioeconomic status (Becker & Krug, 1965), the PARI was included with the two factors deriving from the set of demographic variables employed in this study (the Social Class and the Ethnicity factor) and with mother's IQ in analyses aimed at discovering whether the PARI factors contribute independently in predictions of the outcome variables (see Table 6, Part B). All four of the multiple Rs were statistically significant. Mother's IQ again proved to be the most potent contributor to three of the four outcome variables (P-IQ, FS-IQ, and Bender Gestalt scores), with PARI Control merely tending toward an independent contribution in the case of the Bender Gestalt scores.

TABLE 20.6
Summary of Multiple Regression Analyses Focusing on Childrearing Attitudes as Predictors

Predictor Variables (sets)	Outcome variables							
	WISC-R V-IQ		WISC-R P-IQ		WISC-R FS-IQ		Bender Gestalt	
	t	r	t	r	t	r	t	r
(a)								
PARI: Control	−3.41	−.42***	−2.85	−.36***	−3.62	−.44****	—	—
PARI: Hostility								—
R (2/55)	.43***		.38**		.46***			
(b)								
PARI: Control	—	—	—	—	—	—	2.22	.30*
PARI: Hostility	—	—	—	—	—	—	—	—
Mother's IQ	—	—	2.84	.38***	2.53	.34**	.289	.38***
Social Class factor	—	—	—	—	—	—	—	—
Ethnicity factor	—	—	—	—	—	—	—	—
R (5-49)	.52***		.60****		.64****		.47**	

* $p < .05$
** $p < .02$
*** $p < .01$
**** $p < .001$

Mother's Discomfort

The Discomfort factor was unrelated to any of the WISC-R variables or to the Bender Gestalt scores in bivariate analyses (see Table 20.4). As such, this factor was not included in the multivariate analyses.

Birth and Obstetric Variables and Prematurity (Immaturity)

In the bivariate analyses, only one of the three factors derived from the birth and obstetric variables related to the child's IQ in middle childhood. The first factor, Obstetric History, was significantly related to WISC-R V-IQ ($r = -.29$) but not to P-IQ. It tended toward a significant relationship with FS-IQ ($r = -.26$) and with one of the 10 subtests (similarities, $r = -.26$). Neither of the other two factors, Delivery and Related Variables, and Complications, correlated significantly with any of the WISC-R scores.

The Prematurity factor did not relate in the bivariate analyses to V-IQ but did relate significantly to P-IQ ($r = -.36$) and tended to relate to FS-IQ ($r = -.27$), with prematurely born children having lower IQs. It correlated significantly with three of the five performance subtests: picture completion ($r = -.32$), block design ($r = -.37$), and object assembly ($= -.35$). It also correlated significantly with the Bender Gestalt scores ($r = -.40$), low-birthweight children tending to have poorer visuomotor ability.

Because of the special concern of this research with neonatal prematurity and immaturity, the bivariate correlations between the IQ test scores and each of the four variables comprising the Prematurity factor were also examined.

The variable of birthweight was found to be most closely associated with the IQ variables, being significantly related to P-IQ ($r = .33$) and to the three performance subtests of picture completion ($r = .30$), block design ($r = .37$), and object assembly ($r = .36$). These correlations matched almost identically those obtained for the Prematurity factor.

The three remaining prematurity variables, birth length, head circumference, and gestational age, each tended toward a significant bivariate correlation with P-IQ ($r = .30$, $r = .41$, and $r = .27$, respectively) and with the subtest of block design ($r = .31$, $r = .41$, and $r = .29$, respectively). Birth length also correlated significantly with picture completion ($r = .36$) and tended to correlate significantly with object assembly ($r = .30$), while head circumference correlated significantly with object assembly ($r = .48$). (It should be noted that the N for head circumference was attenuated because of the failure of physicians to report this measure for many of the children.) In addition, birthweight, birth length, and head circumference were significantly correlated with Bender Gestalt visuomotor scores ($r = .41$, $r = .41$, and $r = .53$, respectively); gestational age was not.

The results of multivariate analyses employing the three factors deriving from the 19-variable set of descriptors of birth and obstetric complications are reported in Table 20.7. These factors were utilized alone as a set of predictors

TABLE 20.7
Summary of Multiple Regression Analyses Using Birth Complications and Prematurity (Immaturity) Variables as Predictors

Predictor variables (sets)	Outcome variables							
	WISC-R V-IQ		WISC-R P-IQ		WISC-R FS-IQ		Bender Gestalt	
	t	r	t	r	t	r	t	r
(a)								
Obstetric History factor	—	—	—	—	—	—	—	—
Delivery and Related Variables factor	—	—	—	—	—	—	—	—
Complications factor	—	—	—	—	—	—	—	—
R (3/60)								
(b)								
Obstetric History factor	—	—	—	—	—	—	—	—
Delivery and Related Variables factor	—	—	—	—	—	—	—	—
Complications factor	—	—	—	—	—	—	2.25	.28*
Prematurity factor	—	—	−2.39	−.30**	—	—	−3.87	−.45***
R (4/59)			.42**				.49***	

(c)

Obstetric History factor	−2.48	−.33**	−2.20	−.30*	−2.88	−.38***	−3.12	−.41***
Delivery and Related Variables factor	—	—	—	—	—	—	—	—
Complications factor	—	—	—	—	—	—	—	—
Prematurity factor	3.74	.47****	4.41	.53****	—	—	—	—
Mother's IQ	—	—	—	—	5.31	.60****	2.23	.30*
R (5/49)	.55***		.64****		.67****		.55***	

(d)

Obstetric History factor	−2.23	−.31*	—	—	−2.57	−.35**	−3.10	−.41***
Delivery and Related Variables factor	—		—	—	—		—	—
Complications factor	—		—	—	—		—	—
Prematurity factor	—		−2.03	−.28*	—		—	—
Mother's IQ	—		2.72	.37***	3.19	.42***	—	—
Social Class factor	—		—		−2.12	−.30*	—	—
Ethnicity factor	—		—		—		—	—
R (7/47)	.59***		.69****		.72****		.56***	

$* \ p < .05$
$** \ p < .02$
$*** \ p < .01$
$**** \ p < .001$

of the four outcome scores and then in conjunction with the Prematurity factor and demographic variables.

Table 20.7 (Part A) shows that the three birth and obstetric factors did not, as a set, relate significantly to the WISC-R or Bender Gestalt (Koppitz) data.

As may be seen in the table (Part B), when the Prematurity factor was added to the three birth and obstetric factors, there were significant relationships with P-IQ and the Bender Gestalt scores. In both significant analyses, the Prematurity factor made a significant independent contribution. The Complications factor tended toward a significant independent contribution to the Bender Gestalt scores.

In the next analyses (Table 20.7, Part C), mother's IQ was added to the set of predictor variables. In all four analyses, the multiple Rs were statistically significant. The additional variable, mother's IQ, made significant independent contributions to the three analyses involving the WISC-R and tended toward an independent contribution to the Bender Gestalt scores. The Prematurity factor also made a significant independent contribution to the Bender Gestalt scores. In these analyses (which involved a somewhat smaller number of subjects because of missing data), the Obstetric History factor was now found to make significant independent contributions to both V-IQ and FS-IQ and to tend toward a significant independent contribution to P-IQ.

In the fourth set of analyses, summarized in Table 20.7 (Part D), the two demographic factors of Social Class and Ethnicity were added to the foregoing set of predictor variables. Once again, all four analyses were statistically significant. Mother's IQ made significant independent contributions in two of the analyses, to P-IQ and FS-IQ. The Prematurity factor made a significant independent contribution to the Bender Gestalt scores and tended toward a significant independent contribution to a second outcome variable, P-IQ. The Obstetric History factor made a significant independent contribution to FS-IQ and tended toward a significant independent contribution to V-IQ. The Social Class factor tended toward a significant independent correlation with FS-IQ.

One-Year Developmental Status

In the bivariate analyses, the Cattell DQ was significantly related to P-IQ ($r = .34$) and FS-IQ ($r = .30$) but not to V-IQ. It was significantly related to two performance subtests (picture completion, $r = .34$; and object assembly, $r = .32$) and tended toward a significant relationship with a third (picture arrangement, $r = .27$). The corrected DQ was unrelated to any of the WISC-R scores, indicating that it was not as good a predictor of IQ in middle childhood as was the uncorrected DQ.

The Gesell motor basal score was not significantly related to any of the WISC-R scores.

The Gesell personal–social basal score was significantly related to V-IQ ($r = .38$), tended toward a significant relationship with P-IQ ($r = .33$), and was significantly related to FS-IQ ($r = .39$). The score was significantly correlated with one verbal subtest (vocabulary, $r = .46$) and tended toward a significant correlation with another (information, $r = .31$). It also tended toward a significant correlation with one performance subtest (picture completion, $r = .33$).

Bivariate analyses employing ratings of the child at 1-year of age highlighted the relationship between certain of the ratings and later IQ. Social development scores at 1 year were related to V-IQ ($r = -.46$) but not to P-IQ and tended to relate significantly to FS-IQ ($r = -.36$). These scores related significantly to one verbal subtest (comprehension, $r = -.48$) and tended toward a significant relationship with two others (similarities, $r = -.33$; and arithmetic, $r = -.33$) but were not significantly related to any of the performance subtests. Thus social development as judged herein predicted, primarily, verbal IQ.

Sensorimotor development, another 1-year score based on ratings, was not significantly related to any of the outcome scores.

Mother's evaluation of baby's potency at 1 year tended to relate to P-IQ ($r = .28$) and was unrelated to both V-IQ and FS-IQ in bivariate correlations. It related significantly to two performance subtests (picture completion, $r = .36$; and object assembly, $r = .41$) but not to any verbal subtests.

Mother's evaluation of baby's activity at 1 year was unrelated to V-IQ, P-IQ, or FS-IQ. It was significantly related to one verbal subtest (vocabulary, $r = .33$) and tended to relate significantly to another (comprehension, $r = .26$); it was unrelated to any of the performance subtests.

None of the 1-year ratings was found to relate to Bender Gestalt scores.

Since the 1-year ratings were generally poor predictors of later outcome, only one of them, social development, was included in the multiple regression analyses. In these analyses, the tests of 1-year infant status, the Cattell, the Gesell, and the social development scores were considered as predictors of WISC-R IQ and Bender Gestalt performance in middle childhood.

In the first set of analyses, a set of predictors consisting of the Gesell personal–social basal score and the Gesell motor basal score yielded multiple correlations that only tended toward significance with V-IQ and FS-IQ (see Table 20.8, Part A).

When the Cattell DQ was combined with the two Gesell scores as predictors, none of the multiple Rs was statistically significant (see Table 20.8, Part B). This result is in contrast with the bivariate correlations involving the Cattell DQ. In the bivariate analyses, however, the number of subjects with available data was considerably larger ($N = 64$) than in the multivariate analyses ($N = 42$).

Since the Gesell personal–social basal score and the social development rating score predicted some of the outcome variables in bivariate analyses, they were combined as a predictor set to determine their relative importance. As summarized in Table 20.8 (Part C), the multiple correlations with V-IQ

TABLE 20.8

Summary of Multiple Regression Analyses Using 1-Year Status and Demographic Variables as Predictors

Predictor variables (sets)	Outcome variables							
	WISC-R V-IQ		WISC-R P-IQ		WISC-R FS-IQ		Bender Gestalt	
	t	r	t	r	t	r	t	r
(a)								
Gesell personal–social basal	2.38	.36*	—	—	2.53	.38**	—	—
Gesell motor basal	—	—	—	—	—	—	—	—
R (2/39)		.38*				.39*		
(b)								
Cattell DQ	—	—	—	—	—	—	—	—
Gesell personal–social basal	—	—	—	—	—	—	—	—
Gesell motor basal	—	—	—	—	—	—	—	—
R (3/38)								
(c)								
Gesell personal–social basal	—	—	—	—	—	—	—	—
Social development score	− 2.60	− .40**	—	—	—	—	—	—
R (2/36)		.53***				.47***		

* $p < .05$
** $p < .02$
*** $p < .01$

and FS-IQ were statistically significant, the social development score contributing independently to V-IQ.

Also computed were additional analyses in which mother's IQ and mother's education are added to the two Gesell variables as predictors. This set related significantly to the three WISC-R variables. For two of the analyses (P-IQ and FS-IQ), mother's IQ made significant independent contributions. The Gesell personal-social score tended to contribute significantly to V-IQ and FS-IQ.

Discussion

The purpose of the present research is to compare the utility of various classes of descriptors of the status and milieu of infants during the perinatal period and at 1 year for predicting the intellective and perceptuomotor functioning of these middle-class, relatively intact individuals in middle childhood, that is, at a mean age of approximately 8 years.

Among the perinatal and 1-year descriptors that significantly predicted WISC-R IQ in middle childhood, two are well established in the literature, the highly intercorrelated measures for social class and mother's IQ. The bivariate correlation ($r = .50$) between the Social Class factor and WISC-R full-scale IQ found in the present study is somewhat higher than that ($r = .38$) found by Broman et al. (1975) for their white, preschool subjects. A more definitive relationship between social class and IQ might be expected for the subjects in the present study, since they were older than those in the Broman et al. sample. Hindley (1968) concluded that this relationship increases with age in younger children; in addition, the reliability of childhood IQ assessments increases with age (Terman & Merrill, 1937; Wechsler, 1974). Rubin and Balow (1979) reported that socioeconomic status was a better predictor of IQ at ages 4 and 7 than an infant development scale administered at 8 months.

The bivariate correlation ($r = .55$) between mother's IQ and the WISC-R FS-IQ for the children in the present study is similar to that ($r = .51$) reported by McCall et al. (1973) between IQ scores of mothers and their $9\frac{1}{2}$–$10\frac{1}{2}$-year-old offspring and to the correlation of .50 expected on the basis of the work of Erlenmeyer-Kimling and Jarvik (1968).

Of the 10 standard WISC-R subtests administered, only the arithmetic and comprehension subtests failed to relate either to mother's IQ or to the Social Class factor in the bivariate analyses. Arithmetic, in fact, was not significantly related to any of the predictor variables. Kaufman (1975), in a factor analytic study of the WISC-R, documented that the arithmetic subtest is somewhat anomalous among the WISC-R subtests. Apparently, the comprehension subtest may be unique as well.

In the bivariate analyses, both mother's IQ and the Social Class factor correlated significantly with V-IQ, P-IQ, and FS-IQ. When mother's IQ and the Social Class factor were combined in a multiple regression analysis it became evident that although the two predictor variables were highly intercorrelated ($r = -.49$), they related differently to V-IQ and P-IQ. Mother's IQ made a significant independent contribution to P-IQ, whereas the Social Class factor tended toward a significant independent contribution to V-IQ. If mother's IQ is considered a crude index of the biological anlage of intelligence, then it is this putative biological contribution that seems to relate more definitively to perceptuomotor cognition in middle childhood. This conclusion is buttressed by the finding of a unique contribution of mother's IQ to the Koppitz score on the Bender Gestalt, which is also a measure of perceptuomotor functioning. On the other hand, the Social Class factor, presumably an indicator of the quality of the developmental environment of the child, tended to relate to verbal cognitive skills in middle childhood but failed to contribute independently to either of the perceptual–cognitive measures.

When a number of the major components of the Social Class factor were considered along with mother's IQ, the data indicated that none of the three social class variables made an important unique contribution to any of the outcome variables (although mother's IQ continued to do so). Apparently, then, the importance of the Social Class factor is dependent on the combined influence of a number of demographic indicators and not on any of these alone, insofar as intelligence and perceptuomotor functioning in middle childhood are concerned.

Of course, these results cannot be construed as a definitive statement on the nature–nurture controversy as it applies to IQ. Mother's IQ may relate strongly to the child's IQ because high-IQ mothers may structure an environment conducive to the development of high IQ in their children. The elements of this environment may not be reflected in the descriptors of socioeconomic status employed in this study or in the PARI childrearing attitude variables mentioned earlier.

Second, the bivariate correlations between mother's IQ and the child's IQ are no higher, in this study, than .55; thus, some 70% of the variance of IQ in middle childhood is explained by factors other than mother's IQ. Another obvious lacuna in the present research is the absence of data on father's IQ.

Somewhat unexpectedly, the PARI Control score was found to be strongly predictive of IQ in middle childhood in the bivariate analyses. However, the large intercorrelations between this score and both mother's IQ and the Social Class factor devalue the importance of the relationship, as seen in the multiple regression analyses. The association between socioeconomic status of mother and PARI scores has been documented by Becker and Krug (1965). Thus, maternal childrearing attitudes, as measured by the PARI, do not appear to make an important independent contribution to cognitive functioning. This view is indirectly supported in previously reported findings by the present authors regarding the PARI scales (Goldstein, Taub, Caputo, & Silberstein, 1976). It was noted that mother's PARI scores on Control and Hostility, assessed at the birth of the infant and when the infant was 1 year old, were highly intercorrelated and were not at all influenced by the infant's characteristics at birth or at 1 year. Instead they related strongly to demographic descriptors, such as socioeconomic status and mother's IQ.

Among the three factors summarizing the categories of birth and obstetric variables, only the Obstetric History factor predicted the child's later IQ in the bivariate analyses. This factor related significantly to V-IQ and tended to relate to FS-IQ. Similarly, in the multiple regression analyses involving the birth and obstetric complications factors with other variables, the Obstetric History factor continued to show significant independent relationships with middle childhood IQ. Ironically, the two other factors derived from this set of variables, Delivery and Related Variables and Complications, had been found in an earlier report by the present authors to relate significantly to 1-year Cattell DQ, whereas the Obstetric History factor had not (Goldstein, Caputo, & Taub, 1976). Thus, although variables descriptive of delivery and of complications seemed to exert powerful effects on the adaptive functioning of the infant at 1 year, these effects were nil for the same subjects in middle childhood. Yet, apparently incongruously, the "sleeper factor" of Obstetric History suddenly became relevant.

The seminal research of Zajonc (Zajonc, 1976; Zajonc & Markus, 1975) provides a cogent explanation of the sleeper effect of this factor. Most of the descriptors found to load on the Obstetric History factor are simply variants of family size, that is, estimates of the number of children already in the family at the time of birth of the study subject (e.g., N children, N full-sized births, N premature births—living). In the Zajonc confluence model, family size is, of course, one of the critical variables contributing to the intellectual environment within the family, a large number of siblings serving generally to dilute or debase the intellectual environment of the developing child.

Thus, the significant negative relationship between the Obstetric History factor and IQ appears to be based on the possible attenuation of the child's cognitive development with increasing family size.

The confluence model may also explain, at least tenuously, the failure of the Obstetric History factor to predict Cattell DQs at 1 year of age, while the two factors clearly relating to delivery and complications did. The Obstetric History factor, despite its name, may reflect critical aspects of the milieu of the developing child (i.e., the intellectual environment) that were not yet salient at the time of the infant's first birthday. The other two factors in this group, Delivery and Related Variables and Complications, were, by contrast, oriented toward events that had already occurred.

In the bivariate analyses, the Prematurity factor significantly related to both Cattell DQ at 1 year and, in the middle childhood assessment, to WISC-R P-IQ ($r = -.36$). It tended to relate to FS-IQ ($r = -.27$) as well, but not to V-IQ. The performance subtests correlating with the prematurity factor were picture completion ($r = -.32$), block design ($r = -.37$), and object assembly ($r = -.35$). Kaufman (1975), in his factor analysis of the WISC-R data for subjects similar in age to those in the present study, averred that these three subtests loaded most heavily on the factor he termed *Perceptual Organization*. Thus, the asseveration by Lis (1969) and by Phillips (1968) that prematurity (i.e., low birthweight in these studies) is associated with central rather than peripheral visual deficit is supported, especially since peripheral visual problems were not characteristic of the premature subjects in the present study (see Caputo *et al.,* 1974; Taub *et al.,* 1977).

In the multiple regression analyses involving prematurity and the birth and obstetric complications factors, neonatal immaturity or prematurity appeared to be the only anomaly of this genre that related independently to cognitive development beyond the first year of life. In these analyses, the Prematurity factor related independently both to WISC-R P-IQ and to the Koppitz score for the Bender Gestalt test. The addition of mother's IQ to the set of variables served to vitiate the significant independent relationship between the Prematurity factor and later IQ, apparently because of some overlap between these variables. Nevertheless, it is clear that prematurity is strongly and independently related to perceptuomotor functioning in middle childhood, as reflected in the Bender Gestalt score. Thus the hypothesized influence of prematurity on the development of visually mediated behaviors should be further investigated.

In studies by Wiener *et al.* (1968) and by Rubin *et al.* (1973), a Wechsler IQ test (the WISC) was also employed for assessment of cognitive functioning in a longitudinal design. However, unlike the results of the present study, the Wiener *et al.* results showed that low-birthweight subjects and controls were significantly different on both V-IQ and P-IQ. In the Rubin *et al.* research, although low-birth-weight subjects were found to have significantly lower WISC FS-IQ than controls, data for V-IQ and P-IQ were not reported separately. However, since measures of language development, school readiness, and academic achievement administered at ages 4–7 years discriminated low-birthweight subjects from controls, it is likely that, as in the Wiener *et al.* research, these subjects demonstrated verbal deficit as well as deficit in perceptual aspects of cognitive functioning. The vulnerability of verbal functioning in the case of the prematures studied by Wiener *et al.* and by Rubin *et al.* may be a function of the fact that the subject samples employed in those studies contained a relatively high proportion of very low birthweight children (Wiener *et al.*) or of neurologically impaired children (Rubin *et al.*) as compared with the subject sample employed in the present study.

The 10-year longitudinal study by Wright *et al.* (1972) compared the intellective functioning of 65 children of very low birthweight (< 1500 gm) with that of matched full-sized controls. The investigators indicated that for this relatively low SES group, which had high proportions of neurologically impaired children, the low-birthweight children performed significantly more poorly on both verbal and performance WISC IQ measures.

The data herein presented indicated that visual perception was negatively affected by prematurity, whereas the other functions governing cognitive behavior in these relatively intact individuals of moderately low birthweight were not. Rigor in methodology would thereby require that researchers who are assessing cognitive functioning in individuals born at risk employ multifactorial measures of cognitive functioning (including perceptuomotor functioning) rather than tests oriented solely toward general intelligence.

The four variables comprising the Prematurity factor had been selected for further study because of their strong association with 1-year Cattell scores. Of these four, only birthweight unambiguously predicted P-IQ in middle childhood in the bivariate analyses; the others, birth length, head circumference, and gestational age, merely tended toward a significant association with P-IQ. While an attenuated N for head circumference may compromise the predictive efficiency of that variable in the present study, birthweight seems a somewhat stronger predictor of cognitive functioning than the other measures of neo-natal immaturity assessed in the present study. In this regard, Rubin *et al.* (1973) reported that birthweight significantly discriminated their subjects on the Stanford-Binet administered at age 4 and on the WISC administered at age 7 but that gestational age did not. In the longitudinal study by Neligan, Kolvin, Scott and Garside (1976) comparing light-for-date and short-gestation subjects against a control group of subjects born full sized at term, it appears to the present authors that differences found on a variety of cognitive, percep-tual, and anthropometric measures obtained at ages 5 and 7 years covaried with the birthweights of the groups in virtually every instance. The contribu-tion of gestational age to the discrepancies among scores for the groups in that study seems, therefore, moot.

Among the developmental tests administered to the infant at 1 year of age, the bivariate analyses indicated that the Cattell predicted later WISC-R P-IQ ($r = .34$) and FS-IQ ($r = .30$), whereas the Gesell personal–social score predicted WISC-R V-IQ ($r = .38$) and FS-IQ ($r = .39$) and tended to be significantly associated with P-IQ ($r = .33$). (It should be noted that the smaller Ns for the Gesell correlations required larger correlation coefficients to achieve significance.) The Gesell motor scores were not related to WISC-R IQs. Thus, for the Cattell and for the Gesell personal–social scales, there ap-pears to be, to some extent, a division of predictive labor, the former more clearly associated with P-IQ and the latter with V-IQ.

This pattern of associations may be based on the particular array of func-tions tapped by each of the tests. The Cattell test assesses, primarily, activities of a visuomotor nature involving fine motor skills. The test excludes items of a personal–social nature and motor items involving large muscles (Honzik, 1976). The Gesell personal–social schedule, by contrast, consists of both responses to people and self-help items, while the Gesell motor schedule in-cludes both gross skills and fine motor skills (Honzik, 1976).

The two WISC-R subtests that were significantly correlated with Cattell DQ in the bivariate analyses were picture completion ($r = .34$) and object assembly ($r = .32$), the same subtests that related significantly to the Prematurity factor (with the addition of block design) and that loaded heavily on Kaufman's Perceptual Organization factor. Apparently, the Cattell taps, to a significant extent, those infant behaviors that presage later P-IQ (par-ticularly perceptual organization), and it is this skein of emerging cognitive functions that seems to be particularly affected by prematurity.

Neither of the Gesell schedules related to the prematurity factor in bivariate analyses. Thus, the behaviors in infancy that seem, in some degree, to be the precursors of later V-IQ (and V-IQ, per se) were not significantly affected by prematurity. Gross motor development, insofar as it is measured by the Gesell motor schedule, appears to proceed quite apart from both prematurity and later intellective functioning, for the sample studied. It should be noted that the Cattell test and the Gesell personal–social schedule are highly intercorrelated in this study ($r = .54$) yet apparently retain enough uniqueness to allow, to some extent, for differential prediction.

In combining the various 1-year tests in multiple regression analyses, there was no substantial increment in predictive efficiency over that obtained when analyzing the tests individually in the bivariate analyses. This was due, in part, to the high intercorrelations among the 1-year tests. Also, in multivariate analyses involving the Cattell DQ, the reduced N for the variables with which it was combined resulted in a loss of power, effectively eliminating the impact of the Cattell variable.

Interestingly, in combining the two measures that appeared to tap social behavior at 1 year of age (Gesell personal–social basal and the social development scores), a high multiple correlation was obtained for V-IQ ($R = .53$) and also for FS-IQ ($R = .47$). These correlations, based on only two variables, are similar in magnitude to the multiple correlations obtained when six factors (summarizing data from 32 variables) and mother's IQ were employed as predictors. Apparently then, social behavior at 1 year relates strongly to the development of verbal IQ in middle childhood.

Parenthetically, were we to have followed methodological protocol and corrected the Cattell DQs for gestational age in the bivariate analyses, the Prematurity factor would have failed to relate to 1-year DQ but would, of course, have related to WISC-R P-IQ assessed several years later. This would in turn have led to the paradox that prematurity is related to the adaptive functioning of the child when he or she is 8 or 9 years old but not to the adaptive functioning of the same individual when he or she is 1 year old! Rubin et al. (1973), in the aforementioned study, were compelled, for similar reasons, to reject the gestational age correction when they discovered that the corrected developmental test scores for their subjects at 8 months were completely incongruous with later Stanford-Binet and WISC scores for these same subjects. As the present authors have opined previously (see Caputo, Goldstein, & Taub, 1979), the gestational age correction is valid only if "catch up" (not based on compensatory or substitutive mechanisms) occurs on relevant parameters assessed later in the individual's development. As methodologically more sophisticated studies enter the literature, it is becoming evident that the deficits observed among premature infants represent veridical, continuing debility and not simply developmental lag. Application of this correction would, as has been described, becloud the issues involved.

That correction of infancy scores may be required for some functions is, no doubt, reasonable. Suppose, for example, that preterms score lower than full-terms by a given average number of units during some period in infancy but that after that period they catch up to full-terms on that measure. In that case, there is true developmental lag—that is, the deficit has been shown empirically to be a transient one. Then, if one wished to predict the future behavior of a given preterm baby on the function assessed by the measure, a correction might be made (depending on the purpose of the research). But the correction would not be in terms of gestational age; it would be in terms of the known parameters of the developmental lag in that function. Applying such a correction would, it seems to us, require a great many empirical, longitudinal studies of the function, employing preterms and comparable controls. As it is used now, the gestational age correction is often employed to equate the neurological, cognitive, or other functioning of a baby that may not ever function comparably to a full-term infant with respect to the measure involved.

In sum, the question of correcting infancy measures is an empirical one, not a theoretical one. If it can be demonstrated that developmental delay or lag exists in regard to a given function, then infancy scores on that function ought probably to be corrected in consideration of the characteristics and parameters of the lag. That gestational age is involved in developmental lag cannot automatically be assumed. Unfortunately, the gestational age correction seems to have become a convenient deity to which we often irrationally pay obeisance before resuming our scientific stance.

Hunt and Rhodes (1977) provide some infancy data to assess a biological model of development that appears to favor the use of the gestational age correction. However, the authors caution as follows: "An alternative interpretation of the unadjusted scores is that they now reflect the relative risk status of the . . .groups rather than the effects of GA [gestational age]. This question will be resolved in the future by comparing the predictive validity of adjusted and unadjusted 2-year scores with scores earned at later ages [p. 208]." We have assessed the predictive validity of our adjusted and unadjusted early measurements in middle childhood. On the basis of these data, we would subscribe to Hunt and Rhodes's alternative explanation.

The various ratings of the infants made at 1 year of age did not appear to contribute many novel findings. The significant relationship between the social development score obtained at 1 year and WISC-R V-IQ seems to devolve from the fact that this measure, like the Gesell personal–social schedule, assesses the infant's relatedness with others. The sensorimotor development measure, which contains items assaying the neurological integrity of the organism, showed little variability in this study, indicating that the subjects seemed to be relatively free of the blatant sensorimotor deficits often associated with organic brain damage. Nevertheless, this measure did relate strongly to scores on the developmental tests administered at the same time. Apparently, the developmental tests are sensitive to subtle neurological deficits (see Honzik, 1976). However, it would be of interest to determine why the Cattell and Gesell developmental tests predicted aspects of IQ later in life, at least in the bivariate analyses, whereas the sensorimotor development scale, with which these tests were strongly related, failed to do so.

The bivariate correlation of the Bender Gestalt score in middle childhood with the Prematurity factor score ($r = -.40$) serves to affirm the conjecture of the present investigators that it is visually based cognitive functioning that is primarily affected in middle-class prematures. Of the individual measures of neonatal immaturity selected for intensive study, only gestational age failed to predict visuomotor functioning as measured by the Bender Gestalt test. Since gestational age is subject to incorrect estimation, it is possible that the predictive utility of this variable may be compromised in studies in which it is involved. However, the group of relatively well-educated mothers that participated in the present research is, perhaps, less likely than most to err in such estimations. Whether because of susceptibility to measurement error or because of factors intrinsic to the measure itself, gestational age does not appear to be as powerful a correlate of functioning in middle childhood as is birthweight. Mother's IQ was the only other predictor variable relating to visuomotor performance, again reflecting the pervasive influence of this predictor.

Considering the two classes of dependent variables employed in this study, intellective functioning (WISC-R) was more definitively related to the predictor variables assayed in infancy than was visuomotor functioning (Bender Gestalt). This may be due to the superior psychometric properties of the IQ test as compared with the Bender Gestalt test. Or, one may conjecture that intellective functioning is determined by a wider complex of factors operative early in the organism's existence than is visuomotor functioning.

Both verbal and performance aspects of intellective functioning were related to the predictor variables; however, prematurity was the only descriptor of the infant's prenatal or perinatal status (excluding the Obstetric History factor) that predicted cognitive functioning beyond 1 year of life.

References

Aleksandrowicz, M. K., & Aleksandrowicz, D. R. Obstetrical pain-relieving drugs as predictors of infant behavior variability. *Child Development,* 1974, *45,* 935–945.

Ambrus, C. M., Weintraub, D. H., Niswander, K. R., Fischer, L., Fleishman, J., Bross, I. D. J., & Ambrus, J. L. Evaluation of survivors of respiratory distress syndrome at four years of age. *American Journal of Diseases of Children,* 1970, *120,* 296–302.

Ammons, R. B., & Ammons, H. S. *Full-range picture vocabularly test.* Missoula, Mont.: Psychological Test Specialists, 1948.

Anderson, L. D. The predictive value of infant tests in relation to intelligence at 5 years. *Child Development,* 1939, *10,* 202–212.

Bacola, E., Behrle, F. C., de Schweinitz, L., Miller, A. C., & Ma, M. M. Perinatal and environmental factors in late neurogenic sequelae. I. Infants having birthweights under 1500 grams. *American Journal of Diseases of Children,* 1966, *112,* 359–368. (a)

Bacola, E., Behrle, F. C., de Schweinitz, L., Miller, A. C., & Ma, M. M. Perinatal and environmental factors in late neurogenic sequelae. II. Infants having birthweights from 1500 to 2500 grams. *American Journal of Diseases of Children,* 1966, *112,* 369–374. (b)

Bayley, N. Mental growth during the first three years. In R. G. Barker, J. S. Kounin, & H. F. Wright (Eds.), *Child behavior and development.* New York: McGraw-Hill, 1943.

Bayley, N. On the growth of intelligence. *American Psychologist,* 1955, *10,* 805.

Bayley, N., & Schaefer, E. S. Correlations of maternal child behaviors with the development of mental abilities: Data from the Berkeley Growth study. *Monographs of the Society for Research in Child Development,* 1964, *29,* (6, Whole No. 97).

Becker, W. C., & Krug, R. S. The Parent Attitude Research Instrument: A research review. *Child Development,* 1965, *36,* 329–365.

Belmont, L., & Marolla, F. A. Birth order, family size and intelligence. *Science,* 1973, *182,* 1096–1101.

Bender, L. *Instructions for the use of the Visual Motor Gestalt Test.* New York: American Orthopsychiatric Association, 1946.

Benton, A. Mental development of prematurely born children. *American Journal of Orthopsychiatry,* 1940, *10,* 719–746.

Bowes, W. A. Obstetrical medication and infant outcome: A review of the literature. In W. A. Bowes, Jr., Y. Brackbill, E. Conway, & A. Steinschneider, The effects of obstetrical medication on fetus and infant. *Monographs of the Society for Research in Child Development,* 1970, *35,* (4, Serial No. 137).

Brackbill, Y. Obstetrical medications and infant behavior. In J. D. Osofsky (Ed.), *Handbook of infant development.* New York: Wiley, 1979.

Brackbill, Y., Kane, J., Manniello, R. L., & Abrahamson, D. Obstetric meperidine usage and assessment of neonatal status. *Anesthesiology,* 1974, *40,* 116–120.

Broman, S. H. Outcome of adolescent pregnancy: A report from the Collaborative Perinatal Project. Paper presented at the Workshop on Developmental Followup on Infants Born at Risk, 13th Annual Conference of the Association for the Care of Children in Hospitals, Washington, D.C., June 1978.

Broman, S. H., Nichols, P. L., & Kennedy, W. A. *Preschool IQ: Prenatal and early developmental correlates.* New York: Wiley, 1975.

Burton, D. Birth order and intelligence. *Journal of Social Psychology,* 1968, *76,* 199–206.

Cameron, J., Livson, N., & Bayley, N. Infant vocalizations and their relationship to mature intelligence, *Science,* 1967, *157,* 331.

Caputo, D. V., Goldstein, K. M., & Taub, H. B. The development of prematurely born children through middle childhood. In T. M. Field, A. M., Sostek, D. Goldberg, & H. H. Shuman (Eds.), *Infants born at risk.* New York: Spectrum, 1979.

Caputo, D. V., & Mandell, W. Consequences of low birth weight. *Developmental Psychology,* 1970, *3,* 363–383.

Caputo, D. V., Taub, H. B., Goldstein, K. M., Smith, N., Dalack, J., Pursner, J., & Silberstein, R. M. An evaluation of various parameters of maturity at birth as predictors of development at one year of life. *Perceptual and Motor Skills,* 1974, *39,* 631–652.

Cattell, P. *Cattell Infant Intelligence Scale.* New York: Psychological Corp., 1960.

Chorost, S. B. Parental child-rearing attitudes and their correlates in adolescent hostility. *Genetic Psychology Monographs,* 1962, *66,* 49–60.

Churchill, J. A. The relationship of epilepsy to breech delivery. *Electroencephalography and Clinical Neurophysiology,* 1959, *11,* 1–12.

Churchill, J. A., & Colfelt, R. Etiologic factors in athetotic cerebral palsy. *Archives of Neurology,* 1963, *94,* 400–406.

Conway, E., & Brackbill, Y. Delivery medication and infant outcome: An empirical study. In W. A. Bowes, Jr., Y. Brackbill, E. Conway, & A. Steinschneider, The effects of obstetrical medication on fetus and infant. *Monographs of the Society for Research in Child Development,* 1970, *35,* (4, Serial No. 137).

Corrigan, F. C., Berger, S. I., Dienstbier, R. A., & Strok, E. S. The influence of prematurity on school performance. *American Journal of Mental Deficiency,* 1967, *71,* 533–535.

Dann, M., Levine, S. Z., & New, E. V. A long-term followup of small premature infants. *Pediatrics,* 1964, *33,* 945–960.

DeHirsch, K., Jansky, J., & Langford, W. S. Comparisons between prematurely and maturely born children at three age levels. *American Journal of Orthopsychiatry,* 1966, *36,* 616–628.

Douglas, J. W. B. "Premature" children at primary schools. *British Medical Journal,* 1960, *12,* 1008–1013.

Drillien, C. M. Growth and development in a group of children of very low birthweight. *Archives of Disease in Childhood,* 1958, *33,* 10–18.

Elardo, R., Bradley, R. H., & Caldwell, B. M. The relation of infant's home environment to mental test performance from 6 to 36 months: A longitudinal study. *Child Development,* 1975, *46,* 71–76.

Erlenmeyer-Kimling, L., & Jarvik, L. F. Genetics and intelligence. *Science,* 1968, *142,* 1477–1479.

Francis-Williams, J., & Davies, P. A. Very low birth weight and later intelligence. *Developmental Medicine and Child Neurology,* 1974, *16,* 709–725.

Friedman, S. L., Brackbill, Y., Caron, A. J., & Caron, R. F. Obstetric medication and visual processing in 4- and 5-month old infants. *Merrill-Palmer Quarterly,* 1978, *24,* (3), 111–128.

Gesell, A., & Staff. *Gesell Developmental Schedules.* New York: Psychological Corp., 1949.

Goffeney, B., Henderson, N. B., & Butler, B. V. Negro–white, male–female, 8 month developmental scores compared with 7 year WISC and Bender test scores. *Child Development,* 1971, *42,* 595–604.

Goldstein, K. M., Caputo, D. V., & Taub, H. B. The effects of prenatal and perinatal complications on development at one year of age. *Child Development,* 1976, *47,* 613–621.

Goldstein, K. M., Taub, H. B., Caputo, D. V., Silberstein, R. M. Child status and demographic variables as related to maternal child-rearing attitudes. *Perceptual and Motor Skills,* 1976, *42,* 87–97.

Gottfried, A. W. Intellectual consequences of perinatal anoxia. *Psychological Bulletin,* 1973, *80,* 231–242.

Hamburger, M. Realism and consistency in early adolescent aspirations and expectations. Unpublished doctoral dissertation, Columbia University Teachers College, 1958.

Herrnstein, R. J. *IQ in the meritocracy.* Boston: Atlantic–Little Brown, 1973.

Hindley, C. B. Growing up in five countries: A comparison of data on weaning, elimination training, age of walking and IQ in relation to social class from five European longitudinal studies. *Developmental Medicine and Child Neurology,* 1968, *10,* 715–724.

Honzik, M. P. Value and limitations of infant tests: An overview. In M. Lewis (Ed.), *Origins of intelligence.* New York: Plenum, 1976.

Horowitz, F. D., Ashton, J., Culp, R., Gaddis, E., Levin, S., & Reichmann, B. The effects of obstetrical medication on the behavior of Israeli newborn infants and some comparisons with Uruguayan and American infants. *Child Development,* 1977, *48,* 1607–1623.

Hunt, J. V., & Rhodes, L. Mental development of preterm infants during the first year. *Child Development,* 1977, *48,* 204–210.

Jensen, A. R. How much can we boost IQ and scholastic achievement? *Harvard Educational Review,* 1969, *39,* 1–123.

Kang, B. Y., & Cho, S. H. Studies on physical and mental development of low birth weight infants. *Journal of Catholic Medical College,* 1976, *29,* 143–153.

Kaufman, A. S. Factor analysis of the WISC-R at 11 age levels between 6½ and 16½ years. *Journal of Consulting and Clinical Psychology,* 1975, *42,* 135–147.

Kellaghan, T., and Macnamarra, J. Family correlates of verbal reasoning ability. *Developmental Psychology,* 1972, *7,* 49–53.

Koppitz, E. M. *The Bender Gestalt test for young children.* New York: Grune & Stratton, 1963.

Koppitz, E. M. *The Bender Gestalt test for young children* (Vol. 2). New York: Grune & Stratton, 1975.

Lasky, R. E., Lechtig, A., Delgado, H., Klein, R. E., Engle, P., Yarbrough, C., & Martorell, R. Birth weight and psychomotor performance in rural Guatemala. *American Journal of Diseases of Children,* 1975, *129,* 566–569.

Lis, C. Visuo-motor development and its disturbances in a sample of prematures born with birth weight below 2500 grams. *Australian Journal of the Education of Backward Children,* 1969, *16,* 73–84.

Lubchenco, L., Horner, F., Reed, L., Hix, J. E., Metcalf, D., Cohig, R., Elliot, H. C., & Bourg, M. Sequelae of premature birth. *American Journal of Diseases of Children,* 1963, *106,* 101–115.

McCall, R. B., Applebaum, M. I., & Hogarty, P. S. Developmental changes in mental performance. *Monographs of the Society for Research in Child Development,* 1973, *38,* (3, Serial No. 150).

Muller, P. F., Campbell, H. E., Graham, W. E., Brittain, H., Fitzgerald, J. A., Hogan, N. A., Muller, V. H., & Ritterhouse, A. H. Perinatal factors and their relationship to mental retardation and other parameters of development. *American Journal of Obstetrics and Gynecology,* 1971, *109,* 1205–1210.

Murray, C. The effects of ordinal position on measured intelligence and peer acceptance in adolescence. *British Journal of Social and Clinical Psychology,* 1971, *10,* 221–227.

Neligan, G. A., Kolvin, I., Scott, D. M., & Garside, R. F. *Born too soon or born too small: A follow-up study to seven years of age.* London: Spastics International Medical Publications, 1976.

Osgood, C. E., Suci, G. J., & Tannenbaum, P. H. *The measurement of meaning.* Urbana, Ill.: Univ. of Illinois Press, 1957.

Osofsky, H. J. *The pregnant teenager: A medical educational and social analysis.* Springfield, Ill.: Thomas, 1968.

Outerbridge, E. W., Ramsay, M., & Stern, L. Developmental follow-up of survivors of neonatal respiratory failure. *Critical Care Medicine,* 1974, *2,* 23–27.

Pasamanick, B., Constantinou, F. K., & Lilienfeld, A. M. Pregnancy experience and the development of childhood speech disorders: An epidemiologic study of the association with maternal and fetal factors. *American Journal of Diseases of Children,* 1956, *91,* 113–118.

Pasamanick, B., & Lilienfeld, A. M. Association of maternal and fetal factors with the development of mental deficiency. I. Abnormalities in the prenatal and perinatal periods. *Journal of the American Medical Association,* 1956, *159,* 155–160.

Phillips, C. J. The Illinois Test of Psycholinguistic Abilities: A report on its use with English children and a comment on the psychological sequelae of low-birth-weight. *British Journal of Disorders of Communication,* 1968, *3,* 143–149.

Rabinovitch, M., Bibace, R., & Caplan, H. Sequelae of prematurity: Psychological test findings. *Canadian Medical Association Journal,* 1961, *84,* 822–824.

Robertson, A. M., & Crichton, J. U. Neurological sequelae in children with neonatal respiratory distress. *American Journal of Diseases of Children,* 1969, *117,* 271–276.

Rubin, R. A., & Balow, B. Measures of infant development and socioeconomic status as predictors of later intelligence and school achievement. *Developmental Psychology,* 1979, *15,* 225–227.

Rubin, R. A., Rosenblatt, C., & Balow, B. Psychological and educational sequelae of prematurity. *Pediatrics,* 1973, *52,* 352–363.

Russell, J. K., & Millar, D. G. Maternal factors and mental performance in children. In *Perinatal factors affecting human development.* Proceedings of the special session, eighth meeting of the Pan American Health Organization Advisory Committee on Medical Research, Washington, D.C., 9–13 June, 1969.

Schaefer, E. S., & Bell, R. Q. Development of a parental attitude research instrument. *Child Development,* 1958, *29,* 339–361.

Standley, K., Soule, A. B., III, Copans, S. A., & Duchowny, M. S. Local–regional anesthesia during childbirth: Effect on newborn behavior. *Science,* 1974, *186,* 634–635.

Stewart, A., Turcan, D., Rawlings, G., Hart, S., & Gregory, S. Outcome for infants at high risk of major handicap. In *Major mental handicap: Methods and costs of prevention* (Ciba Foundation Symposium 59). New York: Elsevier, Excerpta Medica, North Holland, 1978.

Stott, D. H. Follow-up study from birth of the effects of prenatal stresses. *Developmental Medicine and Child Neurology,* 1973, *15,* 770–787.

Stott, L. H., & Ball, R. S. Infant and preschool mental tests: Review and evaluation. *Monographs of the Society for Research in Child Development,* 1965, *30,* (Serial No. 101).

Taub, H. B., Caputo, D. V., & Goldstein, K. M. Toward a modification of the indices of neonatal prematurity. *Perceptual and Motor Skills,* 1975, *40,* 43–48.

Taub, H. B., Goldstein, K. M., & Caputo, D. V. Indices of prematurity as discriminators of development in middle childhood. *Child Development,* 1977, *48,* 797–805.

Terman, L. M., & Merrill, M. *Measuring intelligence: A guide to the new revised Stanford-Binet Test of Intelligence.* Boston, Mass.: Houghton, Mifflin, 1937.

Thomas, H. Psychological assessment instruments for use with human infants. *Merrill–Palmer Quarterly,* 1970, *16,* 179–223.

Van den Daele, L. D. Natal influences and twin differences. *Journal of Genetic Psychology,* 1974, *124,* 41–60.

Wechsler, D. *Wechsler Intelligence Scale for Children–Revised.* New York: Psychological Corp., 1974.

Wiener, G., Rider, R. V., Oppel, W. C., Fischer, L. K., & Harper, P. A. Correlates of low birth weight: Psychological status at six to seven years of age. *Pediatrics,* 1965, *35,* 434–444.

Wiener, G., Rider, R. V., Oppel, W. C., & Harper, P. A. Correlates of low birth weight: Psychological status at eight to ten years of age. *Pediatric Research,* 1968, *2,* 110–118.

Willerman, L., & Churchill, J. A. Intelligence and birth weight in identical twins. *Child Development,* 1967, *38,* 623–630.

World Health Organization. *Public health aspects of low birth weight.* (WHO Tech. Rep. No. 217). Geneva: Author, 1961.

Wright, F. H., Blough, R. R., Chamberlin, A., Ernest, T., Halstead, W. C., Meier, P., Moore, R. Y., Naunton, R. F., & Newell, W. A controlled follow-up study of small prematures born from 1952 through 1956. *American Journal of Diseases of Children,* 1972, *124,* 506–521.

Zajonc, R. B. Family configuration and intelligence, *Science,* 1976, *192,* 227–236.

Zajonc, R. B., & Markus, G. B. Birth order and intellectual development. *Psychological Review,* 1975, *82,* 74–88.

21

Longitudinal Studies of Preterm Infants: A Review of Chapters 17-20

ARNOLD J. SAMEROFF

The effects of perinatal problems on later development has been an active area of concern for a number of generations of researchers. It has always seemed clear that birth difficulties have a major impact on the child's developmental outcome especially in the realm of intellectual achievement. It is evident that newborn preterm babies look and behave differently from newborn full-term infants. Their needs for clinical interventions are obviously much greater, requiring special environments to protect them until they develop the capacities to survive in a home environment.

There has never been much question that these children can have later problems, but there have been major questions as to the nature of these problems. Are the poor developmental outcomes found for these infants the consequences of the premature birth or are they the consequences of some correlates of the preterm birth? Preterm birth is usually associated with a set of other factors both in the child and in the environment. In the child, especially the very small preterm infant, there are a number of frequently accompanying illnesses, such as respiratory distress syndrome or a variety of perceptual handicaps. Before modern medicine had achieved the high level of sophistication in preventing many of these, the incidence was especially high. From the environmental perspective, preterm birth was frequently associated with poor social circumstance in both the economic and educational realms. Thus, we may ask if the poorer outcomes for preterm births were caused by the prematurity or the accompanying illnesses or the impoverished childrearing environment.

Sameroff and Chandler (1975), in an extensive review of the literature, found little evidence to support the notion that prematurity alone produced

PRETERM BIRTH AND
PSYCHOLOGICAL DEVELOPMENT

poor developmental outcomes. The work of many investigators had found that children with many developmental problems had had birth complications, but prospective studies showed that there was little inevitability in these outcomes. No single birth problem has been shown to have a clear outcome of psychological deficit. Whether the problem was preterm birth, anoxia, or any other specific complication, the range of outcomes often exceeded the range resulting from uncomplicated births.

Despite the variance in the outcome of these longitudinal studies, there were still children from these populations who were not doing well. The question to be answered was why some of the children with early problems had later problems. The critics of the earlier studies found much to be concerned about both in the initial diagnosis of birth complication and in the later assessment of developmental outcome. Possibly, if better techniques of diagnosis or outcome assessment could be devised, clearer connections could be found between the initial health status and later developmental deviancies. Another issue to justify continued research in this area was the changing nature of the preterm population. Whereas 20 years ago there were very few survivors among infants whose birthweights were less than 1500 gm, today there are many. Will studies of these new populations of survivors find clearer evidence of later problems?

The descriptions of four longitudinal studies appear in this volume: the Springfield study reported by Field, Dempsey, and Shuman (Chapter 17); the Los Angeles study reported by Sigman, Cohen, and Forsythe (Chapter 18); the San Francisco study reported by Hunt (Chapter 19); and the Staten Island study reported by Caputo, Goldstein, and Taub (Chapter 20). The contributions from these studies can be assessed in terms of how much light they throw on the issues introduced in the preceding paragraphs:

1. Does preterm birth alone produce developmental problems exclusive of accompanying medical or environmental problems?
2. Will better diagnosis reveal subpopulations of preterm infants that will be at a higher risk for later problems than the preterm population as a whole?
3. Can the use of better assessments of developmental outcome identify problems resulting from preterm birth to which earlier assessments may have been insensitive?
4. Can the poor outcomes that have been thought to be associated with preterm birth be fully explained by environmental factors?

Procedures

The Study Samples

Both the San Francisco and Los Angeles studies included only preterm infants, under 1500 gm for San Francisco and under 2500 gm for Los Angeles.

Both samples were mostly white babies, with a large proportion of Spanish-speaking families in Los Angeles and black families in San Francisco, and represented a range of social statuses.

The Springfield and Staten Island samples were both predominantly white middle-class groups. The Staten Island sample was selected on the basis of a birthweight of under 2500 gm, but a control group of babies with birthweight over 2500 gm was also studied. The most complex sample was in the Springfield study, in which a sample of preterm infants, all of whom had respiratory distress syndrome, was contrasted with a group of full-term infants and in addition with a group of infants with postmaturity syndrome.

Diagnostic Measures

In the Springfield sample, there was a clear diagnosis of respiratory distress syndrome for each preterm infant with a minimum of 12 hours of mechanical ventilation. The San Francisco sample also had a high proportion of respiratory problems, with 40% of the sample having had hyaline membrane disease. Perinatal complication scores were calculated in the Los Angeles and Staten Island studies, while specialized infant behavior or neurological examinations took place in the Springfield and Los Angeles studies. The range of perinatal assessments was from actual observations and specialized testing to notations from the medical records.

Outcome Measures

The outcome measures shared by all the studies centered on intelligence testing. Infant assessments included the Bayley, the Cattell, and the Gesell. In early childhood, the Stanford-Binet and the WISC-R were used. The oldest children at follow-up were the school-aged children in the Staten Island group, and the most differentiated assessment was for these children. A combination of the WISC-R and the Bender Gestalt permitted the separate evaluation of a number of intellectual functions. In addition, behavior ratings were made for the children by their parents. The oldest children in the San Francisco study were given a clinical diagnosis so that school disabilities were an outcome in that sample.

Environmental Assessment

In contrast to most of the earlier studies in this area, the present four studies were all concerned with the impact of environmental factors on the child's development. At a minimum, parents' education or social class were considered. In addition, parental attitudes were assessed in the Staten Island sample, while actual observations of parent–child interactions were made in the Springfield and Los Angeles studies.

Results of the Studies

The four studies represent varying degrees of diagnostic sophistication and of outcome assessment. Can we draw any conclusion from the pattern of results that will permit us a fair evaluation of the effects of preterm birth on developmental outcomes?

San Francisco Study

At 4–6 years of age almost one-half of this group of babies with birthweight under 1500 gm were judged to have some abnormality in functioning that would interfere with their school functioning. However, when attempts were made to find neonatal differences between those that had later difficulties and those that did not, no conclusions could be drawn.

Infants who had suffered hyaline membrane disease were in both the normal and abnormal groups. Hunt found that prediction from infancy to early childhood was unreliable even in gross diagnostic categories. Even extreme scores could not guarantee positive or negative outcomes. By way of contrast, Hunt reported that at 4–6 years the factor that correlated the most with intellectual outcome was parental educational level. The conclusion from this study appears to be that while low-birthweight infants are well represented in samples of children with later school difficulties, their newborn status is not a determining factor in their deviancy. There must be some mediating influences. The best candidate for these are caretaking conditions, which were not assessed in this study but were in two of the other studies.

Springfield Study

The Field, Dempsey, and Shuman study specialized in preterm infants who had had a clear episode of respiratory distress syndrome. These preterm infants were found to differ as a group from full-term infants matched for gestational age in areas of medical, physical, mental, motor, and behavioral development. By 2 years of age, however, these differences seem to have diminished, although there had been some suggestion of differences in 4-year-old language performance in an earlier study by these investigators.

Within this middle-class sample, general environmental factors did not seem to differentially affect outcome. However, there were clear differences in the parent–child interactions. The mothers of the preterm infants were much more active in their interactions with the children, and may have been more overprotective as the infants grew older.

Although no attempt was made to test individual predictions in this study, the closeness of the mean developmental scores and the overlap in distributions suggest that, as in the San Francisco study, no reliable predictions can be made from newborn status.

Los Angeles Study

Sigman, Cohen, and Forsythe make the preceding point quite clearly in their presentation. They argue that any consistency in developmental status from early infancy will not be found in the newborn status, but rather from the consistency in the interaction of caregiver and child. The most effective predictors to developmental status at 2 years of age did not include any of the early behavioral or medical factors. It was only at 8–9 months that infant variables began to be related to developmental outcome, and even these effects may have been mediated by caretaker interactions. The caretaking environment, by playing a major role in the developmental transformations that characterize the early growth of intelligence, has the power to reduce or amplify earlier problems. Thus, although newborn status may not have a direct impact on later intellectual status, it affects the caretaking environment, which does have a direct impact.

Staten Island Study

The many variables that went into the data analysis of the Caputo, Goldstein, and Taub chapter were factor analyzed to reduce the data set to a manageable size. In the case of birth and obstetric condition, 19 variables were reduced to three factors, Obstetrical History, Delivery and Related variables, and Complications. When the full set of variables was related to intellectual outcome at school age, the Social Class factor and maternal educational level were the strongest correlates. Of the medical factors, only Obstetrical History related significantly to full-scale WISC IQ. Low birthweight did show a significant relationship to performance but not verbal IQ. In contrast to other longitudinal studies of prematurity that extended into the school years, this study did not include many infants of very low birthweight or with many neurological problems. As a consequence, these investigators concluded that visually based cognitive behavior is especially sensitive to the effects of prematurity alone.

The results of the Staten Island study do not take us much farther than earlier reports of deficits associated with prematurity. The strong relation of intellectual outcome with social status and parental education requires the investigators to control for these influences when seeking for effects of birth status alone. We are continually left with the unanswered question: Are the later developmental problems associated with prematurity the effect of prematurity or of the fact that poorer and less educated groups are more likely to have preterm babies?

Summary and Conclusions

Taken as a group, the four studies reported here do much to enrich our understanding of the relation of perinatal complications to later developmental outcomes. This enrichment is equally divided between negative and positive findings, that is, the identification of factors that do not seem to have an impact on outcomes as well as those that do. The single most potent factor influencing developmental outcome turns out to be the cultural environment of the child, as expressed in socioeconomic status and parental educational level. This result was found in three of the four studies. The one study that did not report this result had a relatively homogeneous middle-class sample.

This standard finding requires investigators to control for the environmental factors in their attempts to find special effects of birth conditions. Since previous studies have found interactions between social status and birth condition in producing developmental outcomes, a factorial design is necessary to separate these variables. If one merely uses matched preterm and control groups, the problem will not be solved. If the populations are primarily middle class, few differences will be found between the preterm and the control groups. If the populations are primarily lower class, then many differences will be found between the groups.

The second finding of major import for experimental design is that in all the studies there was a significant overlap between the outcomes for the preterm groups and the control groups. No single factor, either birthweight alone or accompanying physical problems, clearly predicted a specific developmental outcome.

The conclusion that emerges from these two facts—the large impact of environment and the small impact of birth status—is that an understanding of the developmental relationship between birth and outcome requires a study of the actual interaction of the two variables. Two of the studies provided us with such an opportunity, the Springfield and the Los Angeles reports. Field (1980) has analyzed developmental outcomes as an interaction between the continuum of reproductive casualty suggested by Pasamanick and Knobloch (1961) and the continuum of caretaking casualty suggested by Sameroff and Chandler (1975). She has suggested that, depending on which continuum is operative, the nature of the parent–infant interaction will be changed. Mothers of preterm infants, a sample with reproductive risk, tend to be overactive in their interactions with their children. Mothers from lower social status groups, a sample with caretaking risk, tend to be underactive in their interactions. If developmental predictions are to be made, the quality of these interactions must be considered.

Empirically, the moderating effect of caretaking behavior was best demonstrated in the Los Angeles study. Sigman *et al.* argue that early infancy is a period in which both the behavior of the infant and the caregiver are in states of rapid change. It is only after the relationship between the partners in the developmental process is stabilized that developmental prediction becomes possible. Outcomes in that study tended to show the clear mediating effects of those interactions.

In conclusion, it must be said that, whether or not preterm birth has a specific identifiable impact on later intellectual outcome, many preterm babies do end up with developmental problems. The previous study of this problem has raised important questions not only about the effects of birth complications in particular but about the developmental process in general. The continued study of this problem may help us to find better descriptions of the dynamic processes by which early problems are overcome and later ones created.

References

Field, T. M. Interactions of high risk infants: Quantitative and qualitative differences. In D. B. Sawin, R. C. Hawkins, L. O. Walker, & J. H. Penticuff (Eds.), *Exceptional infant* (Vol. 4): *Psychosocial risks in infant-environment transactions*. New York: Brunner/Mazel, 1980.

Pasamanick, B., & Knobloch, H. Epidemiologic studies on the complications of pregnancy and the birth process. In G. Caplan (Ed.), *Prevention of mental disorders in children*. New York: Basic Books, 1961.

Sameroff, A. J., & Chandler, M. J. Reproductive risk and the continuum of caretaking casualty. In F. D. Horowitz, M. Hetherington, S. Scarr-Salapatek, & G. Siegel (Eds.), *Review of child development research* (Vol. 4). Chicago: Univ. of Chicago Press, 1975.

22

Biomedical and Psychosocial Interventions for Preterm Infants

CRAIG T. RAMEY
PHILIP SANFORD ZESKIND
ROSEMARY HUNTER

Intervention can be a presumptuous, intrusive, and ineffective endeavor. It can also be the handmaiden to improvements in therapeutic practices. Because intervention into life processes is a highly controversial activity, because of its potentially negative as well as positive impact, we would like to specify four major premises that we share concerning early intervention into human lives in general. Although these premises apply directly to therapeutic strategies for premature infants, we think that they also apply to a wider range of developmental problems. Our first assumption is that intervention strategies that concentrate on and measure developmental processes are to be preferred to ones that focus only on outcome measures. Such an approach is more likely to discover the causal pathways whereby effective therapeutic interventions have their impact. Our second assumption is that the earlier intervention treatments are implemented after the identification of a supposedly detrimental condition, the greater the likelihood of affecting relevant underlying causal processes and mechanisms while they are most malleable. Third, a multifaceted, interdisciplinary treatment-evaluation strategy is to be preferred to a unidimensional, unidisciplinary evaluation strategy. The preferred strategy can be especially sensitive to possible negative effects on development as well as provide a more thorough documentation of positive effects. And fourth, to be fully helpful to those individuals it seeks to serve, intervention should be firmly grounded in explicit theory as well as in good research practices. Such grounding will facilitate a strategic approach to problems of development rather than a more characteristic ad hoc approach.

PRETERM BIRTH AND
PSYCHOLOGICAL DEVELOPMENT

Identification of Target Populations

Intervention is not an option to but a necessary step in the kinds of experiments necessary to advance our understanding of prematurity and to treat its consequences. However, intervention itself goes beyond the observation of infant capabilities and group comparisons; intervention is an alteration of ongoing life processes in which painful errors such as the retrolental fibroplasia experience cannot be totally prevented. For this reason, one first concern of the interventionist is the accurate identification of the infant at risk.

Although numerous studies and reviews indicate the premature infant is at risk for adverse developmental sequelae (e.g., Caputo & Mandell, 1970; Cornell & Gottfried, 1976; Knobloch & Pasamanick, 1966; Wiener, 1962), the developmental outcome may not necessarily be below average (Francis-Williams & Davies, 1974; Phillips, 1972; Rabinovitch, Bibace, & Caplan, 1961) and the individual may meld successfully into the general population (Taub, Caputo, & Goldstein, 1975). Are all infants who are judged to be preterm appropriate targets for intervention, and if not, by what criteria do those who will provide intervention base their decisions?

The different definitional criteria of prematurity, such as from measures of gestational age, birthweight (e.g., Caputo & Mandell, 1970), gestational age derived from birthweight (e.g., Braine, Heimer, Wortis, & Freedman, 1966), or the combination of both measures (e.g., Rubin, Rosenblatt, & Balow, 1973), have led to heterogeneous populations with a myriad of attributes and courses of development. The complexity of the definitional issue needs to be underscored. For example, the shorter the infant's period of gestation, the greater is the infant's risk status (Lubchenco, 1976). Similarly, the lower the infant's birthweight, the greater is the infant's risk status (Drillien, 1964). Paradoxically, however, the *least* preterm infants may have the *greater* intellectual deficits when a group of low-birthweight infants are studied (Douglas, 1956), just as the *lowest* birthweight infants may have the *least* adverse effects when a group of preterm and full-term infants are compared (Rubin *et al.,* 1973). In these studies, infants who are low birthweight for their gestational age (small for gestational age, or SGA) had the greatest deficits. Thus, a preterm low-birthweight infant who is appropriate for gestational age (AGA) may have a better prognosis than a full-term, low-birthweight infant who is SGA. For this reason, some suggest that we must include weight-for-age measures in order to understand the attitudes of the preterm infant. However, although some researchers find differences in attributes of SGA and AGA preterm infants (Fitzhardinge & Stevens, 1972; Lubchenco, *et al.,* 1963), others do not (Weiner, 1970). The point is that any number of anthropometric indexes of maturity (e.g., Caputo, *et al.,* 1974) are measures of conditions that may act independently or in various combinations to affect the attributes of the preterm infant.

Further, in the identification of those infants who are at risk, the situation is not that the attributes of preterm infants are static between or within cohorts. We must ask, for example, are the attributes of preterm infants of 20 or even 10 years ago the same as those of preterm infants of today or tomorrow? With improvement of medical care, the attributes of small preterm infants changed significantly in the past (Hess, Mahr & Bartelme, 1939). Changes in the nursery intensive care unit (NICU) have increased infant survival rates as recently as between the late 1960s and the early 1970s (Hunt, Harvin, Kennedy, & Tooley, 1974). Differential survival rates may affect the attributes of the populations from which samples are drawn. Similarly, as development progresses within a cohort, attributes of the preterm infant may change relative to the term infant. Preterm infants may show markedly deficient performance, at an early point in time yet show average performances or better relative to their peers at later stages.

The important points to be made from these remarks, and ones that will be emphasized throughout this chapter, concern the concept of being at risk. First, the concept of being at risk is a probabilistic one based on projected outcomes and attributes of infants born with a complex system of identifying factors that may differentially affect infant development. Thus, specific interventions must conform to specific developmental attributes. Second, the probability of developing a specific attribute is dynamic as medical practices change. Thus, intervention programs of today and tomorrow cannot rely solely on yesterday's studies. A conceptualization of the attributes of the population as it exists today is important if one is to understand which interventions are appropriate. Third, the attributes of the individual infant develop and change over time. Intervention must therefore be based on meticulous observation, flexibility to meet changing demands, and constant attention to possible side effects. For these reasons, identification of infant biomedical and behavioral attributes and the processes by which they develop and change may be more salient to those who provide intervention than global categories of estimates of gestational age and anthropometry. In the biomedical context immediately following birth, this empirical approach is a necessity.

Biomedical Context for Intervention

The guiding principles of biomedical interventions are survival and simultaneous minimization of damage. However, born too soon, the preterm infant presents a dilemma to those seeking theoretical guidelines for his care. The preterm infant is a baby who should not yet be, but is. And it is not merely that the infant is a compact version of a full-term baby. The general organ immaturity presents many qualitative as well as quantitative differences. For example, the lungs not only are smaller but are lacking in the production of chemical lubricants necessary for adequate ventilation. Because of such functional maturational differences, standards for normal newborns often lack application in the premature baby.

The temptation, then, is to turn to a fetal model. In a way, the many monitoring and support lines to the modern premature infant can be seen as a replacement for some of the surveillance functions of the placenta and maternal systems. Yet any attempt to recreate an intrauterine environment will be severely limited by practical considerations. Some compromise between the fetal and newborn model must be struck. Yet, there are no norms. A general objective of the medical care of preterm babies is to provide the supplies and environment necessary for optimal growth and maturation. But what is optimal growth for a premature infant—the growth rate of the fetus or of the newborn, or something in between? An how should the preterm infant be fed—with constituents available to the fetus, the periodic filling of the stomach with breast milk as in the newborn, or something in between? The same set of questions can be raised for every aspect of care for preterm infants.

In response, for example, to such respiratory problems as respiratory distress syndrome, asphyxia at birth, apneic spells, and chronic pulmonary disease, active intervention is required and accounts for much of the medical paraphernalia surrounding the tiny premature infant in a modern NICU. Cardiac and respiratory monitoring lines, taped to the chest and sounding an alarm when problems arise, are standard. Oxygen supplied by a plastic hood surrounding the baby's head or through a tube placed in the trachea is often required. An arterial catheter inserted through the umbilicus is also fairly standard equipment for frequent blood sampling. Active babies require restraints on their extremities to assure this line is not inadvertently pulled. Mechanical assistance for ventilation, either by continuous positive airway pressure to maintain adequate lung inflation or by a respirator, necessitates additional bedside machinery, tubes, and monitors.

Temperature instability in preterm infants was recognized by turn-of-the-century physicians and prompted work on the incubator. The lack of maintenance of constant body temperature is highly related to mortality and morbidity statistics in prematures (Silverman, Fertig, & Berger, 1958). This thermal need is still met by the incubator or isolette for many babies but increasingly is supplied through radiant heat above an open crib.

Nutritional care is another area in which changes have occurred. Earlier practices of withholding feeding to lessen the chance of regurgitation and aspiration are now recognized as dangerous, and every effort is made to supply the preterm infant with the nutrients necessary for normal growth. In the extremely premature infant with poor sucking, swallowing, and gag reflexes, and a stomach that will hold only 2 cc at a time, providing adequate nutrition represents a real challenge. Intravenous therapy (requiring an additional attachment to the baby) is often required in the early days. Extremely premature infants are biochemically unable to tolerate and metabolize milk feedings in the concentrations required for adequate growth. Intravenous supplements are used to augment nutrition supplied through a dilute formula fed in small amounts via a tube running from the nose to the small intestine—yet another support line to the infant. The immature bowel of extremely premature infants may not be able to handle even this modified feeding regimen, and it may be necessary to resort to total parenteral nutrition. In this method, a solution of protein derivatives, carbohydrates, vitamins, and minerals is supplied via an indwelling catheter surgically placed through the jugular vein in the neck.

Jaundice (due to the reduced metabolic capacity of the immature liver) is another disorder frequent in prematures and demanding continuous assessment and intervention. Since the discovery by Cremer, Perryman, and Richards (1958) and Franklin (1958) that exposure of infants to visible light resulted in a fall in bilirubin levels, this has been the treatment of choice for all but the most severe cases of neonatal jaundice. High-energy flourescent lights used for these treatments have the potential for causing retinal damage, and occlusive padding of both eyes during the period of treatment is a standard precaution.

In each of these examples, we find that the preterm infant presents a case where intervention must provide an avenue for the immature organism to adapt to an environment for which it may not yet be prepared. The infant is neither fetus nor newborn, but "something in between." The infant's care, then, cannot be that of the fetus or newborn, but "something in between." Although seemingly simplistic, this is of considerable weight when posing questions about intervention with premature infants. Both the fetus and the newborn are part of natural reciprocating systems that appreciate and respond to their needs—and that are available for study and description. By virtue of its anachronous birth, the premature infant is thrust into a position that has no naturally occurring support system. The knowing and responding must be fabricated and, by definition, are artificial approximations based on trial and error. Empiricism is thus a necessity and characterizes the currently operating, inductive theoretical approach that organizes the medical approach to the care of most premature infants. This empirical approach, with its frequent monitoring of infant attributes, may provide the basis for the approach to continued intervention once the infant leaves the nursery.

Environmental Context

Once the baby who is prematurely born successfully passes the initial task of neonatal survival, we must ask, is further intervention necessary, and if so, for whom and to what end? There is good reason to believe that the detrimental effects of prematurity are exacerbated in nonsupportive and ameliorated in supportive postnatal caregiving environments (Drillien, 1964, 1970; Sameroff & Chandler, 1975). Traditionally, these different caregiving environments have been defined in terms of the socioeconomic status (SES) of the child's parents. The role of the postnatal caregiving environment, however, is not clear cut. For example, beyond possible nonsupportive postnatal conditions, the poor outcome of premature infants in low SES environments may be partly due to prenatal and perinatal histories that may include less optimal nutritional and birth conditions that may also adversely affect developmental status (Birch & Gussow, 1970). Some investigators suggest that the influence of SES contributes to impairment only in the least intact groups and only in quite extreme levels of underprivilege (Braine *et al.*, 1966), whereas others aver that later cognitive performance is related to birthweight and neurological impairment, independent of SES level (e.g., Wiener, Rider, Oppel, Fischer, & Harper, 1965). Perhaps the description of the postnatal caregiving environment solely in terms of SES characteristics may preclude the level of analysis required to untangle the fundamental processes of development that may account for the seemingly discrepant findings.

At another level of analysis, specific nonsocial and social parameters of the environmental contexts can be evaluated for their differential effects on the development of preterm infants. But here, too, as with the difficulty of finding an appropriate model in early biomedical intervention, we must ask, is a fetal or newborn model appropriate for determining the quality of environmental stimulation? Some suggest simulation of sensory experiences of the womb may be appropriate, such as providing the sound intensity of the maternal heartbeat (Barnard, 1973) or the rhythmical activity simulated in a hammock apparatus (Neal, 1968). Conversely, others have provided sensory experiences more closely approximating those that the full-term infant may obtain, such as tapes of mothers' voices (Segall, 1972), extra handling (Powell, 1974), and enriched experiences (Scarr-Salapatek & Williams, 1973). In a similar debate concerning the stimulatory environment of the hospitalized preterm infant, while some see the premature infant as relatively stimulus deprived and prescribe such interventions as rocking, waterbeds, and tape-recorded simulated heartbeats (Kramer & Pierpont, 1976), others see the preterm infant as being subject to a stimulus bombardment secondary to modern intensive care. Preterm infants staying in the hospital for 7 weeks were found to have to adapt to up to 70 different nurses caring for them (Minde, Ford, Celhoffer & Boukydis, 1975). The NICU is brightly lit and full of activity around the clock. The incubator is known to provide a constant 77 dB hum. As Cornell and Gottfried (1976) suggest in their review of intervention programs with preterm infants, given the variety and amount of sensory experience in modern high-risk nurseries, a sensory deprivation hypothesis for differences between full- and preterm infants is unlikely.

However, beyond specifying the parameters of the environmental context, what is the nature of the relation between the infant and its environment? In the belief that interventions affecting development can most profitably be investigated during periods of rapid change and that theory should guide our intervention efforts, we turn now to a brief sketch of prominent theories of infant development as a means of structuring the process of inquiry. No attempt will be made to provide a comprehensive treatment of specific hypotheses that might be derived from the various theoretical positions. Rather, we intend simply to provide a cursory description of the general theoretical domains that might be of use in understanding forces affecting the development of a preterm infant.

Psychoanalytic Theory

Psychoanalytic and neopsychoanalytic theories, such as those found in the writings of Freud (1953), Ribble (1944), and Erikson (1950), all point to the centrality of the mother–child attachment or bond as an essential process for normal development. Although there are subtle differences among these theorists, the attachment or cathexis of the child to the mother is seen as essentially growing gradually out of the satisfactions that the child derives from the mother's caregiving activities. The orality of the feeding situation is conceived to be particularly important. For Erikson, the orality becomes a metaphor for nurture and caregiving wherein the context is established for the child's sense of basic trust. Whether the orality of the child per se or its metaphorical meaning in infancy is of central importance, it is clear from the psychoanalytic writings that any set of circumstances that interfere with the establishment of a strong mother–child attachment would be detrimental to the child's subsequent development (see, for example, Goldfarb, 1945). As has been noted by several investigators, including Brown and Bakeman (in press), the behavior of premature infants may make these children more difficult to feed and nurture. Hospital routines that exclude the mother from the care of premature infants may exacerbate the infant's fragile condition. Thus, a pattern of nongratification for both the child and his mother may be set up in such a way as to preclude effective attachment. Thus, from a psychoanalytic point of view, significant attention could be devoted to the feeding process and its contribution to development in premature infants.

Learning Theory

Learning theorists, such as Gewirtz (1972), tend to emphasize, as do the psychoanalytically oriented researchers, the centrality of the attachment process in infancy and, like them, assume that any factors that fail to lead to satisfactory attachments will be detrimental to the child's long-term development. The primary difference between the learning theorists as a group and the psychoanalytically oriented theorists lies in the mode of explanation for the attachment process. Learning theorists are likely to emphasize secondary reinforcement as an explanation for why the child's primary caregiver and the child come to have a special relationship.

Theoretical positions by Finkelstein and Ramey (1977) and Ramey and Finkelstein (1978) concerning nonprimary drive reducing response-contingent stimulation emphasize the importance of reciprocal infant–environment interactions in orthogenic development. To the extent that isolettes preclude instrumental responding by the infant, conditions may be established for retarding infant competence.

Organismic Theory

The theoretical work of Piaget (e.g., 1952) also emphasizes the importance of infant–environment transactions during what he calls the period of sensorimotor operations. The central point of Piaget's writings concerning this period is that during human infancy the child's conceptions of the world accrue as a direct result of his manipulations of objects in the physical world and the concomitant sensory feedback that occurs as a result of those direct manipulations. Although Piaget has not addressed himself directly to the issue of development of the preterm infant, it is reasonable to extrapolate from his position that any set of conditions that reduce either the infant's active involvement with the physical environment generally or the range of those experiences would tend to slow and perhaps hinder a normal course of development. Thus, the preterm infant's relatively restricted response repertoire and the environmental constriction due to the use of such devices as isolettes would tend to result in a reduced opportunity to exercise sensorimotor schemata.

Hebb's Theory

Hebb (1949) distinguished between two types of neural tissue available at birth: association tissue and sensorimotor tissue. The ratio of association tissue to sensorimotor tissue, and A/S ratio, he presumed to set the limits of intelligence for a given species. Hebb presumed that the association tissue, which he regarded as underlying higher intellectual functions, is established as a result of sensorimotor experiences occurring in the early part of life. Thus, to the extent that the preterm infant is deprived of significant sensorimotor experiences, he may also be deprived of later associative connections, which will reduce his intellectual abilities. Writing to this point, Wright (1969) argued that "Hebb's emphasis on providing a wealth of sensory motor experience during the early months of life places its emphasis on the *quantitative* aspects of such stimulation, with the *manner* in which the organism is stimulated being less important than the *amount* of stimulation provided through some sense modality [p. 283]."

Ethological Theory

The theoretical work of Bowlby (1958), and its continuation in the research of Ainsworth (e.g., 1972), has emphasized the instinctual responses that comprise the attachment process, namely, the responses of sucking, clinging, following, crying, and smiling. Bowlby has argued that

> to ensure survival of the individual in the species it is necessary for the organism to be equipped with an appropriately balanced repertoire of instinctual responses at each stage of its ontogeny. Not only must the adult be so equipped but the young animal must itself have a balanced and efficient equipment of its own. This will certainly differ in many respects from that of the adult. Furthermore, not only do individuals of different sexes and at different stages of development require specialized repertoires but in certain respects these need to be reciprocal. . . .

It is Bowbly's thesis that

> as in the young of other species, there matures in the early months of life of the human infant a complex and nicely balanced equipment of instinctual responses, the function of which is to ensure that he obtains parental care sufficient for his survival. To this end, the equipment includes responses which promote his close proximity to a parent and responses which evoke parental activity [p. 364].

The extent to which the premature child is an atypical child with respect to his response repertoire, the infant may be hindered from displaying the kinds of instinctual responses that will secure an effective attachment with his primary caregiver.

Previous Intervention Programs with Premature Infants

The history of manipulative experimental research with premature infants can be traced at least back to the research of Hasselmeyer (1964), who increased the handling of one group of premature children while not increasing that for another. The research showed that the extrasensory, tactile, and kinesthetic stimulation resulted in more quiescent behavior, especially before feeding, whereas a low-handled group exhibited more crying behavior before feedings. In 1966, Freedman, Boverman, and Freedman used a group of five co-twin control cases, in which one twin was rocked in a chair twice daily for 30 min beginning 7–10 days after the child began to regain his birthweight. The rocked twins gained weight at a greater rate per day than did control twins. Again, working from an extra-handling hypothesis, Solkoff, Jaffe, Weintraub, and Blase (1969) reported results of an experiment in which five experimental infants were stroked in their isolettes 5 min every hour for 10 days, while five control infants were provided with routine nursery care. The infants who received the extra handling were reported as more active and physically healthier than controls. They also regained their initial birthweights faster and were reported by their mothers at 7–8 months of age to reside in homes characterized by greater intensity and variety of stimulation.

Having noted that low birthweight (a frequent surrogate measure for prematurity) is highly associated with lower-class status and that lower-class children frequently enter school with IQs lower than their more advantaged peers, Williams and Scarr (1971) instituted an intervention program with 120 singletons and sole survivors of multiple births. All infants had birthweights less than 2500 gm, with 75% of the birthweights less than 1500 gm. Random assignment was employed to constitute an experimental and a control group. Within each group, children varied in age from under 1 year to 4 years. In the experimental groups, children were tutored for 4 months, with the exception that infants under 1 year were not tutored directly; rather, home visitors worked with their mothers. A comprehensive assessment battery found that intervention with toys alone (i.e., without tutoring) had no measured treatment effect. Performance on tests measuring motor functions, social maturity, and intellectual ability at the end of the 4-month period revealed that in all cases the tutored group was superior to the untutored and control groups. Further, children with no neurological damage made greater gains than those who were more impaired.

In a second study by these same investigators (Scarr-Salapatek & Williams, 1973), infants below 1800 gm born to lower SES mothers were alternately assigned to experimental and control groups as they entered the premature nursery. Working from a sensory deprivation hypothesis, these investigators instructed nurses in an experimental nursery area to provide special visual, tactile, and kinesthetic stimulation that was thought to approximate good home care for newborn infants. The control group infants received standard pediatric care for low-birthweight infants, which consisted of maintaining them in their isolettes and feeding and changing them with minimal disturbance. After discharge from the hospital, the experimental group infants received weekly visits from a social worker who implemented a stimulation regimen developed by Gordon and Lally (1967). During the lying-in period, the experimental group gained weight significantly faster than did the control group, and at 1 year of age, they had higher scores on the Cattell Infant Intelligence Scale. It is especially important to note that the mean scores for the treated infants approximated that expected of normally developing children.

In a replication and extension of the Scarr-Salapatek and Williams study, Powell (1974) reported essentially the same results for black, singleton infants whose birthweights were between 1000 and 2000 gm. One group of infants received extra handling by practical nurses throughout their stay in the hospital nursery, whereas the subjects in the control group received "ordinary treatment given in a premature nursery." Unlike the Scarr-Salapatek and Williams study, the subjects for this study received less stimulation per day, and their mothers received no follow-up visits except for testing. However, also unlike the Scarr-Salapatek and Williams study, mothers in this group were encouraged to visit and handle the children during their stays in the hospital. Although the differences between the groups were not as dramatic as those reported by the Scarr-Salapatek and Williams study over the first 6 months of life, the Bayley scale performance of the experimental group was higher than that of the control group. The effect of encouraging mothers to visit the hospital was not significant.

In other cases, the encouragement of mothers to interact with their premature infants has resulted in some significant findings. The early developers of the incubator recognized the importance of maintaining parental involvement in the care of premature infants. Budin advised that "it is better by far to put the little one in an incubator by its mother's bedside, the supervision which she exercises is not to be lightly estimated [Kennell & Klaus, 1976 p. 99]." Mothers whose babies were displayed in early incubator exhibits were given free passes to allow frequent visiting with their babies. But somehow this social aspect became lost as incubators were incorporated into nurseries. The glass walls of the incubator became barriers of isolation rather than portholes for attachment. Fear of infection reinforced separation between mother and premature infant. Not until the late 1960s was this fear explored and refuted by scientific inquiry (Barnett, Leiderman, Grobstein, & Klaus, 1970; Silverman & Sinclair, 1967; Williams & Oliver, 1969). Simple handwashing and gown procedures are all that are required in many centers prior to parents touching, holding, feeding, and assisting in the care of their babies.

Barnett et al. (1970) found that mothers allowed in the premature nursery showed more confidence and more skill in stimulating and taking care of their infants than mothers who had limited contact with their premature infants because of traditional hospital routine. Kennell, Trause, and Klaus (1975) randomly assigned 53 mothers of premature infants to an early-contact group or a late-contact group. The early-contact group was allowed contact beginning 1–5 days after birth, whereas the later group only had visual contact through the nursery window until 21 days. Early-contact mothers looked at their female infants, but not their male infants, a greater percentage of the time than the late-contact group. At 42 months, the infants in the early contact group showed significantly higher Stanford-Binet scores than the late-contact group. In a similar study (Seashore, Leifer, Barnett, & Leiderman, 1973), two groups of 22 mothers of premature infants were compared to a group of mothers of full-term infants who acted according to hospital routine. One group of mothers of preterms had visual contact through a nursery window for 3–12 weeks, whereas the other group was allowed full contact once every 6 days beginning in the first 5 days. A week before discharge, all mothers were allowed to be with their infants. Whereas mothers of preterms smiled less often and held their infants less than mothers of full-terms, primiparous mothers of preterms who had been separated were significantly less confident about their ability to take care of their infants than the other mothers at discharge, 1 week, and 1 month later.

A Generalized Model for Evaluating Interventions with Preterm Infants

To a considerable degree, the research on treatment strategies for preterm infants is already characterized by two advantageous features of life science research conducted in therapeutic settings. The recent research has tended to be both interdisciplinary and longitudinal. For example, we see in the research reported by Scarr-Salapatek and Williams (1973) an overlay of psychosocial manipulations onto ongoing biomedical and psychosocial independent variables during the first year of infants' lives, with different dependent variables being measured at different measurement occasions. In conjunction with random assignment to groups, this is a powerful research design, capable of generating intriguing new hypotheses as well as testing already explicitly stated ones.

To the current longitudinal and interdisciplinary features, two additional research features can be emphasized that will increase the explanatory power of future intervention studies with preterm infants: the aptitude × treatment interaction (ATI) designs discussed by Cronbach (1957, 1975) and what Sameroff and Chandler (1975) have called a transactional model of development. A transactional model of development makes use of the concept of bidirectionality of influences between organism and environment. Put simply, they influence each other reciprocally through time. Figure 22.1 is one of

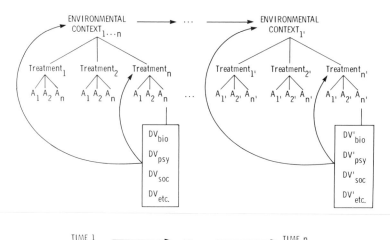

FIGURE 22.1. *A generalized model for evaluating interventions with preterm infants.*

many possible schematic diagrams showing the basic relationships among the four major approaches (longitudinal, interdisciplinary, aptitude × treatment interactions, and transactional processes), or an idealized general intervention design within our framework.

Before commenting on the diagram itself, two terms need to be defined. By *environmental context,* we mean any collection of environmental variables that tend to persist through time. Examples of environmental contexts include mother–child interaction patterns, socioeconomic status of the child's family, and the preterm child's cultural milieu. The level of description can vary from the molecular to the molar, depending upon the purposes of the investigator. For *aptitude,* we invoke Crohnbach's (1975) definition of "any characteristic of the person that affects his response to the treatment [p. 116]," or what we have called "attribute."

The essential point of Figure 22.1 is to provide a simple organizational framework for summarizing and perhaps assisting in the generation of subsequent intervention studies. In Figure 22.1, an alternative set of treatments are conceived to be instituted within a given environmental context for N groups of premature infants who possess given aptitudes. The effects of those treatments on given attributes (A) (e.g., variations in degrees of prematurity) potentially affect a range of dependent variables (DV) in the realms of biology, psychology, sociology, etc. These resulting changes assessed through the dependent variables may in turn alter the environmental context through time, leading to new treatments for altered attributes with new dependent variables. Thus, a cyclic process is potentially activated that needs to be monitored progressively through time.

Within such an approach are two important aspects in the instigation and fulfillment of intervention: (*a*) an attribute-oriented approach based on empiricism; and (*b*) a process-oriented approach based in theory of how the attributes change. As in the biomedical context, attributes that reflect the integrity of the preterm infant can be identified, and intervention can be tailored to fit the significance of possessing those attributes. From psychological theory, the functional salience of attributes as they relate to the environmental context can be ascertained, and intervention can be directed toward the complex infant-environment transactions that guide development.

In this model, then, intervention may not be uniform for all preterm infants. Instead, as mentioned previously in the chapter, specific interventions can be designed for specific infant attributes and environments, as they exist for the infant during the present and as they change and develop. This is not to say, however, that prematurity per se is not a salient attribute. Having a premature baby in itself may establish a differential set of expectations and self-concepts for the parents. For example, the medical problems associated with prematurity are often perceived as a failure to reproduce a normal infant or to be able to care for the baby, especially for primiparous mothers (Caplan, Mason, & Kaplan, 1965; Seashore, *et al.,* 1973). In fact, just calling a normal baby "preterm" elicits in a mother greater autonomic arousal to the infant's cry (Frodi, Lamb, Leavitt, & Donovan, 1978). In this case, the environmental context must include the differential expectations of the parents. But it should be emphasized that the subjective feelings of those who will provide care for the preterm infant change as the caregivers become more familiar with the infant (Corter, Trehub, Boukydis, Ford, Celhoffer, & Minde, 1978), thus setting the stage for changes in the environmental context.

Beyond these changing response sets, though, are the infant's attributes that may affect the quality of care the preterm infant receives. Field (1977) suggests the effects of early maternal separation may contribute less to later maternal–infant interactive failures than specific early behavioral deficits of the preterm infant. For example, preterm infants may be generally difficult to feed (Klaus & Fanaroff, 1973) and less likely to signal feeding readiness by opening the mouth or rooting (Brown & Bakeman, in press). At the mother's first hospital feeding of the baby, a full-term infant may be held more closely than a preterm infant, with a sick preterm infant being held on the mother's lap more often than a healthy preterm infant (DiVitto & Goldberg, 1979). At the second feeding, full-term infants may be talked to and touched more often than preterm infants (DiVitto & Goldberg, 1979). Brown and Bakeman (in press) suggest that black, low SES preterm infants, at the time of hospital discharge, were more difficult to care for and generally less responsive when compared to full-term infants. They were less active and had weaker motor movements, poor head and hand-to-hand control, and poor rooting and sucking. Comparing healthy full-terms, healthy preterms, sick preterms (with RDS), and preterms born to diabetic mothers in a white, middle-class sample, DiVitto and Goldberg (1979) found that the more sick the infant had been, the less likely the infant was to be alert and responsive to stimulation and to have good motor organization.

Field (1977) also found that preterm infants with RDS showed poorer social interactive processes on the Brazelton examination when compared to full-term infants. The social interactive processes comprise the infant's ability to orient, cuddle, be alert, and be consoled with caregivers' attempts at soothing. The unresponsive, lethargic preterm infants who show less well-developed social interactive processes have mothers who employ more active attention-getting procedures (Field, 1977) and initiated more social interactions (Brown & Bakeman, in press) than mothers of full-term infants. Beckwith and Cohen (1978) suggested that the more harzardous the biological course of the preterm infant had been, the more social attention the infant may receive.

Related to the finding that the preterm infant is difficult to console with intervention is the often reported suggestion that the preterm infant is less able to inhibit his level of arousal than full-term infants of the same conceptional age (e.g., Sigman, Kopp, Littman, & Parmelee, 1977). In fact, whereas the motoric processes of infants may be most highly predicted from an infant's birthweight, the strongest predictor of the infant's state control (the infant's ability to organize his states and to shut out disturbing stimuli) is gestational age (Sepkoski, Coll, & Lester, 1977). Infants with lower gestational ages may have more labile states and, with less consolability, may appear to be more irritable.

The suggestions that preterm infants are likely to cry and be irritable (Elmer & Gregg, 1967) and conversely that preterm infants cry less with lower intensities and shorter durations (Brown & Bakeman, in press), or are less likely to give clear distress signals in the form of cries (DiVitto & Goldberg, 1979), have both been reported. The "mewing" cry sound of the preterm infant has been studied for its spectral and perceptual characteristics. Generally, low-birthweight (Michelsson, 1971), especially SGA babies (Zeskind & Stern, 1975), and thin preterm babies (Lester & Zeskind, 1978) can be reliably differentiated from full-birthweight, full-term babies by the high pitch and temporal features of the cry. These authors have also reported the high thresholds for arousal and short durations associated with eliciting cries from preterm or low-birthweight infants. Related to the pitch of the cry is the infant's performance on the Brazelton scale; infants with the highest pitched, aversive cries are the infants with the poorest performances and are the least responsive (Lester & Zeskind, 1978). The cry of the preterm infant elicits greater autonomic arousal in the listener than the cry of a full-term infant (Frodi, Lamb, Leavitt, Donovan, Neff, & Sherry, 1978). Studies of similar cries of infants with prenatal and perinatal complications suggest that, whereas the cries of normal infants may be perceived along one semantic dimension—the "distressing" quality of the sound—the high-pitched cry is perceived along that and a second dimension—the "sick" nature of the infant (Zeskind & Lester, 1978). These perceptions may provide the basis for differential responsivity to infants with these unusual cry features (Zeskind, 1980). Some evidence suggests that the cry features parallel infant recovery such that the high cry pitch disappears with the amelioration of the detrimental condition yet remains in the presence of abnormal neurological sequelae (Michelsson, Sirvio, & Wasz-Hockert, 1977).

Thus, we find that there are a number of attributes that may reflect the changing integrity of both the infant and environment as they respond to one another and as they may be related to later development. For example, infants who were most alert and responsive as newborns later received the most cuddling during feeding, whereas infants who were the least responsive to auditory stimulation continued to get greater levels of auditory and tactile stimulation even after the behaviors of the baby changed (DiVitto & Goldberg, 1979). Perhaps consistent with this finding is the report that, although specific behavioral differences between preterm and full-term infants, in mother–infant interactions evident at 1 month of age may disappear at 3 months of age, differences in overall behavioral style in the interaction remained (Brown & Bakeman, in press). Other investigators have also shown a relation between mother–infant interaction characteristics and preterm infant outcome measures at 9 months. For example, vocalizing during gazing with the mother in the first months is associated with higher Gesell language subtest scores at 9 months (Beckwith, Sigman, Cohen, & Parmelee, 1976). Associated with higher sensorimotor scores at 9 months were more mutual mother–infant gazing at 1 month, more smiling during mother–infant gazing at 3 months, more contingent responses to distress at 3 months, and more attentiveness and more contingent responses to nondistress vocalizations at 8 months (Beckwith, Cohen, Kopp, Parmelee, & Marcy, 1976). Laboratory experiments with normal infants (Finkelstein & Ramey, 1977) and failure-to-thrive infants (Ramey, Starr, Pallas, Whitten, & Reed, 1975) have also implicated response-contingent stimulation as an important factor in normal infant development.

Provision of an appropriately responsive caregiving environment, then, may be a useful mode of intervention. The transaction of infant and environmental attributes during the first 3 years of life can be demonstrated in a study in which biologically at-risk infants were randomly assigned to supportive and nonsupportive caregiving environments as part of an ongoing intervention program (Zeskind & Ramey, 1978; in press). Although fetally malnourished, not preterm, infants were studied, these infants show behavioral attributes similar to preterm infants, such as poor Brazelton scale performances and distinguishing cry features (Lester, 1979; Lester & Zeskind, 1978; Zeskind, 1979). Although fetally malnourished infants showed lower intellectual performances than their well-nourished peers in both the supportive and nonsupportive caregiving environments at 3 months of age, the detrimental effects of fetal malnourishment were ameliorated by 18 months in the group of infants randomly assigned to a day-care center designed to prevent socioculturally caused mental retardation (Ramey & Campbell, 1979). At 18 months, fetally malnourished infants continued to show poorer intellectual performances than their well-nourished counterparts in the nonsupportive caregiving environment. Furthermore, although mothers of all groups of infants showed similar amounts of involvement with their infants at 6 months, the fetally malnourished infants in the nonsupportive environment who did not show recovery obtained less maternal involvement by 18 months than the fetally malnourished infants in the supportive environment and the well-nourished infants in the nonsupportive caregiving environment. These findings were replicated through 36 months of age (Zeskind & Ramey, in press) and showed signs of a worsening condition for the fetally malnourished infants in the nonsupportive environment. Because infants were randomly assigned to environmental groups, we can speculate how the detrimental effects of a biologically at-risk condition, with its concomitant behavioral peculiarities, can lead to reduced caregiving responsivity over time yet be prevented with active intervention designed to provide a responsive environment.

Closing Remarks

The goal of intervention is to provide an optimal set of conditions in which the infant and environment can adapt to one another. Thus, we are concerned with the nature of the relation between the infant's and the environment's ability to respond to each other. Ultimately we must be concerned, then, with the preterm infant's capacity to respond to differential environmental qualities or, in other words, with his ability to benefit from provided intervention. We return to the question of whether the appropriate model for stimulation of the preterm infant is a fetal or newborn one. Blindly providing an extensively stimulating environment to an infant with poor state control may prohibit the infant's existing capacities from taking advantage of environmental attributes by overly arousing the infant into a state that is not optimal for orienting to the environment. Conversely, reduced amounts of response-contingent stimulation may also result in nonoptimal development. This chapter has briefly described an oversimplified idealized model, and particular intervention programs may accomplish only parts of such an ambitious effort. Nevertheless, it is our hope that, through the progressive application of such generalized idealized models, many of the apparent contradictory findings concerning the preterm infant can be clarified, with the ultimate consequence of optimal care for the prematurely born child.

References

Ainsworth, M. Attachment and dependency: A comparison. In J. L. Gewirtz (Ed.), *Attachment and dependency*. Washington, D.C.: Winston, 1972.

Barnard, K. *A program of stimulation for infants born prematurely*. Paper presented at the meeting of the Society for Research in Child Development, Philadelphia, March 1973.

Barnett, C. R., Leiderman, P. H., Grobstein, R., & Klaus, M. H. Neonatal separation: The maternal side of interactional deprivation. *Pediatrics,* 1970, *45,* 197–205.

Beckwith, L., & Cohen, S. E. Preterm birth: Hazardous obstetric and postnatal events as related to caregiver–infant behavior. *Infant Behavior and Development,* 1978, *1*(4), 403–411.

Beckwith, L., Cohen, S. E., Kopp, C. B., Parmelee, A. H., & Marcy, T. G. Caregiver–infant interaction and early cognitive development in preterm infants. *Child Development,* 1976, *47,* 570–587.

Beckwith, L., Sigman, M., Cohen, S. E., & Parmelee, A. H. Vocal output in preterm infants. *Developmental Psychobiology,* 1977, *10*(6), 543–554.

Birch, H. G., & Gussow, J. D. *Disadvantaged children: Health, nutrition, and school failure.* New York: Grune & Stratton, 1970.

Bowlby, J. The nature of the child's tie to his mother. *International Journal of Psychoanalysis,* 1958, *39,* 350.

Braine, M. D. S., Heimer, C. B., Wortis, H., & Freedman, A. M. Factors associated with impairment of the early development of prematures. *Monographs of the Society for Research in Child Development,* 1966, *31,* (4, Serial No. 106).

Brown, J., & Bakeman, R. Relationships of human mothers with their infants during the first year of life: Effects of prematurity. In R. W. Bell & W. P. Smotherman (Eds.), *Maternal influences and early behavior*. Holliswood, N.Y.: Spectrum, in press.

Caplan, G., Mason, E. A., & Kaplan, D. M. Four studies of crisis in parents of prematures. *Community Mental Health Journal*, 1965, *1*, 149–161.

Caputo, D. V., & Mandell, W. Consequences of low birth weight. *Developmental Psychology*, 1970, *3*(3), 363–383.

Caputo, D. V., Taub, H. B., Goldstein, K. M., Smith, N., Dalack, J. D., Pursner, J. P., & Silberstein, R. M. An evaluation of various parameters of maturity at birth as predictors of development at one year of life. *Perceptual and Motor Skills*, 1974, *39*, 631–652.

Cornell, E. H., & Gottfried, A. W. Intervention with premature human infants. *Child Development*, 1976, *47*, 32–39.

Corter, C., Trehub, S., Boukydis, C., Ford, L., Celhoffer, L., & Minde, K. Nurses judgments of the attractiveness of premature infants. *Infant Behavior and Development*, 1978, *1*(4), 373–380.

Cremer, R. J., Perryman, P. W., & Richards, P. H. Influence of light on hyperbilirubinemia of infants. *The Lancet*, 1958, *1*, 1094.

Cronbach, L. J. The two disciplines of scientific psychology. *American Psychologist*, 1957, *12*, 671–684.

Cronbach, L. J. Beyond the two disciplines of scientific psychology. *American Psychologist*, 1975, *30*, 116–127.

DiVitto, B., & Goldberg, S. The effects of newborn medical status on early parent-infant interaction. In T. Field, S. Goldberg, A. Sostek, & H. H. Shuman (Eds.), *Infants born at risk*. New York: Spectrum, 1979.

Douglas, J. W. B. Mental ability and school achievement of premature children at eight years of age. *British Medical Journal*, 1956, *1*, 1210–1214.

Drillien, C. M. *The growth and development of the prematurely born infant*. Baltimore: Williams & Wilkins, 1964.

Drillien, C. M. Intellectual sequelae of "fetal malnutrition." In H. A. Waisman & G. R. Kerr (Eds.), *Fetal growth and development*. New York: McGraw-Hill, 1970.

Elmer, E., & Gregg, G. S. Developmental characteristics of abused children. *Pediatrics*, 1967, *40*, 596–602.

Erikson, E. H. *Childhood and society*. New York: Norton, 1950.

Field, T. M. The effects of early separation, interactive deficits, and experimental manipulations of infant–mother face-to-face interaction. *Child Development*, 1977, *48*, 763–771.

Finkelstein, N. W., & Ramey, C. T. Learning to control the environment in infancy. *Child Development*, 1977, *48*, 806–819.

Fitzhardinge, P. M., & Stevens, E. M. The small-for-date infant. II: Neurological and intellectual sequelae. *Pediatrics*, 1972, *50*, 50–57.

Francis-Williams, J., & Davies, P. A. Very low birthweight and later intelligence. *Developmental Medicine and Child Neurology*, 1974, *16*, 709–725.

Franklin, A. W. Influence of light on the hyperbilirubinemia of infants. *The Lancet*, 1958, *1*, 1227.

Freedman, D. G., Boverman, H., & Freedman, N. *Effects of kinesthetic stimulation on weight gain and on smiling in premature infants*. Paper presented at the annual meeting of the American Orthopsychiatric Association, San Francisco, 1966.

Freud, S. Three essays on the theory of sexuality. *The standard edition of the complete psychological works of Freud* (Vol. 7). London: Hogarth, 1953.

Frodi, A., Lamb, M., Leavitt, L., & Donovan, W. Fathers' and mothers' responses to infant smiles and cries. *Infant Behavior and Development*, 1978, *1*(2), 187–198.

Frodi, A., Lamb, M., Leavitt, L. A., Donovan, W. L., Neff, C., & Sherry, D. Fathers' and mothers' responses to the faces and cries of normal and premature infants. *Developmental Psychology*, 1978, *14*(5), 490–498.

Gewirtz, J. L. Attachment, dependence, and a distinction in terms of stimulus control. In J. L. Gewirtz (Ed.), *Attachment and dependency.* Washington, D.C.: Winston & Sons, 1972.

Goldfarb, W. Psychological deprivation in infancy and subsequent adjustment. *American Journal of Orthopsychiatry,* 1945, *15,* 49–56.

Gordon, I. J., & Lally, R. Intellectual stimulation for infants and toddlers. Gainesville, Fla.: Institute for Development of Human Resources, 1967.

Hasselmeyer, E. G. The premature neonate's response to handling. *American Nurses' Association,* 1964, *11,* 15–24.

Hebb, D. O. *The organization of behavior.* New York: Wiley, 1949.

Hess, J., Mahr, G., & Bartelme, P. F. *The physical and mental growth of prematurely born children.* Chicago: Univ. of Chicago Press, 1939.

Hunt, J. V., Harvin, D., Kennedy, D., & Tooley, W. H. Mental development of children with birthweights ≤ 1500 grams. *Clinical Research,* 1974, *22,* 240.

Kennell, J. H., & Klaus, M. H. Caring for parents of a premature or sick infant. In M. H. Klaus & J. H. Kennell (Eds.), *Maternal–infant bonding.* St. Louis: Mosby, 1976.

Kennell, J. H., Trause, M. A., & Klaus, M. H. Evidence for a sensitive period in the human mother. In *Parent–infant interaction* (Ciba Foundation Symposium, 33). New York: Associated Scientific Publishers, 1975.

Klaus, M. H., & Fanaroff, A. A. *Care of the high-risk neonate.* Philadelphia: Sanders, 1973.

Knobloch, H., & Pasamanick, B. Prospective studies on the epidemeology of reproductive casualty: Methods, findings, and some implications. *Merrill-Palmer Quarterly,* 1966, *12,* 27–43.

Kramer, L. I., & Pierpont, M. E. Rocking waterbeds and auditory stimuli to enhance growth of preterm infants. *Pediatrics,* 1976, *88,* 297–299.

Lester, B. M. A synergistic process approach to the study of fetal malnutrition. *Journal of Behavioral Development,* 1979 *2,* 377–393.

Lester, B. M., & Zeskind. P. S. Brazelton scale and physical size correlates of neonatal cry features. *Infant Behavior and Development,* 1978, *1*(4), 293–402.

Lubchenco, L. O. *The high risk infant.* Philadelphia: Saunders, 1976.

Lubchenco, L. O., Horner, F. A., Reed, L. H., Hix, I. E., Metcalf, D., Cohig, R., Elliott, H. C., & Bourg, M. Sequelae of premature birth. *American Journal of Diseases of Children,* 1963, *106,* 101–115.

Michelsson, K. Cry analysis of symptomless low birth weight neonates and of asphyxiated newborn infants. *Acta Paediatrica Scandinavia,* 1971 [Suppl. 216], 1–45.

Michelsson, K., Sirvio, P., & Wasz-Hockert, O. Sound spectrographic analysis of infants with bacterial meningitis. *Developmental Medicine and Child Neurology,* 1977, *19,* 309–315.

Minde, K., Ford, L., Celhoffer, L., & Boukydis, C. Interactions of mothers and nurses with premature infants. *Canadian Medical Association Journal,* 1975, *113,* 741–745.

Neal, M. V. Vestibular stimulation and developmental behavior of the small premature infant. *Nursing Research Report,* 1968, *3,* 2–5.

Phillips, M. B. Prediction of scholastic performance from perinatal and infant development indices. *Dissertation Abstracts International,* 1972, *33,*1526. (University Microfilms No. 72-25, 648).

Piaget, J. *The origins of intelligence in children.* New York: International Universities Press, 1952.

Powell, L. G. The effect of extra stimulation and maternal involvement on the development of low-birth-weight infants and on maternal behavior. *Child Development,* 1974, *45,* 106–113.

Rabinovitch, M. S., Bibace, R., & Caplan, H. Sequelae of prematurity: Psychological test findings. *Canadian Medical Association Journal,* 1961, *84,* 822–824.

Ramey, C. T., & Campbell, F. A. Compensatory education for disadvantaged children. *School Review,* 1979, *82* (2), 171–189.

Ramey, C. T., & Finkelstein, N. W. Contingent stimulation and competence. *Journal of Pediatric Psychology,* 1978, *3,* 89–96.

Ramey, C. T., Starr, R. H., Pallas, J., Whitten, C. F., & Reed, V. Nutrition response-contingent stimulation and the maternal deprivation syndrome: Results of an early intervention program. *Merrill-Palmer Quarterly*, 1975, *21*, 45–53.

Ribble, M. A. Infantile experience in relation to personality development. In J. V. Hunt (Ed.), *Personality and the behavior disorders*. New York: Ronald, 1944.

Rubin, R. A., Rosenblatt, C., & Balow, B. Psychological and educational sequelae of prematurity. *Pediatrics*, 1973, *52*(3), 352–363.

Sameroff, A., & Chandler, M. J. Reproductive risk and the continuum of caretaking casualty. In F. D. Horowitz (Ed.), *Review of child development research* (Vol. 4). Chicago: Univ. of Chicago Press, 1975.

Scarr-Salapatek, S., & Williams, M. The effects of early stimulation on low-birth weight infants. *Child Development*, 1973, *44*, 94–101.

Seashore, M. J., Leifer, A. D., Barnett, C. R., & Leiderman, P. H. The effects of denial of early mother–infant interaction on maternal self-confidence. *Journal of Personality and Social Psychology*, 1973, *26*, 369–378.

Segall, M. E. Cardiac responsivity to auditory stimulation in premature infants. *Nursing Research*, 1972, 21, 15–19.

Sepkoski, C., Coll, C. G., & Lester, B. M. The effects of high risk factors on neonatal behavior as measured Brazelton scale. In B. M. Lester (Chair), *A panorama of uses and misuses of the Brazelton Neonatal Behavioral Assessment Scale*. Symposium presented at the Biennial Meeting of the Society for Research and Child Development, New Orleans, 1977.

Sigman, J., Kopp, C. B., Littman, B., & Parmelee, A. H. Infant visual attentiveness in relation to birth condition. *Developmental Psychology*, 1977, *13*(5), 431–437.

Silverman, W. A., Fertig, J. W., & Berger, A. P. The influence of thermal environment upon the survival of newly born premature infants. *Pediatrics*, 1958, *22*, 876.

Silverman, W. A., & Sinclair, J. C. Evaluation of precautions before entering a neonatal unit. *Pediatrics*, 1967, *40*, 900–901.

Solkoff, N., Jaffe, S., Weintraub, D., & Blase, B. Effects of handling on the subsequent developments of premature infants. *Developmental Psychology*, 1969, *1*(6), 765–768.

Taub, H. B., Caputo, D. V., & Goldstein, K. M. Toward a modification of the indices of neonatal prematurity. *Perceptual and Motor Skills*, 1975, *40*, 43–48.

Wiener, G. Psychologic correlates of premature birth: A review. *Journal of Nervous and Mental Disease*, 1962, *134*, 129–144.

Wiener, G. The relationship of birthweight and length of gestation to intellectual development at ages 8 to 10 years. *Journal of Pediatrics*, 1970, *76*, 694–699.

Wiener, G., Rider, R., Oppel, W., Fischer, L., & Harper, P. Correlates of low birthweight: Psychological status at 6–7 years of age. *Pediatrics*, 1965, *35*, 434–444.

Williams, C. P., & Oliver, T. K., Jr. Nursery routines and staphylococcal colonization of the newborn. *Pediatrics*, 1969, *44*, 640–646.

Williams, M., & Scarr, S. Effects of short-term intervention on performance in low-birth-weight, disadvantaged children. *Pediatrics*, 1971, *47*, 289–298.

Wright, L. The theoretical and research base for a program of early stimulation, care, and training of premature infants. In J. Hellmuth (Ed.), *The exceptional infant: Studies in abnormalities*. New York: Bruner-Mazel, 1969.

Zeskind, P. S. *Fetal nutritional risk and neonatal cry features*. Paper presented at the meeting of the Society for Research in Child Development, San Francisco, April 1979.

Zeskind, P. S. Adult responses to cries of low and high risk infants. *Infant Behavior and Development*, 1980, *3*, 167–177.

Zeskind, P. S., & Lester, B. M. Acoustic features and auditory perceptions of the cries of newborns with prenatal and perinatal complications. *Child Development*, 1978, *49*, 580–589.

Zeskind, P. S., & Ramey, C. T. Fetal malnutrition: An experimental study of its consequences on infant development in two caregiving environments. *Child Development*, 1978, *49*, 1155–1162.

Zeskind, P. S., & Ramey, C. T. Preventing intellectual and interactional sequelae of fetal malnutrition: A longitudinal, transactional and synergistic approach to development. *Child Development,* in press.

Zeskind, P. A., & Stern, K. Acoustic analysis of the cry response. In B. M. Lester (Chair), Influences on the behavior of the newborn. Symposium presented at the meeting of the Southeastern Psychological Association, Atlanta, March 1975.

23

Intervention during Infancy: General Considerations[1]

JOSEPH F. FAGAN, III
LYNN TWAROG SINGER

This chapter suggests general guidelines for the design of programs that would provide early intervention to offset expected cognitive deficit. We feel that the extension of our guidelines to intervention at any point in development and to deficits in social interaction or difficulties in emotional adjustment is appropriate, but a discussion of such extensions is beyond the scope of the present chapter. Briefly, we see a need for specific, task-related programs of intervention rather than for a general "enrichment" approach. Our second point is that specific intervention requires prior study of processes that provide valid prediction of individual differences, are amenable to theoretical interpretation, and possess alterable components. Finally, we feel that desirable outcomes must be specified along with strategies for choosing candidates for intervention and for assessing the effectiveness of intervention.

The acceleration since the mid-1970s of intervention programs in early infancy has been remarkable. For the most part, such programs have tended to consist of nonspecific enrichment, primarily increased sensory stimulation, directed at infants with a wide variety of risk conditions (Friedlander, Sterritt, & Kirk, 1975). The merit of broad-band, general intervention programs in infancy is debatable. While these programs probably are not harmful, there is little evidence that the majority of existing intervention programs ameliorate the presumed negative consequences of high-risk status early in life. On the basis of a review of a variety of programs for infants and young children at risk, Keogh and Kopp (1978) concluded that, for infant programs, the data

[1] The preparation of this chapter was supported by Multiple Research Project Grant HD–11089 and by a grant from the National Foundation.

base was limited and the theoretical underpinnings were "cloudy." Rationales for the programs they studied seemed derived from the hope that any intervention would benefit development, with the relationship between initial assessment and subsequent intervention remaining largely ill defined. An example of the limited yield obtained from precipitous intervention can be found in the experimental studies of increased stimulation given to premature infants. In their critical review of intervention programs for premature infants, Cornell and Gottfried (1976) noted a trend toward accelerated motor development in infancy for premature infants exposed to a wide variety of types, frequencies, and intensities of sensory stimulation. However, such experimental programs have yielded little information on the relationships between early stimulation and later perceptual–cognitive functioning. Indeed, early differences between preterm and full-term infants in their sensory thresholds and processing capacities are still largely unknown, precluding the development of appropriate intervention programs for those preterm infants who may be at risk for future biological and psychological disabilities. Only a few infant programs have developed a specific plan of intervention following a study of a process. One example is the program that resulted from the work of Fraiberg and her colleagues on object constancy in blind infants (as noted by Keogh & Kopp, 1978). In Fraiberg's research, careful observation, assessment, and hypothesis testing led directly to educational intervention in the blind baby's development and to objective outcome measures for program evaluation. Specifically, Fraiberg's eventual remediation program emerged from a longitudinal study of the sensorimotor development of a group of blind infants, some of whom developed normally and some of whom lagged strikingly in development. Observation of the differences between these groups led to a testable hypothesis that midline hand play early in life appears to be an important forerunner to such later behaviors as object constancy, reaching, and locomotion. Fraiberg altered the components of the processes involved in midline hand play by substituting auditory stimuli for the absent visual stimulation to motivate the hand play of blind infants. She was then able to observe whether the alteration actually influenced the subsequent reaching and walking behavior of the blind infant. While exceptional, Fraiberg's example of specific intervention following empirical exploration of a process should become the rule in designing intervention programs if any progress is to be made.

As Scott (1978) notes in his review of learning theory and mental development, the learning theorist faces three tasks: assessing deficits in learning, identifying (through theory) the processes that impede learning, and generating training procedures (again based on theory) that improve learning. Examples of programs attempting such tasks with older, mentally retarded children include Butterfield; Wambold, and Belmont's (1973) work on short-term memory and the studies of the Zeamans on discrimination learning. Butterfield, Wambold, and Belmont (1973), for example, approached the problem of improving the poor recall of retarded children by training the children to employ particular rehearsal strategies. The emphasis on rehearsal as a remedial device followed from the theoretical position that recall depends on the transfer of information from brief to longer term memory stores, a transfer accomplished by control processes such as rehearsal. An article by Zeaman (1978) is an excellent illustration of the way in which a theory (in this case, a theory of discrimination learning in which selective attention is a major construct) may be searched to identify those theoretical processes (e.g., direction, adjustability, and breadth of attention) that may be linked to the retarded child's poor performance (on discrimination learning tasks).

The tasks faced by the learning theorist in understanding the retarded child are the same tasks confronting those who wish to understand the infant who may be at risk for later cognitive status. Thus, if the aim is to ameliorate later cognitive deficit, our goal should be to explore cognitive processes during infancy that meet three criteria. First, performance resulting from a process should vary with intelligence. Second, the process should be amenable to theoretical interpretation. Finally, alterable aspects of the process should be identified. As an example in the field of infancy, the processes underlying the infant's ability to recognize a previously seen visual target would seem to satisfy all three criteria. Specifically, groups of infants expected to differ in intelligence later in life also differ in the ability to recognize a familiar visual stimulus. Fantz and Nevis (1967), for example, compared home-reared offspring of highly intelligent parents with institution-reared offspring of women of average intelligence, and Miranda and Fantz (1974) compared Down's syndrome with normal infants. In each case, the infants expected to be more intelligent later in life were also superior in visual recognition during infancy. Such group differences early in life are, presumably, indicative of differences in recognition memory among individuals, differences that are also valid estimates of current and of later intelligent functioning. Empirical support for the presumption of individual differences in early cognitive functioning comes from a series of studies by the senior author (Fagan, 1979) aimed at estimating the predictive validity of paired-comparison tests of infant recognition memory as measures of intelligence. Preliminary analyses of the data have been quite encouraging. Specifically, differences in visual fixation to novel stimuli on the part of children tested between 4 and 7 months of age in some of our earlier studies (Fagan, 1971, 1976) are significantly correlated with later intelligence between 3 and 6 years, intelligence operationally defined by performance on vocabulary tests and vocabulary subtests, such as the Peabody Picture Vocabulary Test (PPVT), the Wechsler Preschool and Preliminary Scales of Intelligence (WPPSI), the revised Wechsler Intelligence Scale for Children, and the Stanford-Binet. Validity coefficients range from .37 at 3–4 years to .66 at 6 years, are similar for males and females, and cannot be attributed to variations in socioeconomic status. Moreover, because of less than optimal reliability and various sources of attenuation, the obtained coefficients are probably underestimates of the actual predictive validity of infant visual recognition tests. In short, the results of the earlier work by Fantz, Nevis, and Miranda on differences in early memory on the part of groups expected to vary in later intelligence and the results of current work by the senior author on individual differences in early memory lend strong support to the assumption that variations in early visual memory both reflect and predict variations in intelligent functioning.

The infant's recognition of visual targets has also been subjected to theoretical analyses. Proposed models tend to emphasize either the memorial or the perceptual aspects of the recognition process. Cohen and Gelber (1975) and Olson (1976), for example, propose memory models of infant recognition based on information processing–memory store theories of verbal recall in adults. Such theories focus on transfer of information among memory stores as accomplished by control processes such as rehearsal. Theoretical accounts of infant recognition that emphasize perception include Jeffrey's (1976) account of habituation as a mechanism for perceptual learning and Fagan's (1977) attention model of infant recognition based on variants of attention theories of discrimination learning. While all of these models should be considered preliminary attempts at theoretical interpretation, the main point is that a body of data is sufficiently large to allow theoretical analysis.

Finally, there is some evidence that the infant's recognition of a visual stimulus can be altered. Fagan (1978a, 1978b) has shown that infants' recognition of both faces and abstract patterns can be facilitated by exposing infants to particular related targets during initial study and has also demonstrated some of the conditions controlling such facilitation. Specifically, at 5–7 months, the infant's recognition memory for a man's face was found to be improved by allowing the infant to study various poses of that man. The same facilitation of recognition was found for abstract patterns. It was necessary to present only one associated stimulus along with the to-be-remembered target in order to aid recognition. Such facilitation was most dependent upon the kind of related target shown for study and was more likely to be demonstrated when simultaneous rather than successive exposure to related instances was allowed. Similar instances of facilitation of infants' recognition are contained in a report by Ruff (1978). The value of these demonstrations of facilitation of recognition is twofold. First, it means that models of recognition must be searched for components that may account for facilitation. Second, it means that, whether theoretically explicable or not, certain mnemonic aids for infant recognition exist. In other words, there is a great deal of both theoretical and practical benefit that can come from knowing how to insure that particular information will be encoded by an infant.

But even if we can identify early processes that are related to later cognitive functioning, processes that may be subjected to theoretical analysis and whose output may be enhanced, we must still decide what later outcomes we desire to arise from our understanding of early processes. Our position is that the same degree of specificity that should characterize the investigation of early cognitive processes needs to be extended to the determination of desirable outcomes for intervention. Choice of appropriate outcome is primarily a reflection of political and societal values as well as of practical utility. What constitutes optimal development depends on what people want and what scientists can do. The usual, implied, hope for intervention programs has been an increase in IQ. However, if we assume that IQ represents a stable characteristic, then only some alterable component of perceptual–cognitive functioning can be expected to change in response to intervention. In other words, we must train a child to do more with what he has rather than hold out the hope that he can have more. Thus, instead of attempting to change intelligence per se, we suggest choosing some educationally relevant skill and linking our understanding of that skill to our understanding of early cognitive functioning. Reading, for example, has already been subjected to a considerable amount of process analysis and would seem to be related to processing of visual information very early in life. It seems quite possible to ask, in other words, whether aspects of early visual information processing, such as attention and encoding, may be directed or facilitated early in infancy, thus, in turn, affecting the ability to read later in life. Then we must discover which infants can profit most from early intervention. Early experimental facilitation of visual processing might be tried with various kinds of infants to observe the effects of intervention over time. For example, Down's syndrome infants as compared to normal controls might benefit later in life from longer or from guided exposure in infancy to exaggerated perceptual components of abstract designs that are important to letter recognition. Preterm infants, however, might not show as great a gain as Down's syndrome infants. Other infant groups that would also be expected to perform poorly on school tasks later on, such as failure-to-thrive infants, may have no initial difficulty with visual processing, and appropriate intervention for the failure-to-thrive infant might then be sought elsewhere, for example, in motivational factors. In short, successful intervention depends on linking those cognitive processes that are understood and can be manipulated in infancy with those cognitive skills considered important many years later. Obviously, longitudinal study is necessary to establish the initial links between early and later cognitive processing, for example, between visual recognition and reading. Although often maligned as expensive and hopelessly confounded, longitudinal research is, nevertheless, the only way to acquire knowledge about continuity in processes (McCall, 1977). In the long run, longitudinal research may be less expensive than haphazard, unscientific intervention programs. It does little good, for example, to show that extra stimulation for premature infants promotes accelerated motor development during infancy if early accelerated motor development is itself unrelated to later perceptual–cognitive development. Finally, we must cast our evaluation of the effectiveness of early intervention programs in specific terms. It is scientifically, politically, and morally dangerous to make sweeping claims for the effectiveness of intervention programs. It is more accurate and, in the long run, more helpful to show that children diagnosed as X who enter program Y will show an average gain of N points on a later test of Z.

In summary, the present chapter has argued for a reconsideration of the goals and designs of infant intervention programs. Nebulous goals tied to generalized, nonspecific enrichment that are characteristic of most attempts at intervention in infancy have hindered the acquisition of a reliable data base and the development of effective remediation programs for infants at risk for future cognitive deficit. In our view, successful intervention depends on the linkage of specific, alterable components of cognitive processes in infancy to cognitive skills deemed important later in life. Infants' recognition of visual stimuli has been noted as an example of a widely studied perceptual–cognitive process that might be fruitfully linked to a later cognitive skill, such as reading. Infants' visual recognition memory has been shown to discriminate among groups varying in intellectual ability later in life and is a process that has been subjected to theoretical analysis. There is also some evidence that infants' visual recognition can be facilitated. Whether altering aspects of early visual information processing for particular kinds of infants can affect reading ability later in life is a question that can only be answered through longitudinal research.

References

Butterfield, E. C., Wambold, C., & Belmont, J. M. On the theory and practice of improving short-term memory. *American Journal of Mental Deficiency,* 1973, *77,* 654–669.

Cohen, L. B., & Gelber, E. R. Infant visual memory. In L. Cohen & P. Salapatek (Eds.), *Infant perception: From sensation to cognition* (Vol. 1). *Basic visual processes.* New York: Academic Press, 1975.

Cornell, E. H., & Gottfried, A. W. Intervention with premature human infants. *Child Development,* 1976, *47,* 32–39.

Fagan, J. F. Infants' recognition memory for a series of visual stimuli. *Journal of Experimental Child Psychology,* 1971, *11,* 244–250.

Fagan, J. F. Infants' recognition of invariant features of faces. *Child Development,* 1976, *47,* 627–638.

Fagan, J. F. An attention model of infant recognition. *Child Development,* 1977, *48,* 345–359.

Fagan, J. F. Facilitation of infants' recognition memory. *Child Development,* 1978, *49,* 1066–1075. (a)

Fagan, J. F. Infant recognition memory and early cognitive ability: Empirical, theoretical, and remedial considerations. In F. D. Minifie & L. L. Lloyd (Eds.), *Communicative and cognitive abilities—Early behavioral assessment.* Baltimore: University Park Press, 1978. (b)

Fagan, J. F. Infant recognition memory and later intelligence. Paper presented at the meeting of the Society for Research in Child Development, San Francisco, 16 March, 1979.

Fantz, R. L., & Nevis, S. The predictive value of changes in visual preferences in early infancy. In J. Hellmuth (Ed.), *The exceptional infant* (Vol 1). Seattle: Special Child Publications, 1967.

Friedlander, B. Z., Sterritt, G. M., & Kirk, G. E. *Exceptional infant* (Vol. 3). *Assessment and intervention.* New York: Bruner/Mazer, 1975.

Jeffrey, W. E. Habituation as a mechanism for perceptual development. In T. J. Tighe & R. N. Leaton (Eds.), *Habituation: Perspectives from child development, animal behavior, and neurophysiology.* Hillsdale, N.J.: Erlbaum, 1976.

Keogh, B. K., & Kopp, C. B. From assessment to intervention: An elusive bridge. In F. D. Minifie & L. L. Lloyd (Eds.), *Communicative and cognitive abilities—Early behavioral assessment.* Baltimore: University Park Press, 1978.

McCall, R. B. Challenges to a science of developmental psychology. *Child Development,* 1977, *48,* 333–344.

Miranda, S. B., & Fantz, R. L. Recognition memory in Down's syndrome and normal infants. *Child Development,* 1974, *45,* 651–660.

Olson, G. M. An information processing analysis of visual memory and habituation in infants. In T. J. Tighe & R. N. Leaton (Eds.), *Habituation: Perspectives from child development, animal behavior, and neurophysiology.* Hillsdale, N.J.: Erlbaum, 1976.

Ruff, H. A. Infant recognition of the invariant form of objects. *Child Development,* 1978, *49,* 293–306.

Scott, K. G. Learning theory, intelligence, and mental development. *American Journal of Mental Deficiency,* 1978, *82,* 325–336.

Zeaman, D. Some relations of general intelligence and selective attention. *Intelligence,* 1978, *2,* 55–73.

Subject Index

A

Abortion in nonhuman primates, and stress, 54–57

Acidosis, and atelectasis, 27

Alcoholism, maternal, effect on child, 66

Amniocentesis, in hydrops fetalis, 20

Anemia, in preterm infant, 24

Anesthesia
  and evoked potentials, 79, 80
  and maternal hypotension, 20
  thermogenic response, 25
  use in delivery, 65

Anoxia, 355

Apgar scores
  and gestational age, 346
  in postterm, postmature infant, 303
  in preterm infant, respiratory distress syndrome, 302, 303, 309
  in preterm infant, very low birthweight, 334, 335
  shift in, 334, 337

Apnea
  after feeding, in preterm infant, 28
  and thermoregulation, 26

Asphyxia, neonatal, 21
  and brain injury, 21, 22
  and crib death, 66

Astigmatism, and postnatal age, 294

Atelectasis, 27

Auditory brain-stem responses
  characteristics, 120–122
  and development, 119–122

and lesions, 118, 119
  origin, 118

Auditory development, *see also* Auditory-vocal interactions
  abnormalities, 117
  plasticity, 117
  and responsiveness, 117–122
  sequence, 113, 114
  and speech development, 107, 108

Auditory discrimination, in preterm infant, 129

Auditory feedback
  in birds, 107
  in preterm infant, 109
  and vocalization control, 110–114

Auditory evoked potentials
  and auditory development, 108, 118
  and latencies, 131–134, 138, 140–144
  and maturity, 119–122, 131–134, 138, 140–144
  neural substrates, 118
  in preterm infant, 98, 131–134

Auditory nerve
  myelination, 136
  stimulation, 143

Auditory processing, *see also* Auditory stimulation
  in fetus, 174, 210
  in full-term infant, 161, 163–175
  measurement procedures used, 163–167
  in preterm infant, 161, 163–175, 208–210

Auditory stimulation

425

and preterm infant, development, 179–181

and preterm infant, infection, 405

relationship with infant, 179–183, *see also* Mother–infant interaction

Parity, and low birthweight, 9, 12

Patent ductus arteriosus, treatment, 24

Pediatric complications

and caregiver–infant interaction, 318–320

as developmental outcome measures, 315–320

measurement, 306, 307

in postterm, postmature infant, 307

in preterm infant, respiratory distress syndrome, 307–309

Pediatric complications scale

description, 307

use in postterm, postmature infant, 306–308

use in preterm infant, respiratory distress syndrome, 306–309

Persistent fetal circulation, 23

Phototherapy and hyperbilirubinemia, 31, 32, 399

Pitocin, adverse effects, 20

Polycythemia, 23

Poor pregnancy outcomes

definition, 53

factors affecting, 54–57, 61

in *Macaca nemestrina,* 52–57

prediction, 53

risk, 53–62

and stress, 54–61

types, 53–55

Post-early neonatal period, 6

Postmaturity syndrome

in postterm infant, *see* Infant, postterm, postmature

in preterm infant, 299

Postnatal complications scale

description, 302

use in postterm, postmature infant, 303, 304

use in preterm infant, respiratory distress syndrome, 302, 303

Postnatal medical complications

and caregiver–infant interactions, 316, 318–320

as developmental outcome measures, 315–320

and development in preterm infant, 299, 315–320

and postterm, postmature infant, 303, 304

and preterm infant, respiratory distress syndrome, 303, 304, 309

and later development, 317, 318

measurement, 302–304

Pregnancy, *see also* High-risk pregnancy; Poor pregnancy outcome

complications in, effect on infant, 355, 356

drugs in, effect on infant, 19, 354, 355

mother's weight and low birthweight, 10–14

and stress, *see* Prenatal stress

Premature labor, 18, 19

Prenatal care

importance, 67

and low birthweight, 9

Prenatal stress in nonhuman primates

and abortion, 54–57

effect

on learning, 58, 59

on performance, 59–61

on physical maturity, 57, 58

Prenatal stress and pregnancy rate, 54, 55

Psychometric tests in infants, predictive validity, 219–221

Puerperal fever, deaths from, 68

R

Race, and low birthweight, 6–8, 10–13, 67

Recognition memory, *see also* Visual recognition memory and habituation, 241

Relational information

and component discrimination, 230, 231, 233, 235

and configural discrimination, 230–232, 235

multiple exposures to, in full-term infant, 229–235

perception of, in preverbal infant, 222, 225

and perceptual development, 221, 222

and processing

in full-term infant, 223–237

over time, 224

in preterm infant, 225–237

single exposure to, in full-term infant, 229–235

theory, 223

Resonance, and loudness, 109

Respiration rate, and low birthweight, 49, 50

Respiratory distress syndrome

contribution to prematurity, 310

mild, and developmental deficits, 299, 300

in preterm infant, *see* Infant, preterm, respiratory distress syndrome

severe and developmental deficits, 300

Response-adjusting procedures

and movement inhibition, 91, 92

and response, 114–117, 182, 409
Swaddling, effect on neonates, 174
Symptomatic neonatal plethora, definition, 23
Synapses, 152, 154
Systematogenesis, theory, 74

T

Tactile processing
  in fetus, 174, 210
  in full-term infant, 160, 161, 163–175
  measurement, procedures used, 163–166
  in preterm infant, 160, 161, 163–175, 208–210
Tactile stimulation
  and degree of initial response, 168, 171, 172
  measurement, procedures used, 165, 166
  and quickness of response, 167, 169–172
  and response decrement, 169–171
  and sleep, 170, 171
Term, definition, 3
Thermoregulation
  and hypothermia, 25, 26
  and incubators, 25, 26
  and optimal thermal range, 24, 25
  significance, 24
Tools, use of in infancy, 222
Toxemia, and preterm birth, 19, 20
Transpyloric feeding, 28, 29
Twinning, and morbidity, 355

U

Univeristy of California, San Francisco, Longitudinal Study, 333–348
  characteristics of infants studied, 333, 334
  developmental assessment measures used, 335

V

Vineland social maturity scale
  description, 307, 308
  use in postterm, postmature infant, 307–309
  use in preterm infant, respiratory distress syndrome, 307–309
Visual attention
  and behavioral states, 321
  and caregiver–infant interaction, 321–323, 326
  as developmental outcome measure, 315, 321–324
  and habituation, 241

and later developmental competence, 321–324, 326
  length of, in preterm infant, 321
  and manipulation, 262
Visual cortex, maturation, 154
Visual discrimination
  changes in, with age, 278–280
  as developmental outcome measure, 322–324
  earliest appearance, 276
  factors affecting, 272, 275, 279, 280, 283–287
  and HAS rate, 271–275, 278, 279, 282, 283, 285
  in full-term infant, 278, 279, 294
  measurement, 272
  and prenatal stress, 59
  in preterm infant, 162, 274–276, 280–287, 293, 294
    versus full-term infant, 289–295
  stimuli used as basis, 276
  and subcortical mechanisms, 279, 280
Visual evoked potentials
  and amplitude changes, 87, 88
  and behavioral response, 95
  and constant illumination, 101
  developmental sequence, 77–80, 82, 83, 98, 100
  in kittens, 77–83
  and latency, 77–79, 100, 144
  and maturity, 153, 154
  and monocular deprivation, 82
  and morphogenesis, 154
  in operant conditioning, 87
  pathways, 79, 80
  in preterm infant, 78, 79
  in response-dependent learning, 87, 88, 90
  and visual cortical neuron development, 153
  waveform, 79, 100
Visual habituation
  to color, 242, 243
  and dishabituation, 241, 242, 245
  fixation time, 243–245, 249–251
  and measurement of specific abilities, 242
  pattern, 245
  and preterm, high risk infant, 247–252
  in retarded infants, 242–245, 249, 251, 252
  to shape, 242–245
  and social class, 247–252
  time needed to habituate, 243–245, 249, 250
  usefulness, 241, 242
Visual motor Gestalt test
  correlation with other developmental outcome measures, 362, 364–374, 381, 382
  and low birthweight infant, 361, 362